CHRONIC
WOUND CARE 5
A Clinical Source Book for Healthcare Professionals

Volume I

Co-Edited by
Diane L. **Krasner**
George T. **Rodeheaver**
R. Gary **Sibbald**
Kevin Y. **Woo**

With more than 50 contributors

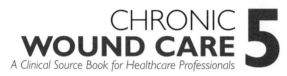

CHRONIC WOUND CARE 5

A Clinical Source Book for Healthcare Professionals

Volume I

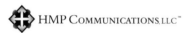

President: **Bill Norton**
Executive Vice President: **Peter Norris**
Vice President/Group Publisher: **Jeremy Bowden**
Managing Editor: **Renee Polvino**
Associate Editor: **Samantha Alleman**
Creative Director: **Vic Geanopulos**
Senior Production Manager: **Andrea Steiger**
Production/Circulation Director: **Kathy Murphy**

Copyright ® 2012
HMP Communications, LLC
83 General Warren Blvd., Suite 100
Malvern, PA 19355

ISBN 978-1-893446-00-7

Dedication

To people with chronic wounds
and their circles of care

Envision and *commit* to
International Interprofessional Wound Caring
to optimize everyone's quality of life.

Acknowledgement

In Appreciation:

To people with wounds and their circles of care
Who inspire all of us.

To the contributors to this fifth edition of *Chronic Wound Care*
Who serve as role models for **International Interprofessional
Wound Caring (IIWC)**.

To the publisher and editors who have supported this
Symposium on Advanced Wound Care 25th Anniversary Volume.

To the entire community whose commitment to wound care
Supports **IIWC.**

Afsaneh Alavi, MD, FRCPC(Derm)
Dept. of Medicine (Dermatology)
Women's College Hospital
University of Toronto
Toronto, Ontario, Canada

Elizabeth A. Ayello, PhD, RN, ACNS-BC, CWON, ETN, MAPWCA, FAAN
Faculty, Excelsior College, School of Nursing, Albany, New York
Senior Adviser, The John A. Hartford Institute for Geriatric Nursing, New York, New York
President, Ayello, Harris & Associates, Inc., Copake, New York

Ruth Anne Baron, BSc ND
North Toronto Naturopathic Clinic
Toronto, Ontario, Canada

Richard Barry, CHT
Vice President of Hyperbaric Services
Diversifed Clinical Services
Jacksonville, Florida

Jennifer A. Berry, FNP-BC
Barnes-Jewish Hospital
Saint Louis, Missouri

Robert E. Burrell, PhD, MSc
Professor and Chair
Dept. of Biomedical Engineering
Faculties of Engineering and Medicine and Dentistry
Professor and Canada Research Chair
Nanostructured Biomaterials Chemical and Materials Engineering
University of Alberta
Edmonton, Alberta, Canada

Karen E. Campbell, RN, PhD
Field Leader MCISc Wound Healing
Western University
Wound Program Manager
ARGC, Lawson Research Institute
St. Joseph's Health Care London
London, Ontario, Canada

Keryln Carville, RN, STN(Cred), PhD
Assoc. Professor Domiciliary Nursing
Silver Chain Nursing Association & Curtin University
Osborne Park, West Australia

Nicole Courchene, MSW
Pittsburgh, Pennsylvania

Linda Cowan, PhD, ARNP, CWS
Evidence Based Practice Coordinator
Associate Investigator, Rehabilitation Outcomes Research Center
North Florida/South Georgia Veterans Health System
Adjunct Clinical Assistant Professor, Adult & Elderly Department
University of Florida College of Nursing
Gainesville, Florida

Jean M. deLeon, MD
Professor, Dept. of Physical Medicine and Rehabilitation
UT Southwestern
Dallas, Texas

Morty Eisenberg, MD, MScCH, CCFP, FCFP
Hospitalist Division Head, Wound Consultant
St. John's Rehab Hospital, Toronto, Ontario, Canada
Assistant Professor, Dept. of Family & Community Medicine
Faculty of Medicine, University of Toronto

Paula Erwin-Toth, MSN, RN, CWOCN, CNS, ET
Director Emerita, Wound, Ostomy and Continence Nursing Education
Cleveland Clinic
Cleveland, Ohio

Robert G. Frykberg, DPM, MPH
Chief, Podiatry
Carl T. Hayden VA Medical Center
Phoenix, Arizona

Laurie Goodman, RN, BA, MHScN
Director
Mississauga Halton Wound Care Initiative
Toronto Regional Wound Clinics
Toronto, Ontario, Canada

Connie Harris, RN, ET, IIWCC, MSc
Senior Clinical Specialist, Wound & Ostomy,
CarePartners ET NOW
SW Regional Wound Care Framework Project Lead
Waterloo, Ontario, Canada

Harriet W. Hopf, MD
University of California, San Francisco
San Francisco, California

Pamela E. Houghton, PT, PhD, MAPWCA
Professor, School of Physical Therapy
Western University Canada
London, Ontario, Canada

David Keast, BSc(Hon), MSc, Dip Ed, MD, CCFP, FCFP
Centre Director
Aging, Rehabilitation and Geriatric Care Research Centre
Lawson Health Research Institute
St. Joseph's Parkwood Hospital
London, Ontario, Canada

John P. Kirby, MD, FCCWS, FACS
Director, Wound Ostomy Center at Barnes-Jewish Hospital
Assistant Professor of Surgery at Washington University
Saint Louis School of Medicine
Saint Louis, Missouri

Diane L. Krasner, PhD, RN, CWCN, MAPWCA, FAAN
Wound and Skin Care Consultant
York, Pennsylvania

Karen Laforet, MCISc-WH, BA, RN, IIWCC
Director of Clinical Services
Calea
Mississauga, Ontario, Canada

Christina Lindholm, PhD, RN
Senior Professor
Karolinska University Hospital/Sophiahemmet
University College
Head of Wound Group
Stockholm, Sweden

Dieter Mayer, MD, FEBVS, FAPWCA
Head of Wound Care
Senior Vascular Consultant
Clinic for Cardiovascular Surgery
University Hospital of Zurich
Zurich, Switzerland

Heather McConnell, RN, BScN, MA(Ed)
Associate Director, International Affairs and Best
Practice Guidelines Centre
Registered Nurses' Association of Ontario
Toronto, Ontario, Canada

WAJ (Jack) Meintjes, MBChB, DOM, FCPHM(SA) Occ Med, MMed(Occ Med)
Division of Community Health
Faculty of Health Sciences
University of Stellenbosch
South Africa

James Merlino, MD, FACS, FASCRS
Dept. of Colorectal Surgery
Cleveland Clinic
Cleveland, Ohio

Linda Norton, BScOT, OT Reg(ONT), MScCH
National Educator
Shoppers Home Health Care, Toronto, Ontario
Director, Interprofessional Team
Canadian Association of Wound Care Institute

Heather Orsted, RN, BN, ET, MSc
Director, International Interprofessional Wound
Care Course
Calgary, Alberta, Canada

Ben Peirce, RN, BA, CWOCN
Regional Director of Performance Improvement
Gentiva Health Services
Fort Lauderdale, Florida

Priscilla Phillips, PhD
Dept. of Oral Biology
University of Florida
Gainesville, Florida

Mary Ellen Posthauer, RD, CD, LD
President, MEP Healthcare Dietary Services, Inc.
Evansville, Indiana

Patricia Price, BA(Hons), PhD, AFBPsS, CPsychol, FHEA
Professor of Health Sciences
Dean of School of Healthcare Studies
Cardiff University
Heath Park, Cardiff, South Wales, United Kingdom

Catherine Ratliff, PhD, APRN-BC, CWOCN, CFCN
University of Virginia Medical Center
Charlottesville, Virginia

George T. Rodeheaver, PhD
Professor and Director, Plastic Surgery Research
University of Virginia Medical Center
Charlottesville, Virginia

Terence J. Ryan, FRCP, DM
Emeritus Professor of Dermatology, Oxford University
Chairman, ISD Task Force, Skin Care for All, Community Dermatology
Marlborough, Wiltshire, United Kingdom

Richard Salcido, MD
William Erdman Professor, Dept. of Rehabilitation Medicine
Senior Fellow, Institute on Aging
Associate, Institute of Medicine and Bioengineering
University of Pennsylvania Health System
Philadelphia, Pennsylvania

Jos M.G.A. Schols, MD, PhD
Professor of Old Age Medicine
Dept. of General Practice and
Dept. of Health Services Research
Caphri - School for Public Health and Primary Care
Maastricht University
Maastricht, The Netherlands

Gregory Schultz, PhD
UF Research Foundation Professor
Dept. of Obstetrics and Gynecology
Institute for Wound Research
University of Florida
Gainesville, Florida

Debra Sibbald, BScPhm RPh ACPR MA PhD
Senior Lecturer, Division of Pharmacy Practice,
Leslie Dan Faculty of Pharmacy
Director, Assessment Services, CEHPEA (Centre for the Evaluation of Health Professionals Educated Abroad)
Toronto, Ontario, Canada

Matthew Sibbald, BSc, MD
University of Toronto
Mississauga, Ontario, Canada

R. Gary Sibbald, BSc, MD, FRCPC(Med, Derm), MACP, FAAD, MEd, MAPWCA
Professor, Public Health Sciences and Medicine
Director, International Interprofessional Wound Care Course and Masters of Science in Community Health
Dalla Lana School of Public Health
University of Toronto
Ontario, Canada

Hiske Smart, RN, MA, PG Dip(UK), IIWCC(Toronto)
Clinical Nurse Specialist and IIWCC Course Coordinator-South Africa
Division of Community Health, Dept. of Interdisciplinary Health Sciences, Stellenbosch University, Stellenbosch, South Africa

Adrianne P.S. Smith, MD, FACEP
Vice President & Medical Director
Regenesis Biomedical, Inc.
Scottsdale, Arizona

Linda A. Stamm, APRN, BC, CWS
Barnes-Jewish Hospital at Washington University
School of Medicine
Saint Louis, Missouri

Joyce Stechmiller, PhD, ACNP-BC, FAAN
Associate Professor of Nursing
College of Nursing
Dept. of Adult and Elderly
University of Florida
Gainesville, Florida

Brenda Stenger, MEd, RN, CWOCN, ET
Cleveland Clinic
Cleveland, Ohio

Nancy A. Stotts, RN, EdD
Professor Emerita
University of California San Francisco
School of Nursing
San Francisco, California

Linda J. Stricker, MSN/ED, RN, CWOCN
Interim Director, WOC Nursing Education
Cleveland Clinic
Cleveland, Ohio

Gordon Sussman, MD, FRCPC(Allergy and Immunology)
Toronto, Ontario, Canada

Gulnaz Tariq, RN, BSN, PG Dip(Pak)
Wound Care Specialist, Sheikh Khalifa Medical City,
Abu Dhabi, United Arab Emirates
IIWCC Course Coordinator-Abu Dhabi

Lia van Rijswijk, RN, MSN, CWCN
Holy Family University School of Nursing and Allied
Health Professions
Philadelphia, Pennsylvania and Newtown,
Pennsylvania

Robert A. Warriner, III, MD, FCCP, FACWS, FAPWCA
Chief Medical Officer
Diversified Clinical Services
Jacksonville, Florida

Katherine T. Whittington, RN, MS, CWCN
Clinical Consultant
Atlanta, Georgia

Laurel A. Wiersema-Bryant, APRN, BC, CWS
Barnes-Jewish Hospital at Washington University
School of Medicine
Saint Louis, Missouri

James R. Wilcox, RN, BSN, ACHRN
Director of Quality Research
Diversified Clinical Services
Jacksonville, Florida

Deidre D. Wipke-Tevis, RN, PhD
Assistant Professor
Sinclair School of Nursing
University of Missouri Columbia
Columbia, Missouri

Kevin Y. Woo, PhD, RN, FAPWCA
Assistant Professor
Faculty of Health Sciences, School of Nursing,
Queen's University, Kingston, Ontario, Canada
Wound Care Consultant
West Park Health Centre
Toronto, Ontario, Canada

M. Gail Woodbury, PhD, BScPT, MAPWCA
Assistant Professor
University of Western Ontario
London, Ontario, Canada
Research Consultant
Canadian Association of Wound Care
Toronto, Ontario, Canada

Continuity and Change in Wound Care

Jeremy Bowden and Peter Norris

We are honored and somewhat surprised to have been asked to write the Foreword to *Chronic Wound Care: A Clinical Source Book for Healthcare Professionals*, 5th edition (*CWC5*), volume 1. As Vice Presidents at HMP Communications, LLC (HMP), the publisher of all 5 editions, our initial reaction was, "Why us?" Forewords to the first 4 editions were provided by esteemed wound care leaders, such as George Rodeheaver, PhD; Evonne Fowler, RN, CNS, CWOCN; Robert Kirsner, MD, PhD; and Allen Holloway, MD. We are embracing this opportunity from a business perspective to address both continuity and change within the field of wound care publishing.

The one constant with every edition of *CWC* has been Dr. Diane Krasner, who has served as editor or co-editor. We at HMP are delighted to celebrate more than 25 years of collaborative efforts with Diane; it is apropos that the first volume of this new edition is launching at the 25th Annual **Symposium on Advanced Wound Care (SAWC)** meeting in Atlanta, Georgia, in April 2012.

Chronic wound care is a fascinating and relatively new healthcare specialty. Many of our thought-leaders, including the hundreds of authors who have published chapters in various editions of *CWC*, have been drawn to the collaborative process of interprofessional care teams that include physicians, surgeons, podiatrists, therapists, and nurses. Although this new specialty is lacking in terms of formal training programs in pre-med, nursing, and therapy schools, these thought-leaders continue to "write the book" on new research advancements and develop evidence-based care regimens for people with chronic wounds. As the dominant healthcare publisher focused on disseminating information on the treatment and care of chronic wounds, we are proud of our ongoing heritage with *CWC*, **SAWC**, and all of our other specialty publications, including *Ostomy Wound Management*, *WOUNDS*, *Podiatry Today*, and *Today's Wound Clinic*.

Now, for the change! The business of publishing is undergoing an epic transition that is both disruptive and challenging. To address these changes, we are introducing a new model for the fifth edition of *CWC*. The past four editions (published in 1990, 1997, 2001, and 2007) involved a long gestation period between each one. With *CWC5,* we are publishing three separate volumes that will launch in April 2012, 2013, and 2014, each timed around the annual **SAWC** spring meetings. In addition, readers may cost-effectively purchase a print and/or digital copy of each volume to fit their personal preferences. Some, like Jeremy, prefer reading books on an iPad; others, like Peter, remain fans of the hard copy publication that can be housed nicely in a bookcase.

As ever, HMP is firmly established as a leader, proactive toward and receptive to the publication and healthcare industries' revolution. This new edition of *CWC* is but one example of our dedication to generating the newest and best information on wound care. We hope you use it well and use it often.

Dr. Diane L. Krasner
Dr. George T. Rodeheaver
Dr. R. Gary Sibbald
Dr. Kevin Y. Woo

The person with a chronic wound may suffer from social isolation, the need for disfiguring bandaging, pain and odor, and mood disturbance. Any combination of these factors can lead to a diminished quality of life. The effects of a chronic wound on the individuals also impact their circles of care, putting stress on sometimes fragile systems. There are often large healthcare system gaps for access to coordinated interprofessional care and supplies.

The theme of the fifth edition of *Chronic Wound Care (CWC5)* — ***International Interprofessional Wound Caring*** — reflects our personal perspectives that the problems faced by people with chronic wounds are universal. These include:
• Limited access to quality wound care teams
• Lack of availability of products, devices, and resources
• Poor quality of life and lack of social support.

The new wound care paradigm prompts us to be evidence-informed and to strive for improved health outcomes by:
• Developing ***International Interprofessional Wound Caring (IIWC)***
• Addressing concerns of people with chronic wounds and their circles of care
• Creating wound care processes — from assessment to health delivery systems
• Translating wound care strategies — from principles to practice to outcomes.

The 23 chapters in volume 1 of *CWC5* are arranged in 4 sections corresponding to the 4 above-identified themes. Each chapter has a section number and a chapter number (eg, 1.2 is Section 1 Chapter 2). Chapters in this edition model **IIWC** with international and interprofessional co-authors, who have collaborated to give the readers multiple perspectives on each topic.

Your challenge is to translate this information to your practice setting, to optimize interprofessional collaboration, and to improve your outcomes for people with chronic wounds.

We hope *CWC5* will inspire you to meet this challenge!

Developing International Interprofessional Wound Caring

International Interprofessional Wound Caring

Diane L. Krasner, PhD, RN, CWCN, MAPWCA, FAAN;

George T. Rodeheaver, PhD;

R. Gary Sibbald, BSc, MD, FRCPC(Med, Derm), MACP, FAAD, MEd, MAPWCA;

Kevin Y. Woo, PhD, RN, FAPWCA

Objectives

The reader will be challenged to:

- Conceptualize the dimensions of the International Interprofessional Wound Caring Model 2012©
- Analyze his or her own practice by comparing and contrasting it to the International Interprofessional Wound Caring Model 2012
- Commit to completing a personal scorecard and construct a personal learning portfolio
- Relate the needs of his or her practice and the needs of the person with wounds to his or her social responsibility for care at community, national, and international levels.

Introduction

A person with a chronic wound often suffers from a myriad of biopsychosocial problems, such as physical disability, pain, social needs, and mental anguish. Addressing these multiple issues properly requires skilled help from knowledgeable wound care professionals; however, wound care expertise and knowledge of the evidence base for practice alone usually are not enough to heal a chronic wound and improve the life of the person with that wound.

In this chapter, the editors of *Chronic Wound Care: A Clinical Source Book for Healthcare Professionals* present the International Interprofessional Wound Caring Model 2012© (Figure 1 and Plate 1 on page 314). Our goals for you are to think about your own work environment and to reflect on whether your environment enables you to practice interprofessional wound care. We challenge you to analyze how your current practice model compares and contrasts with ours. Then ask yourself and other members of your team if you can improve your interprofessional wound caring practice model. Additionally, we challenge you to complete your own personal scorecard and to construct your personal learning portfolio for your continuous professional development and lifelong learning.

In this fifth edition of *Chronic Wound Care*, our new conceptualization of *person*, *patient*, and *circle of care* will be utilized. When the term *person* is used, this refers to an autonomous individual with no specific healthcare relationship for diagnosis and treatment. When the term *patient* is

Krasner DL, Rodeheaver GT, Sibbald RG, Woo KY. International interprofessional wound caring. In: Krasner DL, Rodeheaver GT, Sibbald RG, Woo KY, eds. *Chronic Wound Care: A Clinical Source Book for Healthcare Professionals.* Vol 1. 5th ed. Malvern, PA: HMP Communications; 2012:3–12.

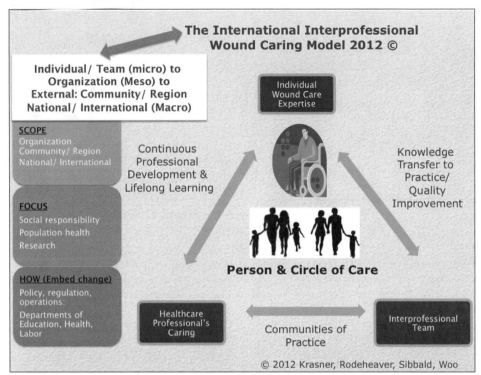

Figure 1. The International Interprofessional Wound Caring Model 2012. © 2012 Krasner, Rodeheaver, Sibbald, Woo.

used, the healthcare provider-patient relationship is implied, including the legal obligation to care. To facilitate expression of all those involved in a person's biopsychosocial environment, we use the expression, *the person's circle of care*. This is not used as a legal term in this textbook as outlined elsewhere. It is utilized as a social term that includes all of the stakeholders in the patient's health and well-being. The circle includes, but is not limited to, the patient, a legal guardian or responsible party, a spouse or significant other, interested friends or family members, caregivers, and any other individual(s) who may have active involvement or interest in the patient's care and well-being.

A person with a wound and his or her circle of care need the wound care expert's professional knowledge and skill, but they also require the expertise of other members of the interprofessional team, including generalist physicians and nurses, physical therapists, dietitians, pharmacists, social workers, discharge planners, and so on. The mix

of professionals that one patient needs will differ from another patient's through individualized patient-centered care.

Each individual healthcare professional's caring behavior is an essential dimension of our model. We sincerely believe that without this commitment to the call to care by all members of the team, wound care cannot be optimized. The human touch — reaching out to the person with a wound and his or her circle of care — builds the trust and the confidence that heals wounds, people, and lives.

Person, Circle of Care, and Population

The first dimension that is central to the model is that of the person with a wound and his or her circle of care. Several key factors often contribute to the development of chronic wounds. People with chronic wounds are often older — the average age is 70 years for venous leg ulcer sufferers and 60 years for people with diabetic neuropathic foot ulcers. These individuals frequently have coexisting medical conditions that can impair healing. Oral drugs prescribed for patients' medical needs often interfere with the wound healing process. Chronic wound patients often experience pain that has not been adequately addressed by their healthcare team. Several international pain surveys have demonstrated that pain is the third to fifth most important component of care for healthcare providers and may be the first priority for patients.[1] This disconnect emphasizes the need to address individualized patient-centered concerns as part of any chronic wound treatment plan. You will find numerous chapters in this fifth edition of *Chronic Wound Care* that focus on particular aspects of the chronic wound experience that must be addressed for the patient, family, and caregiver.

Chronic wounds usually interfere with a person's quality of life and activities of daily living. Imagine the social isolation that a person with a leg ulcer feels when he or she cannot eat with the rest of the family because the odor from the wound is offensive. The person with a diabetic neurotrophic foot ulcer can lay awake for hours because of burning and shooting neuropathic pain in both feet at night. The chronic pain, suffering, and diminished quality of life often lead to depression. Depression is particularly common in persons with diabetes due to multiple complications, including neuropathy as well as ischemia, infection, and deformity. Individuals suffering from chronic wounds often have decreased capacity for the activities of daily living. They often lack the physical stamina for employment, leading to a high number of absentee days, or even can be trapped into long-term disability. Frequent dressing changes may interfere with employment opportunities, and the cost of supplies may not be covered by the healthcare system. Affected individuals often are unable to walk long distances or stand for any prolonged period of time. They may have difficulty sleeping and even maintaining an adequate level of self-care. We must address all of these patient-centered concerns.

Historically, patients often are given instructions on how to treat a wound with minimal discussion to explain the cause(s) or address patient-centered concerns. The patient may not comprehend the pathophysiology of the wound and the importance of his or her cooperation

(and his or her family's and caregiver's cooperation) to promote wound healing. This is typical of the concept of **compliance**, which is the act or process of obeying an order or command. This is very provider-centered care — not patient-centered care. Recent literature has emphasized the concept of **adherence** or the ability of a patient to follow through on a treatment or regime.[2] The emphasis shifts away from provider-centered care and refocuses on the patient's perspective. To increase the collaborative network even further, the term **coherence** refers to frank discussion between the healthcare professional and the person with a wound, allowing both points of view to be considered and a negotiated treatment plan that incorporates both perspectives to be developed.

We must work toward collaboration to include persons with chronic wounds and their circle of care. We must acknowledge the fact that every person who has a social network of caregivers, family, friends, and concerned acquaintances is likely to have far better outcomes than those individuals who are socially isolated.[3]

Wound Care Expertise

Wound care expertise consists of evidence-based wound care knowledge of the skills and expert knowing gained from clinical experience and of the attitudes and values that we bring to practice as individuals. Healthcare providers can acquire knowledge of the evidence base for wound care by reading or by attending formalized courses, conferences, and seminars. Novice healthcare professionals transition to expert practitioners with time and experience as described by Benner[4] and others. As healthcare providers, we need to treat the whole patient and not just the hole in the patient (Figure 2). Our knowledge base should include expertise about the cause(s) of common chronic wounds, such as venous leg ulcers, pressure ulcers, diabetic neurotrophic foot ulcers, and nonhealing surgical wounds. We also need to know about uncommon chronic wounds, palliative wounds, and deteriorating wounds. This knowledge needs to be complemented with the ability to assess and treat pain, other patient-centered concerns, and local wound care expertise.

Traditional wound care has often been delivered with saline wet-to-dry gauze dressings. Removal of these dressings can cause local bleeding and

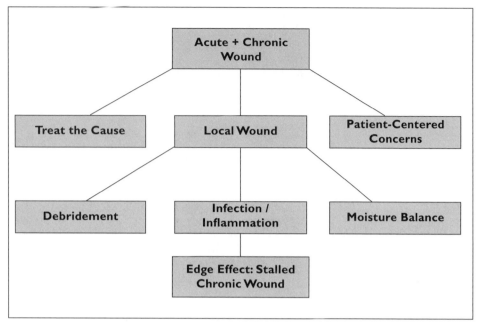

Figure 2. Wound bed preparation paradigm for holistic patient care. Sibbald et al. 2000, 2003, 2006, 2007, WHO 2010, 2011.

pain, and the procedure is nursing time-intensive. Since the classic work of Winter[5] in 1962, several advantages for moist wounds have been identified and include a faster healing rate with occlusion and enhanced re-epithelization with removal of eschar. To translate this into everyday practice, several newer, moist, interactive wound dressings have been added to our therapeutic toolkit.

Local wound care expertise goes well beyond the selection of the appropriate dressing to look at criteria to benchmark healing and when to use advanced products, including growth factors, skin substitutes, complementary therapies, and other procedures, such as skin grafting. We often teach the principles of local wound care with the mnemonic: *DIM* before *DIME* for adequate Debridement, Infection and Inflammation control, and Moisture balance before the Edge effect, signaling stalled healing and the need for active local therapy. The optimal wound care practices outlined in the preparing the wound bed algorithm are essential before advanced and often expensive therapies are considered (see Chapter 4.15).[6–8] If a wound with the ability to heal is not 30% smaller at Week 4, despite optimal local wound care, it is unlikely

to heal by Week 12, and advanced therapies should be considered.[9] Clinicians are reminded that if a wound is unlikely to heal (eg, due to inadequate vasculature or coexisting illness), advanced therapies are seldom indicated and their chance of success is minimal (nonhealable wound). In addition, a maintenance wound does not heal at the expected rate because the patient may refuse to wear the compression that is required to correct venous disease or because the healthcare system does not provide plantar pressure redistribution for a person with a neurotrophic foot ulcer and the patient cannot afford the treatment.

There is a need to link our new knowledge and research findings in wound care to the improved outcomes of patients with wounds worldwide. This process involves the inclusion of evidence from 3 different perspectives:[10]

- *Efficacy* — it works in idealized patients
- *Efficiency* — it works in usual patients
- *Effectiveness* — it has benefit at a reasonable cost.

The current organization of the evidence base for wound care may not encompass all 3 perspectives. One of the pitfalls of randomized controlled trials (RCTs) in wound research is the strict subject selection, eliminating most "usual" patients, and the disadvantage when attempting to extrapolate the RCT results to the real world of clinical practice for patients who would not meet the entry criteria of the study. Efficacy studies compare strictly controlled patients without confounding variables to a placebo. These conceptual studies are necessary for proof of concept. These studies need to be complemented with RCTs comparing the new treatment to usual practices or evidence-informed practice in a clinic that includes usual current treatment for all patients assessed with wounds that have the ability to heal. This treatment must be cost neutral or cost saving for the practice to be translated into day-to-day care by obtaining reimbursement within a healthcare system (effectiveness). There is a need to build economic models to test the feasibility of integrating a new treatment that may be expensive but have cost savings or may be cost neutral to the healthcare system.

Sackett et al[11] emphasized the importance of combining clinical expertise and the best available external evidence, expert knowledge, and patient preference. Without clinical expertise, practice risks becoming tyrannized by evidence — even excellent external evidence may be inappropriate for an individual patient. Without current best evidence, clinical practice rapidly will be out of date, to the detriment of patients. This combination of the scientific evidence base with expert opinion contextualized to local practice is referred to as *evidence-informed practice*. We also must remember the central needs of the patient and the consultation with patients to determine their preferences for treatment. The person's experiences with illness and the experiences of his or her circle of care are often forgotten in the rush for RCTs and other levels of evidence.

To translate the evidence-based paradigm, we can develop a clinical practice guideline. However, all guidelines are not created equal. The methodological quality of a guideline can be assessed through the Appraisal of Guidelines for Research & Evaluation (AGREE II) Instrument (www.agreetrust.org). This instrument examines 6 domains: scope and purpose, stakeholders, rigor, clarity, applicability, and editorial independence. Through this process, we can identify high-

quality guidelines and recommendations for translation into practice without continually creating new guidelines or reinventing the wheel.

The Interprofessional Team

Professionals involved in wound care come from diverse professional backgrounds. Each professional brings unique expertise, adding strength to the team. Team collaboration helps fill knowledge gaps, broadens perspectives, and optimizes patient care delivery. Many of the contributors to the fifth edition of *Chronic Wound Care* have shared their collaborative experiences working in teams. This teamwork has presented both benefits and challenges that need resolution.

Teams are not created overnight. Individuals in a multiprofessional network need to respect each other's expertise and work toward improving patient outcomes. The next step is to form an interprofessional team with group care plans and sharing of situational learning from experience. In some cases, this may even evolve to a transprofessional team. Advanced practice team members can often perform the functions of more than one team member when required. Highly functioning teams have a flattened structural framework with shared care of patients and do not exemplify the pyramidal structure of a dominant leader and followers that have little to do with key patient care decisions.

Each of us as individuals requires a network of other individuals with complementary expertise in wound care. Let us conceptualize our team for this chapter. George Rodeheaver, PhD, as the basic scientist, brings us new perspectives, treatments, or diagnostic procedures from the laboratory or clinical investigations for consideration. Diane Krasner, RN, as a nurse and allied healthcare professional, focuses on prevention, local treatment, and allied healthcare issues across the continuum of care. Gary Sibbald, MD, as the physician key opinion leader, evaluates innovative treatments or procedures and trials them before identifying the strengths and weaknesses as well as the advantages and disadvantages for patient care before translating a new modality into everyday clinical practice. Kevin Woo, RN, as a nurse researcher and educator, shares his passion for knowledge generation, synthesis, and translation. These 4 distinct professional perspectives broaden our base and strengthen our team.

By practicing as a team, healthcare professionals are able to balance the amount of responsibility and the workload, particularly in challenging cases. It is imperative that all team members share their knowledge and experience in order to provide better care. Tuckman[12] has defined 4 stages to team development: forming, storming, norming, and performing. Several aspects are more likely to be found in successful teams, including clear communication, flexibility, adaptability, openness, shared leadership, and mutual respect.

Healthcare Professional's Caring

Wound care experts must realize that working in a silo even with individual caring cannot offer the person and his or her circle of care optimal treatment. Many individuals who have become healthcare professionals do so because they truly want to help others. The journey to successful healthcare professional status requires a formalized training program that often supplies the basics of nursing, medicine, podiatry, physical therapy, occupational therapy, and other healthcare professional disciplines. It is important to complement professional knowledge with skills to work within a healthcare system. Professionals in health disciplines need to develop communication, collaboration, and management skills. A caring healthcare professional must have a patient-centered approach. This can be exemplified by the Keller and Carroll model[13] to patient communication:

- Engage
- Empathize
- Educate
- Enlist.

For each patient, we should know something about him or her other than the reason for the visit (*engagement*). This information may include hobbies, important family events, or milestones in his or her life. We need to be good listeners, and we need to *empathize* with patients' pain and suffering and not dismiss their concerns with trivial sympathetic comments. Establishing patients' perspectives on their disease processes allows healthcare professionals to *educate* individuals from current beliefs to a negotiated treatment plan, taking patients' wishes into account and having a consensus on the next steps. We then need to *enlist* the patient to be an active participant and take personal responsibility for the diagnostic and treatment process.

As individuals, healthcare professionals need to be in tune with their own belief systems and have a balance with attention to their physical, spiritual, psychological, and social needs. Professionalism refers to the behavior of a professional to uphold ethical and interpersonal values. Healthcare professionals are expected to demonstrate respect for others and uphold appropriate boundaries between themselves, coworkers, and patients.

We should create a comfortable work environment with compassion for others and commitment to improving illness and promoting wellness. There is a need to be a health advocate and to promote a healthy living style and wellness by setting a good example. Other ways to advocate for health include developing new and better healthcare systems with universal access, treating illness early, educating the general public, and supporting wellness.

Continuous Professional Development and Lifelong Learning

Continuous professional development (CPD) refers to lifelong learning that is learner- and workplace-centered. This is also referred to as situational learning because it is determined by practice and problems with patient care. Continuous professional development relates to day-to-day activities. The outcomes from CPD are more likely to change behavior and improve patient care outcomes than an accredited classroom event or traditional continuing education programs.

Single educational events without secondary enabling or reinforcing strategies to bring the information back to the workplace are often unsuccessful in changing practice. Enablers, reference guides, and toolkits are examples of products that can be utilized to change practice. An enabler or quick reference guide is a 20-second to 2-minute reading time summary of relevant strategies for bedside or patient care. An educational toolkit is designed for the implementation of best clinical practices and may consist of educational materials, measuring guides, monofilaments, and other useful aids to clinical practice. Mentorship after an educational event or small learning groups and educational outreach visits (during which an expert may translate the information learned in the formalized setting for the workplace) can also facilitate the integration of new knowledge into practice.

As healthcare professionals, we also must commit to lifelong learning through experience. We learn from the literature, but we also must learn from our experiences and dialogues with colleagues. The first step is to create a network of individuals with whom we can consult when we do not have an answer to a clinical question. We may need to involve a preceptor to learn a skill or task that is important to our job or clinical activities. Preceptorships are often time-limited and driven by specific goals and objectives. Beyond preceptorships, we also may need a mentor. A mentor is an individual who, in a nonjudgmental, comfortable manner, can provide guidance for job-related, personal, and other decisions to achieve life goals and balance as well as to advance a career and promote wound care expertise. Some mentorship relationships have a time-limited spectrum, while others can evolve into a co-mentorship relationship. A younger mentee may be a computer "native" and can teach a computer "immigrant" mentor tricks of the new technologies. At the same time, the senior mentor can continue to add contextual knowledge from lifelong experience, solving difficult situational clinical problems for the younger mentee.

We often learn from relaying case studies or case series and then discussing diagnoses and management. Another dimension to a case history is storytelling. In storytelling, the emotional and situational components of the history and the sequence of events are related with a personal analysis or honesty that may not be contextualized in the formal case history dominated by facts in the sequential history, physical, investigation, and treatment process. Storytelling and the personal anecdote remain critically important methods — even with the current trend of evidence-informed healthcare.

Knowledge Transfer into Practice

Knowledge transfer into practice refers to the link between scientific evidence and the need to change clinical practice. This is a conceptual framework of moving new knowledge from the laboratory bench to the literature/classroom and ultimately to the bedside in order to improve patient care outcomes. This concept requires the transfer of knowledge from efficacy or proof-of-concept

RCTs in idealized patients to the trial of the same principles in usual everyday wound care clinics in order to demonstrate that the integration of the concept improves patient care outcomes.

Wikipedia, the Internet's free encyclopedia, describes 3 related concepts in the health sciences: knowledge utilization, research utilization, and implementation. These concepts describe the process of bringing a new idea, practice, or technology into consistent and appropriate use in a clinical setting.[14] The study of knowledge utilization and implementation is a direct outgrowth of the movement toward evidence-based or evidence-informed healthcare. Research to demonstrate efficacy of a new treatment is often completed in idealized patients, and this research needs to be repeated with usual patients to confirm that the same treatment will make a difference in everyday practice settings on usual patients.

Informal Communities of Practice

The concept of a community of practice (CoP) refers to the process of social learning that occurs when people who have a common interest in some subject or problem collaborate over an extended period to share ideas, find solutions, and build innovations. Do you have a wound care CoP?

A previous version of Wikipedia noted, *"The term [community of practice] was first used in 1991 by Jean Lave and Etienne Wenger [to describe] situated learning as part of an attempt to 'rethink learning' at the Institute for Research on Learning. In 1998, the theorist Etienne Wenger extended the concept and applied it to other contexts, including organizational settings…Some of the aims and goals of a community of practice include: the design of more effective knowledge-oriented organizations, creating learning systems across organizations, improving education and lifelong learning, rethinking the role of professional associations and a design of a world in which people can reach their full potential…[a community of practice is] a group of individuals participating in a communal activity, and experiencing/continuously creating their shared identity through engaging in and contributing to the practices of their communities."*

Following are questions to ponder:
- Do you participate in one or more CoP?
- Can you describe their membership and essential components?

Concept	Strength	Weakness	Threats	Opportunities	Next Steps: Personal Portfolio
Wound care knowledge					
Patient and circle of care					
Interprofessional team relations and new partnerships					
Caring clinician and personal growth					
Continuous professional development/ lifelong learning					
Knowledge transfer projects					
Community of practice					

Figure 3. Personal scorecard.

• How could you optimize your participation to maximize your social learning and improve your wound care knowledge?

• Could and should you foster a CoP?

Local to Global, Micro to Macro

Persons with chronic wounds do not always receive the expert professional healthcare that they require. Professor Terence Ryan outlines several examples of this in Chapter 1.2. There is a social responsibility to increase collaboration within interprofessional teams on community, national, and international levels. The World Health Organization (WHO) document, "Transformative Scale Up of Health Professional Education,"[15] highlights the active strategies of healthcare personnel, especially in developing countries, including Sub-Saharan Africa where millions of people are without health services. More providers are needed, and these providers require training that is more relevant to the population's health needs. Education of individual professions needs to include a greater emphasis on interprofessional communication and collaboration. There is also a gap between the needs of private and public healthcare systems and the social responsibility to these countries that must be balanced with improved personal finances that accompany immigration to a developed country. Policies from the WHO will be welcomed to assist developing countries (national authorities) in working with local communities, development partners, and educational institutions.

Conclusion

The fifth edition of *Chronic Wound Care: A Clinical Source Book for Healthcare Professionals* is a compilation of the evidence base for chronic wound care with expert opinion from key wound care leaders around the world. It is the starting point for your personal journey to improve outcomes for people with chronic wounds. Figure 3 presents a personal scorecard for you to copy and update on a regular basis for your personal self-assessment and evaluation of the journey. This is also a way to identify personal needs and plan your future educational portfolio. We challenge you to be:

- More effective communicators and collaborators with your patients and their circle of care
- Patient-centered (Do you practice the 4-E model?)
- Better distillers of *wound care knowledge* through:
  - Examining the evidence base presented in this book
  - Reviewing guidelines with good methodological quality
  - Seeking the opinions of others in your own personal network in order to develop your *wound care expertise*
  - Building your own wound care network or *community of practice* within or outside your organization or workplace.

Have you also personally:

- Become a more dedicated *interprofessional team member* by listening, sharing, and collaborating with passion and commitment
- Developed a *knowledge translation* strategy for your workplace to improve the efficacy, efficiency, and effectiveness of your care
- Improved your *personal caring?*

Regarding your current physical, psychological, spiritual, and mental scorecard:

- Where are your strengths and weaknesses, and can you improve?
- Do you have an action plan?

Can you be more effective in your commitment to *continuous professional development and lifelong learning*? Do you learn personally from a situational *continuous professional development* model, or do you still rely on conferences and formal educational opportunities to obtain continuing education credits as your major method of learning?

In closing, we challenge you to complete your own personal scorecard and to construct your personal learning portfolio. We urge you to reach out to patients, families, and caregivers in order to build the trust and the confidence that heal wounds, patients, and lives.

We wish you every success in *International Interprofessional Wound Caring!*

Diane L. Krasner
George T. Rodeheaver
R. Gary Sibbald
Kevin Y. Woo

References

1. World Union of Wound Healing Societies. *Principles of Best Practice: Minimising Pain at Wound Dressing-related Procedures.* A Consensus Document. London, UK: MEP Ltd; 2004.
2. Osterberg L, Blaschke T. Adherence to medication. *N Engl J Med.* 2005;353(5):487–497.
3. Snyder RJ. Venous leg ulcers in the elderly patient: associated stress, social support, and coping. *Ostomy Wound Manage.* 2006;52(9):58–68.
4. Benner P. *From Novice to Expert: Excellence and Power in Clinical Nursing Practice.* Menlo Park, CA: Addison-Wesley Publishing Co; 1984.
5. Winter GD. Formation of the scab and the rate of epithelization of superficial wounds in the skin of the young domestic pig. *Nature.* 1962;193:293–294.
6. Sibbald RG, Williamson D, Orsted HL, et al. Preparing the wound bed—debridement, bacterial balance, and moisture balance. *Ostomy Wound Manage.* 2000;46(11):14–37.
7. Sibbald RG, Orsted H, Schultz GS, Coutts P, Keast D; International Wound Bed Preparation Advisory Board; Canadian Chronic Wound Advisory Board. Preparing the wound bed 2003: focus on infection and inflammation. *Ostomy Wound Manage.* 2003;49(11):23–51.
8. Sibbald RG, Goodman L, Woo KY, et al. Special considerations in wound bed preparation 2011: an update©. *Adv Skin Wound Care.* 2011;24(9):415–436.
9. Woo K, Ayello EA, Sibbald RG. The edge effect: current therapeutic options to advance the wound edge. *Adv Skin Wound Care.* 2007;20(2):99–117.
10. Price P. The challenge of outcome measure in chronic wounds. *J Wound Care.* 1999;8(6):306–308.
11. Sackett DL, Straus SE, Richardson WS, Rosenberg W, Haynes RB. *Evidence-based Medicine: How to Practice and*

Teach EBM. 2nd ed. Edinburgh, Scotland: Churchill Livingstone; 2000.

12. Tuckman BW. Developmental sequence in small groups. *Psychol Bull*. 1965;63:384–399.

13. Keller VK, Carroll JG. A new model for physician-patient communication. *Patient Educ Couns*. 1994;23(2):131–140.

14. Greenhalgh T, Robert G, Macfarlane F, Bate P, Kyriakidou O. Diffusion of innovations in service organizations: systematic review and recommendations. *Milbank Q*. 2004;82(4):581–629.

15. World Health Organization. Transformative Scale Up of Health Professional Education. Available at: http://www.who.int/hrh/resources/transformative_education/en/index.html. Accessed January 8, 2011.

International Chronic Wound Caring

Terence J. Ryan, FRCP, DM

Objectives
The reader will be challenged to:
- Provide insight into the globalization of wound care
- Discuss experiences of treating wounds more common in the tropics and currently without access to the skills of a wound healing team
- Provide insight into other systems of healthcare to which the patient has access.

Introduction and the Development of Wound Healing Interventions

That it is possible to write about international chronic wound caring is a consequence of a number of historical events. Wound care of the armed forces fighting in many foreign lands dates from the crusades through the Napoleonic wars and the two World Wars. Interventions and policies to prevent wound bed infection gradually developed from Lister's use of carbolic acid through the discovery of antiseptics, such as Eusol and Dakin's solution, in World War I and then penicillin in World War II. The prevalence and focus on the care of leg ulcers, pressure ulcers, diabetic foot ulcers, and post-mastectomy lymphedema of the upper arm have increased since about 1960, especially with the formation of societies and associations built to manage these wounds. Often stimulated by patient demand or the devices industry, the medical profession frequently led interventions that were then carried out by nursing or other allied health professionals, such as the chiropodist/podiatrist. Once these interventions were established, increasing opportunities surfaced in the form of national and international meetings, focus groups, publications, and, most recently, the Internet. There have always been individual or bands of missionaries taking expertise to less accessible lands to manage leprosy, for example, but globalization has resulted in the possibility of the most expert practitioner's knowledge reaching the previously inaccessible. Self-help has become available at a low cost. National and international organizations have given increasing support to developing world interventions. Wound

Ryan TJ. International chronic wound caring. In: Krasner DL, Rodeheaver GT, Sibbald RG, Woo KY, eds. *Chronic Wound Care: A Clinical Source Book for Healthcare Professionals*. Vol 1. 5th ed. Malvern, PA: HMP Communications; 2012:13–24.

healing, which in the past had been insufficiently identified for its capacity to benefit, is now on the bookshelves of the United Nations' agencies.[1]

The Skin as the Focus of Wound Healing

How important would wound healing be if it did not involve the accessible skin most of the time? This chapter draws attention to repair of the skin in a global context and a never-ending war against a threatening environment from which we are protected by an effective barrier when in good health. Though the skin is large and exposed, the concept of it failing like other organs has been discussed less often. Failure of its 4 main functions has to be remedied if complete wound healing is to be attained.

Thus, there must be concern about 1) the loss of barrier function between the body and a threatening environment; 2) the inability to manage overheating or excessive cooling; 3) sensory impairment causing itch, pain, or numbness; and 4) the disfigurement and consequent faulty communication of the "look good, feel good" factor.

The author is a dermatologist and Chairman of the International Society of Dermatology's task force for **Skin Care for All: Community Dermatology**.[2] This endeavor seeks for dermatology physicians, who have had several years of additional training in the diagnosis and management of skin diseases, to be wound healers, lymphedema managers, and custodians of neglected tropical diseases (eg, leprosy, leishmaniasis, lymphatic filariasis, yaws, and Buruli ulcers). Dermatologists must have knowledge of essential drugs and devices as well as access to patients.

In 2011, discussions at the World Health Organization (WHO) initiated the view that "Health for All," which is inclusive of well-being and ultimately must include complete healing, would be more appropriately named if it were to focus on the individual's capacity to adapt and self-manage.[3] Thus, the endpoint of wound healing would be a disfigured person who is coping well with self-management and who feels healthy.

It is important not only to estimate needs, such as the burden of disease — so clearly illustrated by the chronic wound or by the stage of lymphedema known since Roman times as elephantiasis — but also to show that any organization with

which one works has a clear capacity to benefit.[2] For example, one must make the benefit clear by demonstrating how to prevent wounds in the first place, how to administer first aid, and how to heal wounds and manage lymphedema so that there is a reduced burden of unhealed wounds lasting many years. Additional benefits include limiting costs and establishing ways to share the load through teams, partners, and collaborations. From an international perspective, the aim will be to have at least one team practicing gold standards in a tertiary hospital or training school in every nation or state. This will be a source of knowledge for district hospitals and then primary care where, at this wider level, the healthcare practitioner should be equipped and able to cope with most common problems. One must plan to protect the national hospital from being overloaded with patients who could be managed at a lower level.

Epidemic Versus Patient-Centered

As advocated by Gandhi (Figure 1), being patient-centered is a requirement when any one person or team treats a chronic wound, but international wound care sees epidemics. When these epidemics involve obesity, diabetes, HIV/AIDS, tropical diseases, or landmine injuries to the legs, priorities change from one-to-one care with kindness and the delivery of gold standard practice to the acquisition of access to care over inhospitable terrain with a focus on plan-

---

The following text is adapted from a commentary by Gandhi and taken from the entrance of the General Hospital in Mumbai, India:[17]

A patient is the most important person in our hospital. The Patient is not an interruption to our work; the patient is the purpose of it. The patient is not an outsider in our hospital, but a part of it. We are not doing a favour by serving him or her; the patient is doing us a favour by giving us an opportunity to do so.

Figure 1. Gandhi's statement on patient-centered care.

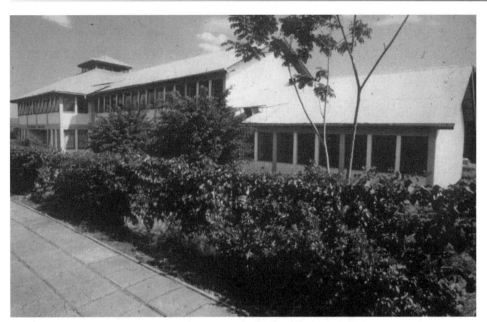

Figure 2. The Regional Dermatology Training Centre in Moshi, Tanzania.

ning, training, and delivering essential drugs and devices to an appropriate but minimally skilled workforce. The difference in knowledge base is illustrated by an endemic problem, ***podoconiosis*** (a form of elephantiasis/lymphedema caused by small soil particles that penetrate the skin and wreck the lymphatics), affecting more than a million persons in Ethiopia.[4] Here, physicians and nurses must know how to obtain and fit footwear for a million people in need. In Ethiopia, this can be the most important knowledge for a population disabled by swollen and affected feet due to not wearing shoes in an irritant soil.

As an example of public health planning inclusive of wound healing, the profession of dermatology should be examined. Over the last few decades, the dermatology profession has set up hundreds of wound healing centers to serve the developing world. The International Foundation for Dermatology (IFD) chose to set up a training school and to develop a curriculum on "Healthy Skin for All" in Sub-Saharan Africa.[5]

The Regional Dermatology Training Centre (Figure 2) in Moshi, Tanzania, was founded in 1992 as a response to nations without advice from governments, universities, and hospitals. The center provides training over 2 years. It initially focused on the development of allied health professionals who had only a few years of general medical training but had significant skills through extensive practice in primary care. The number of specialist doctors (MDs) in training is increasing. It is a WHO collaborating center for dermatology, sexually transmitted infection (STI), and leprosy. The curriculum includes skin diseases, STI, and leprosy inclusive of wound healing. A diploma equivalent to a Master's Degree has been issued to more than 200 persons who are able to take up senior management and practitioner roles and provide leadership, often at the highest level, in 12–14 African nations. The wound healing instructions given are based on developed world practice, including plastic surgery skills, but there is also instruction on locally available low-cost practices, such as larva therapy and the collection and use of honey. The author's teaching has ranged from toenail cutting to first aid of spinal injuries to pressure ulcer prevention.

A 2-year attempt to set up a regional dermatology training center in China was initiated in response to surveys of village doctors on the old Silk Road in West China who were greatly in need of updated skills in the face of the HIV/AIDS epidemic spread by lorry drivers. The proj-

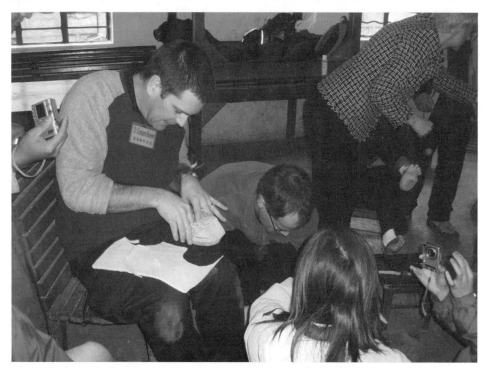

Figure 3. A visiting footwear team provides updated wound care in a leprosy village in Yunnan, China.

ect was to be based on district hospitals. There are more than 50 ethnic minorities and languages besides Tibetan in China. The project was withdrawn because of lack of government support and corruption — both recurrent impediments to international wound care. However, among many points learned relevant to international work is the need to communicate with ethnic communities. Interpreting and learning the language is key to successful practice based on education. All the major nations with large populations have tribes who only speak local languages. Almost all international wound healing projects will fail unless this key need is met. A rider is that, sadly, the many young doctors and elective medical students who want to visit such projects become an impediment if they cannot speak the language and have no relevant skills to offer. One may add that the role of the wound healing organizer is to provide some training before departure, and often, small handbooks can include guidance on minimal skills and local language.

Emphasis must be placed on self-help and the upgrading of whatever system of medicine is available locally and sustainable at low cost. For example, the gold standard treatment of a snakebite is immobilization to prevent lymphatic spread of the poison,[6] immediate identification of the snake, and the injection of specific antivenom. In practice, help will come from a ***traditional health practitioner (THP)*** who will scarify the area and apply a tourniquet. A drive over rough terrain to more expert help may severely shake the patient and mobilize the venom. Patients can die of fright, and this is one aspect of snakebites that THPs manage well by understanding patients' fears about causes, such as witchcraft, and exorcising the evil spirit believed to live in the snake.

A group of wound healers (2 dermatologists, 1 from the United Kingdom and 1 from South Africa, 1 plastic surgeon from the United Kingdom, a nurse from Australia, and 3 podiatrists from the United Kingdom), hosted by a Christian charity (careful to hide its religious identity), toured the best military wound healing services in Yunnan,

China. The tour revealed that costly gold standard care is only available to a class that can afford it. At a leprosy village, one could see an adequately housed and fed community, all of whom had wounds labelled as leprosy when they were clearly venous leg ulcers and wounds caused by undetected nails sticking into numb skin and by lack of attention to footwear. Institutions providing kindness, many of which are affiliated with religious orders, exist throughout India, Africa, and South America. One should be aware that many governments are grateful for help but have regulations preventing import of overt religious symbolism. Quite often, the patients become institutionalized and sit immobile, doing very little and developing gravitational disease of the lower leg. The wound healer has to persuade those affected to become more mobile, with the expectation that they will be able to hold jobs and work. On this China expedition (Figure 3), in a farmhouse some miles from the border of Tibet, a paraplegic with pressure ulcers benefited from the local purchase and transport of a rubber mattress and from instruction on how to use charcoal to manage odor.

Managing beggars with wounds in India has required teaching not only wound care but also how to replace the begging and the use of the wound to attract sympathy. For example, providing someone with a goat may foster ownership of an animal friend that needs looking after, raise self-esteem, and restore dignity, which may result in community respect. Sometimes the wound carers, doing well by dressing the wound, ignore a simple intervention, such as removing from outside the household a thorn bush from which a numb foot with no footwear will incur another wound. As this chapter is written, the author is days away from outreach visits to Indian communities with severe lymphedema from filariasis. With the author mentoring a program of care[7] and with Indian community physicians auditing a government-sponsored 18-month program to provide morbidity control at 2 distant outreach sites, the capacity to benefit was clearly demonstrated by smaller limbs and less frequent episodes of high fever due to cellulitis. Model teams recruited 13 members, including an administrator; a doctor; a nurse; locally recruited, accredited social health activists (Asha); and sometimes patients who have themselves fully responded to the regimen for managing elephantiasis. Empty buildings were rid of litter and bats and were washed and painted. Many camps were held with well publicized 1-day demonstrations. Two series of more than 600 patients with elephantiasis, one a fishing community and another an agricultural community, were taught self-help and the use of Indian systems of medicine, such as yoga to mobilize the lymphatic system and Ayurvedic herbals to manage the overload from skin infection (Plate 2, page 315).

Collecting Data to Inform Resource Providers

Collecting data to inform potential or past resource providers is essential work if funds are to be recruited. Some countries, such as the United States and the United Kingdom, have much improved the accuracy and approach to data collection on skin disease and its assessment and expression as a burden with unmet needs.[8] Assessment and management in resource-poor environments are now improving but still inadequately funded. It is not just the dermatology medical professionals leading advocacy. The International Skin Care Nursing Group (ISNG), initiated in the United Kingdom and affiliated with both the International Council of Nurses and the International League of Dermatological Societies (ILDS), is providing nursing leadership[9] and has always emphasized skills in wound healing and amplified its public health approaches.

Empowerment of Women

Those involved in wound care, including dermatologists, allied health professionals (principally nurses), and, most often, family members, are more likely to be women than men. For the task force for Skin Care for All, the empowerment of women to improve their effectiveness has the backing of an organization founded in the memory of Maria Duran, a Columbian dermatologist who helped organize the first meeting on the Advancement of Women in Dermatology in Turkey.[10] The meeting was chaired by Turkan Saylan from Istanbul, a protagonist for leprosy control and management of disability. Dr. Saylan also encouraged a British group of teenagers, led by the author of this chapter, to demonstrate ac-

Table 1. The minimal requirements for wound healing and lymphedema[16]

Wound healing:

1) Manage systemic conditions, such as diabetes, anemia, HIV, and AIDS.

2) Protect the wound from trauma, such as sustained pressure.

3) Promote a clean wound base and control infection.

4) Maintain a moist environment.

5) Control periwound edema.

Lymphedema:

1) Enhance movement of lymph.

2) Reduce overload from the venous system.

3) Reduce overload due to inflammation from entry points for irritants and bacteria.

cident prevention and first aid at the University of Istanbul.

Chronic Wounds in the Developing World

In the developing world, the chronic wound is often due to trauma. Road accidents are most prevalent where new roads allow higher speed and become a quicker route even for pedestrians.[11] Infective causes are also common. Recently, a mycobacterial cause of huge chronic ulcers in young people, named the *Buruli ulcer*, has increased throughout West Africa and can be found in other regions in the tropics. Early treatment of the ulcer was by excision, but now that its bacterial cause has been identified, rifampicin and streptomycin are given. An American wound healing team clearly demonstrated that wound healing skills, including managing associated lymphedema, made a huge difference in achieving complete healing. See Table 1 for the minimum interventions in any wound healing and lymphedema program. Buruli ulcer has recently benefited from improved instruction on wound healing technology. The WHO's need for wound healing expertise for Buruli ulcer led to the formation of the World Alliance for Wound & Lymphedema Care (WAWLC) and the publication of a white paper (a document prepared by

experts for advice to governance). As a handbook, it is now on the shelves at the WHO.

Other Systems of Health and the Local Scenario

Learning to collaborate with local systems of healthcare is an important objective in international healthcare. For example, the author learned from personal experience in Sierra Leone that there is no alternative in rural areas. Even a large 400-bed hospital had no anesthetist and sought untrained recruits from a local village to give ketamine for operations on typhoid-induced perforated intestines in children. The THPs performed much scarification of the wounded, which introduced infection, and one aim is to prevent this practice through education of THPs, best done by finding a leader to organize an association of THPs to whom one can provide education. On the other hand, the use of bark-derived soaps, which are good antiseptics, is threatened by policies that regard all traditional health as witchcraft or by complete deforestation in certain environments. Preserving forests by educating local people to value them for their medicines is a worthwhile occupation for the wound healer.

In Asia, where written traditions of medicine extend back some 3000 years, an international approach has included recognizing the use of plant-based wound healing agents. A scheme of collaboration with wound healers in Vietnam brings their prescribers to a UK laboratory where their prescriptions can be tested for antibacterial activities or actions, such as collagen gel contractility, or epithelization of *in-vitro* preparations of skin models wounded by a scratch test. Helping to publish such interventions[12] in good English is another example of globalization.

All such aforementioned programs are a development of public health interventions, but they will succeed only if distributed alongside other public health programs. Indeed, Western biomedical practice cannot intervene successfully without awareness and a degree of partnership and effective integration with other systems of healthcare. These include Indian and Chinese systems of medicine as well as traditional health practice in Africa.[13] In an era of evidence-based medicine, written traditions that are several thousand years old can be subjected to systematic review.[14]

One problem that has to be faced is the need to get each patient to the right resource of healing activity. This resource may be the accessible low-cost THP who will be favored more when the local government hospital is unattractive, over-crowded, rat infested, and surrounded by litter. The overwhelming number of patients waiting to be seen in any health center often includes many who could be treated elsewhere. The author has experienced 2 situations in which unattractive-ness was resolved and more time was made avail-able for wound and lymphedema care. In India, training nurses to be experts has been successful. In one such situation, the nurses transformed the health center into a clean, well painted facility with a flourishing herbal and blooming garden. Adding a crèche for local tribal people has in-creased familiarity. In such a location, wounds and lymphedema can be given the attention they need.[15]

Another program was based in Mali,[16] a West African country with a French-speaking popu-lation. This was a 1-day training of all health center personnel to recognize and manage the 3 most common conditions resulting from bac-terial, fungal, and parasitic invasion of the skin: namely, *impetigo*, *tinea*, and *scabies*. The aim was to prevent the health services from being over-whelmed by common diseases and to allow the healthcare worker to give more attention to more serious skin conditions, such as *leprosy*, or *wounds* and *burns*. It also reduces wrong diagnoses that contribute to ineffectiveness and higher cost pre-scribing. Other programs now exist in Mexico, Mali, Patagonia, and Cambodia, all administered or supported by the IFD.

In the field of wound healing, the curriculum includes improving techniques of making wounds — for example, incision and suturing after biopsy. In resource-poor regions, effective low-technology interventions are promoted, including the use of herbal remedies, such as honey, and biosurgery em-ploying maggots to aid wound healing.

Other Programs of the Task Force for Skin Care for All

Public health approaches to wound care and lymphedema are underfunded. Compared to the billions of dollars expended by The Global Fund each year for malaria, HIV, and tuberculosis, the resources for international skin care are mini-mal. It is possible that there has been too much emphasis on the disfigurement and disablement of a poverty stricken, odorous population. Such emphasis over many years, now known as the burden of disease, has lacked the appeal of evi-dence for capacity to benefit. Donors want their funding to generate achievement. The task force for Skin Care for All: Community Dermatology has produced a CD, "Capacity to Benefit," of 43 achievements and is collecting more. The task force's publications appeared in the May 2010 edition of the *International Journal of Dermatology*. It will add "how to do it," emphasizing the pro-vision of skin care in a public health framework and listing the leading organizations making up an alliance in the fields of wound healing, burns, lymphedema, or the neglected tropical diseases, such as leprosy. Almost every relevant condition has an affiliation of experts. Government minis-ters prefer interventions that bring them billions of dollars. A self-help low-cost program does not bring in that sort of money, and it is necessary to demonstrate altruism. Plenty of it exists.

The task force is the public health face of skin care and it looks at populations. One population is mobile. The morbidity and health issues fac-ing mobile populations forced to move due to strife, climate change, or economic migration has been extensively studied and supported by the dermatologist Aldo Morrone[17] through the es-tablishment of the National Institute for Health, Migration, and Poverty in Rome. The immigrant without skin ailments before migrating is very likely to develop them during a difficult migra-tion. Some of the wounds are due to torture; many are due to strife.

Dermatology also overlaps and embraces ve-nereology, ie, the study of STI, including HIV/AIDS. HIV and AIDS both present frequently in the skin, and resulting therapy can commonly produce adverse skin reactions. Tissue viability also may be generally impaired. For example, skin grafting more often fails in immunocompromised patients.

Information technology, including telehealth, is advancing in expertise and becoming more avail-able as mobile phone technology and distribution expand.[18] Telehealth is used by all levels of health-care, including THPs in rural Africa. The skin is easily photographed and easily biopsied. Samples can be posted and histopathological analysis sent back to guide the management of skin lesions.[19]

Climate Change

Climate change makes Skin Care for All more difficult to achieve.[20] When considering how skin carers can contribute to its mitigation, there are several entry points. *Reducing fuel consumption and deforestation through clean water technology* is one. Those who care for the skin have developed expertise in the management of hazards from sun, flood, and cold exposure. An example of the climate change causing wounds and lymphedema is the induction of cancer through sun exposure. *Cancer prevention and treatment* must be on the agenda of international wound healing. At the Regional Dermatology Training Centre, severe cancers occur in those affected by albinism who have no protection from the sun.[21]

Where possible, we have taught excision to allied health professionals, and now many experienced surgeons have visited and fellowships have been provided to expert centers. This has resulted in even large cancers being excised with minimal disfigurement.

Programs to protect the skin from the hazards of climate are well developed in the United States and in Australia with their Slip Slop Slap sunscreen application campaign. In Tanzania, the albino program focuses on seeking shade and wearing hats, and along the western mountain ranges of the Americas, the American Indian, who is genetically prone to polymorphic light eruptions, is protected. Many conditions like these, which are influenced by climate, may worsen unless the experience of skin carers is fully appreciated and funded.

As an example of the globalization of key interventions, a memorandum of understanding between Procter & Gamble, the IFD, and the ISNG provides *water fit for drinking* and for washing, distributing sachets named PUR®, each one cleaning 10 L of water within 30 minutes. Procter & Gamble also gives *glycerine as an emollient*, and this can be seen as a collaborative initiative promoting the lowest level of technologies used in skin care.[22] Water and emollients are the lowest technology.

Social marketing[23] of concepts, such as "Black

is Beautiful" or "Natural is Beautiful," is important in reducing the damage done with skin-lightening creams containing harmful agents, such as strong steroids or mercury. Also, tattoos, body piercings, smoking, and even graffiti can be initiated by a desire to raise self-esteem. The Community Dermatology Task Force believes that understanding these issues and anything that encourages the carer of the skin to understand the need and to develop *interventions to raise self-esteem* are keys to managing skin well-being. People with disfigurements due to scarring and consequences of burns, in particular, need help and support in this way. Millions of individuals in their youth have had interventions for reasons of self-esteem. Later in their lives when they no longer feel good about these interventions, these individuals fall into a program of wound healing. Many previously local charities, such as Changing Faces, are becoming global to add dignity and self-esteem to the disfigured and rejected.[24]

All programs need to be patient-centered to ensure effective patient engagement that will uphold treatment adherence and empower people to self-manage. Even in the delivery of community management, awareness of individual needs has to be preserved but recognized as a part of the community profile. Where possible, the *self-management dimension for care* needs to be supported through planned education and support to enhance treatment adherence and prevention of skin barrier deterioration; nurses have a key role here. The extent to which the absence of skin care leads to morbidity and indeed at times mortality[25] should be emphasized through educational initiatives. Morbidity needs the backup of formal quality-of-life scoring so that the burden is fully realized and the basis of community participation and income generation can be developed.[25]

The Future of Community Care

The future of community care depends on effective alliances and collaborations. As previously stated, the International Society of Dermatology task force for Skin Care for All: Community Dermatology writes about the scope and range of public health program needs. Following this background work describing successful interventions as a service need both in terms of workforce and of materials required, the task force is pre-

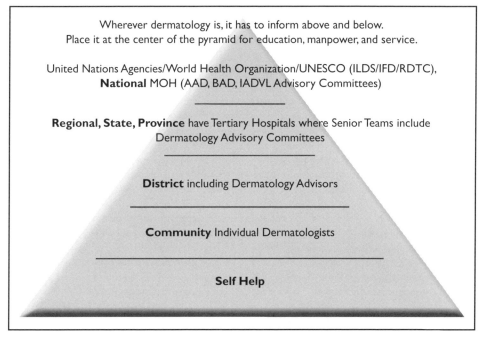

Wherever dermatology is, it has to inform above and below.
Place it at the center of the pyramid for education, manpower, and service.

United Nations Agencies/World Health Organization/UNESCO (ILDS/IFD/RDTC),
National MOH (AAD, BAD, IADVL Advisory Committees)

Regional, State, Province have Tertiary Hospitals where Senior Teams include
Dermatology Advisory Committees

District including Dermatology Advisors

Community Individual Dermatologists

Self Help

Figure 4. Pyramid distribution of advice provided by skin carers must be both to governance above and to practitioners below.
Legend: ILDS = International League of Dermatological Societies; IFD = International Foundation for Dermatology; RDTC = Regional Dermatology Training Centre; MOH = Ministry of Health; AAD = American Academy of Dermatology; BAD = British Association of Dermatologists; IADVL = Indian Association of Dermatologists, Venereologists, and Leprologists.

paring the A-B-Cs of how to promote community dermatology. It will work with organizations managing wounds, burns, and lymphedema and will work with the WHO to contribute to its interventions on skin care for the **neglected tropical disease (NTD)** programs. Leprosy is one of these. Hopes for the elimination of this disease have not been fulfilled, but the healthcare workers managing its vertical program are far fewer than in the past. It remains the prototype of stigma from disfiguring disease. Podoconiosis has recently been added to the list of NTDs and current simple nongovernmental organization projects are already helping thousands of patients.[4] Leishmaniasis is another common disease that results in disfigurement and is greatly in need of techniques to prevent or treat scarring.

Experts working in the framework of a pyramid of care (Figure 4) with the most needy at its base and governance at the top must give equal atten-

tion to both. No amount of effort to provide care to communities by those who are locally available will succeed if management at higher levels is uneducated about best practice. At the bottom, there is a need to provide locally available, sustainable, low-cost care, mainly through primary care initiatives. The support of the nursing profession is crucial to this service delivery model.

The significant lack of experts worldwide, most of whom are based in the secondary and tertiary hospital sectors, means that expertise in skin care cannot always be delivered to those who need it. An article written by the ISNG[9] outlines initiatives by nurses and examines the development of the nurse within the dermatology field and the need to cascade dermatological expertise from specialist to generalist community-based healthcare workers. It logically follows that there is an expectation to adopt a strategic approach that identifies the educational needs of nurses, harnesses the appropriate expertise, shares good practice, and operates in close interprofessional collaboration with dermatologists. As written by its recent chairman:

Work led by the International Skin Care Nursing Group (ISNG) has sought to stimulate and develop the capacity of nursing to respond to these widespread needs through promoting service delivery models that operate interdependently with dermatologist-led care. Such health professionals are well placed to work with community workers in resource poor countries and manage core clinical issues, including skin barrier protection and maintenance and the management of chronic wounds, applying preventative and educative strategies where possible. Evidence of such work is seen in South Africa with the development of a new Postgraduate Diploma in Dermatological Nursing to adequately prepare a cadre of nurses who can work in peripheral community based clinics addressing issues of skin and wound integrity. To realise this potential there is a need for the development of inter-professional team working, support for nursing development and complement their expertise.[9]

In this context, diagnosis is based on focusing on the common diseases. Attention to better diagnosis and the availability of essential drugs must include awareness and reminders of diseases, such as the NTDs. Reducing the prevalence of ineffective remedies, often bought at the roadside, is also a part of the program.

Wounds, Burns, and Lymphedema

For several decades and especially during the development of the task force for Skin Care for All: Community Dermatology, there has been emphasis on extending care of the skin beyond dermatology to include wounds, burns, and lymphedema. The public health territory of global injury epidemiology points to injury as a leading cause of death, highest in middle income and lowest in lower income groups. Head injury from a motorbike accident resulting in instant death, being an acute event, cannot be included as part of the remit of the task force for Skin Care for All, while trauma resulting in chronic nonhealing skin wounds should be. As mentioned by Escandon et al,[26] these wounds, such as pressure ulcers in the paraplegic, can lead to death and add to the little emphasized statistic of mortality due to skin conditions. Its prevalence is underestimated in data describing the scale of the injury problem.

The literature of classification and coding of injury tends to focus on anatomical sites, such as the head, trunk, or limb, but an injury severity score separately identifies external sites, meaning the skin, and includes much that is written about the economic and social burden. The care of the person living with an amputation stump, the pressure ulcer in the paraplegic, and of course burns are just a few examples in the literature relating to injury. Preventing the consequences of injury from becoming a top cause of loss of disability-adjusted years and managing those consequences require interventions from the skin carer.

The field of burns is an appropriate subject for a task force providing care for people with skin conditions who arrive in the primary care health center or require self-help. Topics for education include **accident prevention, first aid**, and **management** as well as **rehabilitation of the disfigured**. Education provided by skin carers has the capacity to benefit when factors are acknowledged, such as the greater susceptibility of the skin without sensation to burns; the importance of the availability of clean water fit for drinking; the need to avoid inflammable clothing and furnishings; child-to-child programs to prevent the youngest child from approaching the fireplace; safe firework displays (especially in China); and the whole question of disfigurement restoration and the "look good, feel good" factor that permeates the management of all skin disease. These require environmental, engineering, legislative, and educational approaches with rules on inflammable clothing and bedding as well as whole-country teaching of first aid. If, as debated at the WHO, the definition of health is to be altered — meaning the capacity to adapt as an agency to effectively self-manage — those who care for the skin are well in the lead to contribute to health for all through promoting skin health.

Conclusion

International chronic wound caring under the heading of Skin Care for All and a community program inclusive of wounds, lymphedema, and burns must pervade all health systems. Its principle themes must be written about in all relevant publications so that the diagnosis is correct and the interventions are available and affordable. Health promotion must prevent the deterioration of the skin barrier and the development of chronic wounds. While the management of HIV/AIDS, malaria, and tuberculosis receives billions of dollars per annum, data must be collected on disease prevalence, access to interventions, the size of the work force, and essential drugs and devices lists to inform resource providers. Donors have yet to be persuaded of the benefits of skin care, and wound healers must learn to value the public health relevance of skin health.

The task force for Skin Care for All: Community Dermatology can demonstrate in its recent publications its "capacity to benefit." It will seek alliances to explain how to approach the problem, but solving very common public health problems requires a strategic approach to ensure that resources are provided to enlarge the work force and equip it to aid effective self-management. Effective management requires a carer with knowledge who carries appropriate therapies (essential drugs and devices) and has access to the patient (Plate 3, page 315).

Practice Pearls
- Wound healers must learn to value the relevance of public health.
- Management of the skin integrity is integral to good wound prevention and care (including burns and lymphedema).
- The interprofessional wound care team needs to be patient-centered and connected to prevention strategies and public health programs.
- Enabling community health workers with common diagnostic and treatment principles can free tertiary care facilities to optimize the management of complex wound care patients.
- Globalization has allowed expert practitioner knowledge to reach inaccessible persons with chronic wounds, but to be successful, interventions must be focused on self-help with ethnic and local contextual relevance.
- International agencies need to develop effective alliances with each other and with local healthcare systems.

Self-Assessment Questions
1. Skin health is linked to:
   A. Wounds
   B. Burns
   C. Lymphedema
   D. Skin cancer development
   E. All of the above

2. Funding for research and patient care is most likely to be available for:
   A. HIV/AIDS
   B. Tropical diseases
   C. Lymphedema
   D. Wound care
   E. Skin care

3. Buruli ulcer:
   A. Is caused by a mycobacterium focusing on adipose tissue
   B. Can only be cured with extensive surgical excision
   C. Almost always responds to a combination of rifampicin and streptomycin
   D. Is found in the tropics except for West Africa
   E. Both A and C

Answers: 1–E, 2–A, 3–E

References
1. Macdonald JM, Geyer MJ, eds. *Wound and Lymphoedema Management.* Geneva, Switzerland: WHO Press; 2010:1–122.
2. Ryan TJ. The International Society of Dermatology's Task Force for Skin Care for All: Community Dermatology. *Int J Dermatol.* 2011;50(5):548–551.
3. Huber M, Knottnerus JA, Green L, et al. How should we define health? *BMJ.* 2011;343:d4163.
4. Davey G. Podoconiosis, non-filarial elephantiasis and lymphology. *Lymphology.* 2010;43(4):168–177.
5. Ryan TJ. Healthy skin for all. International Committee of Dermatology. *Int J Dermatol.* 1994;33(12):829–835.
6. Howarth DM, Southee AE, Whyte IM. Lymphatic flow rates and first-aid in simulated peripheral snake or spider envenomation. *Med J Aust.* 1994;161(11-12):695–700.
7. Narahari S. Treating lymphoedema patients in Indian villages. *J Lymphoedema.* 2011;6(2):87–90.
8. Hay RJ, Fuller LC. The assessment of dermatological needs in resource-poor regions. *Int J Dermatol.* 2011;50(5):552–557.
9. Ersser SJ, Kaur V, Kelly P, et al. The contribution of the nursing service worldwide and its capacity to benefit within the dermatology field. *Int J Dermatol.* 2011;50(5):582–589.
10. Murrell DF, Ryan TJ, Bergfeld WF. Advancement of wom-

en in dermatology. *Int J Dermatol.* 2011;50(5):593–600.

11.   Ryan TJ. Wound healing in the developing world. In: Macdonald JM, Geyer MJ, eds. *Wound and Lymphoedema Management.* Geneva, Switzerland: WHO Press; 2010:3–6.

12.   Phan TT, Lee ST, Chan SY, Hughes MA, Cherry GW. Investigating plant-based medicines for wound healing with the use of cell culture technologies and *in vitro* models: a review. *Ann Acad Med Singapore.* 2000;29(1):27–36.

13.   Ryan TJ, Hirt HM, Willcox M. Collaboration with traditional health practitioners in the provision of skin care for all in Africa. *Int J Dermatol.* 2011;50(5):564–570.

14.   Narahari SR, Ryan TJ, Bose KS, Prasanna KS, Aggithaya GM. Integrating modern dermatology and Ayurveda in the treatment of vitiligo and lymphedema in India. *Int J Dermatol.* 2011;50(3):310–334.

15.   Ryan TJ. Community dermatology inclusive of leprosy: its past present and future. *Lepr Rev.* 2007;78:7–10.

16.   Mahé A, Faye O, N'Diaye HT, et al. Definition of an algorithm for the management of common skin diseases at primary health care level in sub-Saharan Africa. *Trans R Soc Trop Med Hyg.* 2005;99(1):39–47.

17.   Ryan TJ, Morrone A, Hay R, Fuller LC, Naafs B, Sethi A. Guidelines on the role of skin care in the management of mobile populations. Based on a workshop Rome 24th-25th March 2011 *International Journal of Dermatology.* In press.

18.   Schmidt-Grendlemier P (2011) in CD, "Capacity to Benefit," www.intsocderm.org and update in press in *International Journal of Dermatology.*

19.   Bertramelli H (2011) in CD, "Capacity to Benefit," www.intsocderm.org and update in press in *International Journal of Dermatology.*

20.   Andersen LK. Global climate change and its dermatological diseases. *Int J Dermatol.* 2011;50(5):601–603.

21.   McBride SR, Leppard BJ. Attitudes and beliefs of an albino population toward sun avoidance: advice and services provided by an outreach albino clinic in Tanzania. *Arch Dermatol.* 2002;138(5):629–632.

22.   Brooks J. Water fit for drinking is fit for washing wounds! A case study at a Ugandan hospital. *Community Dermatology.* 2011;7(12):17–32.

23.   Karelas GD. Social marketing self-esteem: a socio-medical approach to high-risk and skin tone alteration activities. *Int J Dermatol.* 2011;50(5):590–592.

24.   Changing Faces. Available at: www.changingfaces.org.uk. Accessed February 11, 2012.

25.   Basra MK, Fenech R, Gatt RM, Salek MS, Finlay AY. The Dermatology Life Quality Index 1994–2007: a comprehensive review of validation data and clinical results. *Br J Dermatol.* 2008;159(5):997–1035.

26.   Escandon J, Vivas AC, Tang J, Rowland KJ, Kirsner RS. High mortality in patients with chronic wounds. *Wound Repair Regen.* 2011;19(4):526–528.

Science of Wound Healing: Translation of Bench Science into Advances for Chronic Wound Care

Linda Cowan, PhD, ARNP, CWS;
Joyce Stechmiller, PhD, ACNP-BC, FAAN;
Priscilla Phillips, PhD;
Gregory Schultz, PhD

Objectives

The reader will be challenged to:

- Assess the basic concepts of molecular regulation in normal wound healing and identify common alterations that may lead to chronic wounds
- Analyze evidence for state-of-the-art approaches to correct molecular imbalances in chronic wounds
- Formulate basic concepts regarding the implication of biofilms in contributing to chronic inflammatory states of nonhealing wounds
- Identify potential diagnostic tools that may assist the clinician in rapid detection of important biomarkers indicating impaired wound healing.

Introduction

Traditionally, most acute skin wounds heal without clinically significant complications, and the resulting scar tissue functions similarly enough to un-wounded skin that the repaired wound does not cause substantial problems. However, some acute skin wounds fail to heal in an expected or predicted manner and become chronic, which invariably leads to a wide range of complications, including infection, poor quality of life, increased risk of lower limb amputation, and, ultimately, death from systemic sepsis. Although much is understood about the basic science of normal skin wound healing, only recently has research begun to unravel the molecular and cellular reasons why some wounds fail to heal. Fortunately, these discoveries are constantly being translated into new therapies that selectively target the bacterial, molecular, and cellular abnormalities that impair healing, correct imbalances, and convert the chronic wound into a healing wound.

Overview of Normal Skin Wound Healing

The process of normal healing within acute skin wounds involves a distinct 4-phase sequence that results in the creation of a scar: hemostasis, inflammation, repair, and remodeling (Plate 4, page 316).[1–3] During the initial hemostasis phase, fibrinogen is proteolytically converted to fibrin by thrombin, leading to formation of the fibrin clot, which stimulates platelets to degranulate, releasing numerous growth factors and proinflammatory cytokines

Cowan L, Stechmiller J, Phillips P, Schultz G. Science of wound healing: translation of bench science into advances for chronic wound care. In: Krasner DL, Rodeheaver GT, Sibbald RG, Woo KY, eds. *Chronic Wound Care: A Clinical Source Book for Healthcare Professionals.* Vol 1. 5th ed. Malvern, PA: HMP Communications; 2012:25–35.

in the wound. These important regulatory molecules chemotactically draw in neutrophils and macrophages, initiating the inflammatory phase. As shown in Plate 5 (page 316), a key function of the inflammatory cells is to engulf invading bacteria and fungi and kill them by generating reactive oxygen species (ROS) inside the endosomes. A second key function of inflammatory cells is to secrete proteases, including the matrix metalloproteinases (MMPs) and elastase, which remove (debride) extracellular matrix (ECM) molecules like collagen that were damaged during the injury.[4] Inflammation continues to increase, reaches a maximum by about 5 to 7 days after injury, and, in the absence of continued inflammatory stimulation, decreases to low levels by about 14 days after injury. Acute inflammation stimulates the wound to enter into the repair phase, which is characterized by proliferation and migration of fibroblasts from the adjacent uninjured dermis into the provisional fibrin wound matrix, where the fibroblasts synthesize large amounts of new collagen and other ECM proteins that replace the fibrin matrix.[5] Vascular endothelial cells in the surrounding vasculature also proliferate and migrate into the fibrin matrix to form new capillaries (neovascularization) that provide essential nutritional support for the rapidly metabolizing fibroblasts. Epithelial cells from the edge of the injury and especially from the stem cell niches in the hair follicles and sweat glands proliferate and migrate across the new scar matrix that is being generated by the fibroblasts. Some fibroblasts in the wound matrix differentiate into myofibroblasts and contract the newly forming scar matrix, reducing the wound area by ~20% in human skin wounds. When the epithelial cells have resurfaced the wound, the first 3 phases of wound healing are completed, but the initial scar matrix is not static. Over the next 6 to 12 months, the initial scar matrix is slowly remodeled by proteases that remove the highly irregular scar tissue, which is replaced by new collagen that is organized into a much more normal, basket-weave structure found in uninjured dermis.[4]

Normal skin wound healing is a highly integrated process that involves platelets, inflammatory cells, fibroblasts, epithelial cells, and vascular endothelial cells. The actions of these wound cells are closely regulated by key proteins including pro- and anti-inflammatory cytokines, growth factors, receptors, proteases, inhibitors, and ECM proteins that dictate the activities of these cells. As normal wound healing proceeds, the regulatory proteins and the responses of the individual cells interact ultimately to result in repair of the injury.

Overview of Molecular and Cellular Abnormalities in Chronic Wounds

All chronic wounds begin as acute wounds, but acute wounds become chronic wounds when they fail to progress through the sequential phases of healing as expected.[4,6] A key question to ask is, are there common molecular and cellular patterns in chronic wounds that indicate the stage of the wound healing sequence where most chronic wounds stall? The simple answer is yes. Cellular and molecular data from numerous clinical studies suggest that most chronic wounds get "stuck" in a prolonged inflammatory phase that is due to the presence of both planktonic (free flowing) and biofilm bacteria in the wound (Figure 1).[7,8] The bacteria stimulate production of proinflammatory cytokines like tumor necrosis factor-alpha (TNF-α) and interleukin 1 (IL-1), which act as chemotactic factors (chemical messengers) to recruit neutrophils, macrophages, and mast cells into the wound. The inflammatory cells that are drawn into the wound secrete proteases (MMPs, neutrophil elastase, and plasmin) and ROS in an attempt to kill bacteria and detach biofilm colonies that are tightly attached to the wound bed. However, because bacterial biofilms are tolerant to ROS as well as antibodies and even antiseptics, the biofilms persist and continue to stimulate inflammation. This results in chronically elevated levels of proteases and ROS that eventually begin to destroy essential proteins that are necessary for healing, including growth factors, their receptors, and ECM proteins. These "off-target" effects of proteases and ROS combine to reduce cell proliferation, migration, and generation of functional scar matrix.[1,9–11] The "biological sum" of this prolonged inflammatory state is a distorted molecular and cellular wound environment that prevents wound healing. In the simplest terms, the molecular and cellular environment between acute

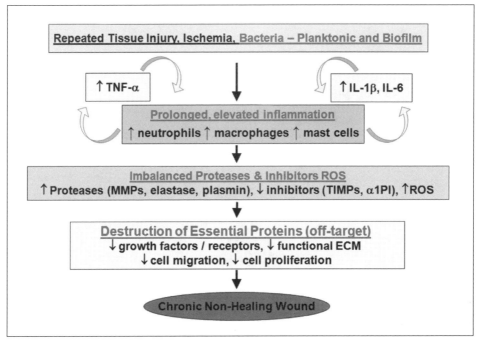

Figure 1. Molecular and cellular pathology of chronic wounds. Acute wounds that become critically colonized by planktonic and biofilm bacteria develop chronic inflammation that is characterized by high levels of proteases and ROS that destroy "off-target" proteins that are essential for healing, resulting in a chronic wound.

healing wounds and chronic wounds is totally different. As shown in Figure 2, these "imbalances" must be corrected by clinical therapies or the wound will not progress to healing. Strategies designed to reverse these imbalances would be expected to promote healing, and indeed, innovative new treatments are being developed and tested, and some have already been shown to clinically improve healing of chronic wounds. Of utmost importance is attention to evidence-based wound care, adequate wound bed preparation, appropriate management of underlying disease, and correction of other contributing factors (such as too much or too little moisture, excessive friction and shear, and inadequate nutrition) that may impair wound healing.[4]

Repeated Tissue Injury

Clinical observations indicate that acute wounds that develop into chronic wounds are frequently subjected to repeated episodes of tissue injury leading to ischemia, such as prolonged

pressure in spinal cord-injury patients (pressure ulcers), vasculopathies (venous leg ulcers), or blunt trauma that occurs on plantar foot surfaces of people with diabetic neuropathy.[4,6] This causes the epidermis to break down, generating an open wound that quickly becomes colonized with planktonic bacteria.

Bacterial Bioburden and Biofilms

Decades of clinical and laboratory research have conclusively shown that high concentrations of planktonic bacteria found in clinically infected wounds can impair wound healing, primarily by stimulating inflammation and by secreting exotoxins, proteases, and virulence factors that impair inflammatory cell functions and break down host tissue to promote dissemination of the bacteria and to provide nutrients for the rapidly proliferating bacteria. Historically, many nonhealing wounds were not reported to have high levels of planktonic bacteria when assessed by standard clinical microbiology as-

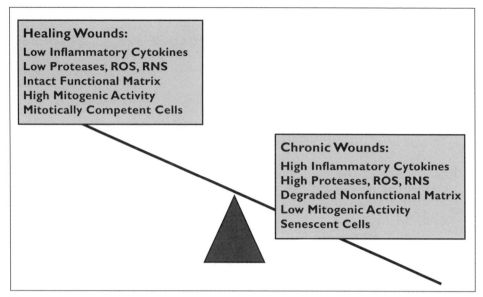

Healing Wounds:

Low Inflammatory Cytokines
Low Proteases, ROS, RNS
Intact Functional Matrix
High Mitogenic Activity
Mitotically Competent Cells

Chronic Wounds:

High Inflammatory Cytokines
High Proteases, ROS, RNS
Degraded Nonfunctional Matrix
Low Mitogenic Activity
Senescent Cells

Figure 2. Imbalanced molecular and cellular environments of healing and chronic wounds. The molecular and cellular environment of acute healing wounds is dramatically different than that of chronic wounds and must be "rebalanced" to approximate the environment of healing wounds before healing can progress. Adapted with permission from Mast BA, Schultz GS. Interactions of cytokines, growth factors, and proteases in acute and chronic wounds. *Wound Repair Regen.* 1996;4(4):411.

says. However, serial aggressive debridement and systemic and topical treatments designed to reduce bacterial bioburden were frequently found to improve healing. This led to the concept of *critical colonization*, which was an attempt to recognize that something about the bioburden was impairing healing (Plate 6, page 317). New data suggest that the critical factor determining wound bioburden is usually the presence of bacteria in polymicrobial biofilm communities.[5]

A *biofilm* is a community of microorganisms surrounded by an extracellular polymeric matrix (EPM), which attaches to a surface.[12] Recent studies demonstrate that biofilms are becoming a significant component of infections in humans.[12-14] The Centers for Disease Control and Prevention and the National Institutes of Health project that biofilms are associated with 65% of nosocomial (hospital-acquired) infections and up to 80% of all human infections in the United States. In addition, treatment of biofilm-associated infections costs billions of dollars and results in hundreds of thousands of

deaths annually in the United States.[12] Both acute and chronic wounds are susceptible to the development of biofilms within the wound bed.

Open wounds provide a perfect environment for opportunistic organisms, such as bacteria, to reside and reproduce. Analyses of the microflora of chronic wounds (such as pressure and diabetic foot ulcers) demonstrate a phenomenon known as *chronic wound pathogenic biofilms*.[12-14] Typical mechanisms by which biofilms impede wound healing progress involve heightening the level of inflammation; increasing the amount of ROS and proteases in the wound bed; stimulating overly aggressive immune responses; producing detrimental exogenous toxins within the wound environment; and impairing normal chemokine signalling pathways.[15] Aerobic organisms within biofilms use oxygen and help to create anaerobic niches within the biofilm matrix that support the development of anaerobes within the biofilm.[12] Importantly, the presence of biofilms in a wound may affect the wound healing process without visible clinical signs of infection. However, there may be indications of bacterial imbalance (eg, change in wound color or odor together with the presence of devitalized tissue and ischemia).[15]

Studies suggest that certain bacterial groups, which by themselves are considered essentially harmless (such as Corynebacterium spp), tend to form symbiotic communities with other bacteria and fungi in chronic wounds. These polymicrobial groups in biofilms are termed *functional equivalent pathogroups* because they have been shown to have functionally detrimental effects on wound healing similar to other well known pathogens, such as *Staphylococcus aureus*.[12] In addition, biofilm colonies may extend 2 mm beneath the wound bed and into surrounding healthy tissue, making them difficult to eradicate by many traditional bedside debridement methods. Treatment options to consider include debridement and the use of a broad-spectrum topical antimicrobial agent directly after debridement to control the planktonic bacterial load and to reduce the progression into biofilms. Importantly, recent data indicate that mature biofilm communities can re-establish in wounds within 3 days following debridement.[5] If control of microbial progression from planktonic to mature biofilms is not achieved, a change from an early stage biofilm to a polymicrobial "complex" mature wound biofilm may develop and ultimately lead to a compromised state. [15]

Biofilm experts suggest that traditional culturing methods, which involve inoculating a culture medium with a cotton swab sample obtained from the patient, are insufficient to identify true components of the polymicrobial mature biofilm colonies.[12,15] The exact microbial composition of biofilms is largely undetectable by traditional cotton swab culture techniques due to the protective polymeric coating that biofilms produce. This self-protective coating encapsulates the colony and is also impervious to most systemic and topical antimicrobials/antibiotics. Other limitations of the traditional clinical swab sampling approach include the following:

- Cotton swab cultures typically query only the most common aerobic organisms
- Culture results are often unavailable for 2 to 3 days
- The culture is naturally biased toward identifying only those cultivable bacterial species

that are easily cultured under standard laboratory conditions on standard growth media.[12]

Recent literature suggests that the polymerase chain reaction (PCR) assay is a cost-effective, rapid, and more sensitive method to detect microbial pathogens (particularly biofilm microbes) in clinical specimens. The diagnostic value of PCR may be clinically superior to traditional swab cultures as well as other modern options, such as pyrosequencing techniques. Pyrosequencing essentially generates millions of short ~100 nucleotide sequences, and software scans the entire bacterial and fungal DNA databases for matches of DNA sequences. Thus, pyrosequencing can identify all bacterial and fungal species present in a biopsy, but it is more expensive and requires about a week to generate the data. The PCR identification of bacteria and fungi in wound biopsies is a more focused and limited approach that uses primer sequences that "probe" for unique DNA sequences of ribosomal RNAs. This real-time PCR testing specifically probes for ~30 bacteria and fungi species in a wound sample. However, it is less expensive and rapid (costs ~$100 and is completed in less than 24 hours).[15]

Elevated Proinflammatory Cytokines

Closely linked to the bacterial bioburden in a wound is the proinflammatory cytokine profile. In general, fluids from acute healing wounds tend to have an early peak of major proinflammatory cytokines, TNF-α and IL-1β, and their natural inhibitors, P55 and IL-1 receptor antagonist, within the first few days after injury, which corresponds to the rapid increase in inflammatory cells in the acute wound.[16] The levels of proinflammatory cytokines begin to decrease after 6 to 7 days as the inflammatory stimuli in acute wounds decrease. However, in a study of chronic leg ulcers, the levels of inflammatory cytokines, IL-1β, IL-6, and TNF-α were significantly higher than in acute healing wounds, and as the chronic ulcers began to heal, the levels decreased.[8] These findings indicate that chronic wounds have persistently elevated levels of proinflammatory cytokines, but as chronic wounds heal, the molecular environment changes to a less proinflammatory wound environment.

Elevated Proteases

Another major concept to emerge from wound fluid analyses is that levels of proteases, especially MMPs and neutrophil elastase, are much higher in chronic wounds than in acute wound fluids.[6,16,17] During the early phase of acute wound healing, the average level of protease activity in mastectomy fluids was found to be low, suggesting that protease activity is tightly controlled during the early phase of wound healing.[9] However, in chronic wounds, the average level of protease activity was found to be approximately 116-fold higher than in acute mastectomy wound fluids. Furthermore, as chronic venous ulcers began to heal, the levels of protease activity decreased.[9] Similar results were reported for fluids or biopsies of chronic pressure ulcers, where levels of MMP-2, MMP-9, and MMP-1 were 10 to 25 times higher than levels in acute surgical wound fluids.[18,19] Levels of the tissue inhibitors of metalloproteinases (TIMPs), which are the natural inhibitors of MMPs, were found to be decreased in wound fluids from chronic venous ulcers compared to acute mastectomy wound fluids.[20]

In nonhealing chronic pressure ulcers, MMP-8, the neutrophil-derived collagenase, was elevated, indicating that there may be a persistent influx of neutrophils releasing MMP-8 and elastase, which could contribute to the destruction of ECM proteins and growth factors that are essential for healing.[21] Chronic venous ulcers were found to have 10-fold to 40-fold higher levels of neutrophil elastase activity and to have degraded α1-antitrypsin. Elevated MMP-2 and MMP-9 levels in chronic venous ulcers also were observed to coincide with degradation of fibronectin in the wound bed.[22,23] Fibronectin is an important multidomain adhesion protein that is present in the ECM and granulation tissue and is important in promoting epithelial cell migration. Proteases in chronic wound fluids were shown to rapidly degrade exogenously added growth factors, such as transforming growth factor-alpha (TGF-α), epidermal growth factor (EGF), or platelet-derived growth factor (PDGF), using *in-vitro* laboratory tests. In contrast, exogenously added growth factors were stable when added to acute surgical wound fluids.[1,9–11]

Reduced Mitogenic Activity of Chronic Wound Fluids

Another key concept that emerged from laboratory analysis demonstrates that the mitogenic activity of chronic wound fluids is dramatically less than levels in acute wound fluids. For example, fluids from chronic leg ulcers did not stimulate DNA synthesis of cells in culture, while acute wound fluids strongly stimulate proliferation of cells in culture. Furthermore, when acute and chronic wound fluids were combined, the mitotic activity of acute wound fluids was inhibited.[7,24,25] These results show that the proteases in chronic wound fluid degrade growth factors that are normally present in acute wound fluids, and without the essential actions of these growth factors, wound healing will not progress.

Factors Affecting Cell Senescence

In chronic wounds, the capacity of the wound cells to respond to cytokines and growth factors is altered. Research suggests that fibroblasts (cells that manufacture collagen and perform other essential functions in wound healing) have a diminished response to growth factors in chronic wounds. For example, fibroblast cultures established from chronic venous leg ulcers proliferated slowly and formed less dense confluent cultures when compared to normal fibroblast cultures established from uninjured dermis.[26] In another study of chronic venous leg ulcers that were present for more than 3 years, fibroblasts proliferated poorly in response to PDGF added to the culture medium and rapidly approached senescence compared to fibroblasts cultured from venous ulcers that had been present for less than 3 years.[27]

The molecular environments of acute and chronic wounds are dramatically different (Figure 2). Healing wounds have low bacterial bioburden and no biofilms, low levels of inflammatory cytokines, low levels of proteases, high levels of growth factors, and cells that divide rapidly in response to growth factors. The molecular and cellular environment of chronic wounds is exactly the opposite. Chronic wounds have high levels of bacterial biofilms, elevated levels of inflammatory cytokines, high levels of proteases, low levels of growth factors, and cells that are approaching senescence.[27–29] With this in mind, new treatment strategies should be designed to re-establish in

Table 1. TIME and wound bed preparation assessment tool

TISSUE	Debridement assessment: • Color assessment • Tissue perfusion • TCP02 (color Doppler angiography)
INFECTION	Wound bed and surrounding skin: • Temperature • Odor • Color • pH
MOISTURE	Assess maceration or desiccation, leg volume transepidermal water loss (TEWL)
EDGE	2D evaluation • Acetate tracing • Digital photography • Digital tools and PC software • 3D evaluation • Probes, molds • Scanning systems

Adapted with permission from Dowsett C, Ayello E. TIME principles of chronic wound bed preparation and treatment. *Br J Nurs.* 2004;13(15):S16–S23.

chronic wounds the balance of bacterial bioburden, cytokines, growth factors, proteases, their natural inhibitors, and competent cells found in healing wounds. Chronic wounds fail to heal because of molecular and cellular abnormalities in the wound environment. For example, studies have shown altered signaling pathways and levels of gene expression (eg, elevated c-myc and beta-catenin, altered intracellular localization of EGF receptor) that reflect the stalled migration of keratinocytes at the edge of chronic wounds.[30] Several innovative approaches to identifying and managing chronic wounds are being developed and are based on identifying and correcting these types of molecular and cellular abnormalities.

Innovative Approaches for Correcting Molecular Abnormalities of Chronic Wounds

Debridement. Clearly, proper wound debridement is a key element of wound bed preparation. This was demonstrated by Steed et al[29] who performed a clinical study that showed that healing of chronic diabetic foot ulcers (treated at 10 different centers) was closely correlated with the frequency of debridement. The benefit of wound debridement was seen in both patients who received standard care and patients who were treated with topical PDGF. It is possible that frequent sharp debridement of diabetic ulcers may reduce the level of inflammation in the wound by mechanically removing biofilms as well as by converting the chronic wound into a pseudo-acute wound molecular environment. Therefore, appropriate wound debridement should be considered a vital component in the care of patients with chronic diabetic foot ulcers.

TIME to heal wounds. A second category of approaches to correcting the molecular imbalance in chronic wounds is targeted at the elevated levels of inflammatory cytokines. The simplest approach to correcting this condition is to prepare the wound bed using debridement and moisture control. This concept has been more thoroughly described in an article that unites wound bed preparation under a *TIME* acronym that stands for **T**issue debridement, **I**nfection/inflammation, **M**oisture balance, and **E**dge effect (Plate 7, page 317). Correctly applying the concepts of wound bed preparation to the care of a patient's wound requires a tool that helps assess when each of the 4 components has been optimized. As shown in Table 1, assessment of the TIME components involves good clinical judgment and objective measurements of wound parameters, as described by Dowsett and Ayello.[31]

Proteases. Another important clinical approach to correcting molecular imbalances in chronic wounds is to lower the levels of MMPs and other proteases. Several therapeutic approaches are currently used. Innovative wound dressings that contain denatured collagen (gelatin) and oxidized regenerated cellulose (Promogran, Systagenix Wound Management, Quincy, Massachusetts) are available. The gelatin in the dressing acts as a substrate sink for proteases, especially MMPs, and has been shown to reduce levels of protease activities in fluids from chronic human wounds measured *in vitro*.[32] One study of chronic diabetic plantar surface ulcers found that 31% of 51 patients treated with Promogran added to conventional dressings had complete wound closure compared with 28% of 39 patients treated with conventional dressings (P = .12).[33] Analysis of healing rates in subcategories of patients suggested that the effect of Promogran was more dramatic in healing in ulcers of less than 6 months' duration.

Another clinical approach that has been used to correct elevated levels of proteases, especially MMPs, is applying topical protease inhibitors. One study investigated topical treatment of diabetic foot ulcers with doxycycline.[34] Doxycycline is a member of the tetracycline family of antibiotics and is an effective inhibitor of metalloproteinases, including MMPs and the TNF-α converting enzyme (TACE).[35] A randomized controlled trial of 1% topical doxycycline treatment of patients with chronic diabetic foot ulcers found that all 4 ulcers treated daily with doxycycline in a carboxymethyl cellulose vehicle healed in less than the 20-week treatment period, while only 1 of 3 ulcers treated with vehicle healed in 20 weeks. Importantly, no adverse events attributable to the doxycycline treatment occurred.[34]

Other methods of wound care can be used to lower levels of proteases in wound beds. For example, negative pressure wound therapy (NPWT) removes wound fluid containing high levels of proteases from the wound bed while drawing fresh plasma that contains protease inhibitors (α2 macroglobulin, α1-antitrypsin) into the wound bed.[36] In addition, dressings that absorb large amounts of wound exudate, especially dressings that contain highly charged polymers (eg, negatively charged polyacrylic acid or carboxymethylated cellulose or positively charged polyquats), can ionically bind the charged protease proteins and sequester the proteases in the matrix of the dressing, thus sparing the proteins in the wound bed that are essential for healing.[37]

Optimal use of advanced therapies to reduce the elevated levels of proteases would ideally depend on actually measuring the levels of proteases in a patient's wound. Thus, clinicians may find a rapid, point-of-care (POC) detector that measures levels of MMP activities in a wound fluid sample useful. Two prototype MMP detectors are currently under final development. Both MMP detectors would enable clinicians to assess the level of MMP protease activity in wound fluid samples collected at the bedside in approximately 10 minutes. One device utilizes lateral flow strip (LFS) technology like that used in early pregnancy test kits that are performed at home on urine samples. This LFS detector for MMPs produces a line on the test strip when MMP activities in a wound fluid sample are low and no line on the test strip when the MMP activities are high, which is opposite from how LFS detectors typically indicate if a biomarker is present in a sample. A second prototype MMP detector generates a fluorescent signal that is proportional to the level of MMP activities in wound fluid that is collected on a swab and added to the MMP substrate solution. Gibson et al[38] used the fluorescence POC detector prototype to measure MMP levels in samples of acute and chronic wound fluids collected by swabs at the bedside. After 10 minutes of reaction, MMP levels were almost 6 times higher in chronic wounds (n = 6) than the average level measured in acute wounds (n = 3). Assessing the level of MMPs in wounds should help clinicians determine if the level of proteases is so high that healing would not likely occur and could help clinicians determine if the wound should be debrided and treated with dressings that reduce protease activities and/or reduce bacterial bioburden.

Growth factors. The application of recombinant growth factors to the wound is another approach to correcting the abnormal molecular environment of chronic wounds. Several clinical studies have reported improved healing of various types of chronic wounds with recombinant human growth factors and cytokines, including PDGF,[39,40] keratinocyte growth factor-2 (KGF-2),[41] transforming growth factor beta (TGF-β),[42] basic fibroblast growth factor (bFGF),[43,44] and granulocyte-macrophage colony-stimulating factor (GM-CSF).[43] It is important to recognize that growth factors can only function well in chronic wounds when the environment is similar to that found in acute wounds. In other words, growth factors cannot convert a chronic wound to an acute wound and do not function in a necrotic, inflamed, protease-laden wound. Thus, the principles of wound bed preparation must be used in conjunction with topical growth factor treatments.

A logical extension of the principles of wound bed preparation is to combine therapies that address more than one aspect of TIME. Indeed, combining topical growth factor treatment (Regranex®, Healthpoint, Ltd., Fort Worth, Texas) with protease inhibiting dressings (Fibracol Plus® collagen-alginate, Systagenix Wound Management, Quincy, Massachusetts, or Oasis® small intestinal submucosa, Healthpoint, Ltd.) rapidly healed 34 of 36 chronic wounds that had failed to heal by other wound care techniques, including when these therapies were used alone.[45] However, combining therapies should be used with caution because some combinations of topical treatments can inactivate or impair active components of one or more of the treatments.[46] For example, combining microbicidal dressings that contain PHMB, ionic silver, or iodine with Santyl® debriding ointment reduces the enzymatic activity of the collagenase enzyme in the Santyl.[47]

Conclusion

Wound healing occurs through 4 phases. These phases are sequentially regulated by the actions of cytokines, growth factors, ECM proteins, and proteases. If an acute wound fails to move through a phase of healing, molecular imbalances will occur, leading to a chronic wound. Chronic wounds are characterized by bacterial biofilms, elevated

Practice Pearls
- Moist wound healing is evidence-based. Avoid using products or therapies in chronic full-thickness wounds that dry out the wound bed at any time. Remember, balance is important. Keeping the wound bed moist but not too moist (as evidenced by periwound maceration or dressings that need to be changed more than 2 or 3 times per day) is sometimes a challenge.
- Always attempt to include the patient's preferences, values, and any unique patient limitations (cognitive, physical, and psychosocial/emotional) in your treatment plan. For example, a patient or his or her caregiver is not likely to be compliant with a daily treatment plan that requires him or her to manually "milk" and discard bloody drainage from tubing left in a surgical wound if he or she faints at the sight of blood.
- Start with the simple and most cost-effective products and therapies for chronic wound care that address TIME principles. Always recheck wound progress within 2 weeks of starting or changing wound treatments. If wound healing is the goal (not palliative wounds) and no improvement is seen within 2 to 4 weeks of initiating a wound treatment, 1) verify that all TIME principles are being addressed, 2) verify patient/caregiver understanding/compliance with treatment orders, 3) assess and address comorbid conditions that may impair wound healing (unrelieved friction/shear/pressure; inadequate nutrition), and 4) consider tissue biopsy to rule out other pathology (eg, malignancy, pyoderma gangrenosum). If all of these factors have been satisfactorily addressed, consider changing wound treatment modalities, possibly including the initiation of advanced therapies.

inflammatory cytokines and proteases, low levels of mitogenic activity, and senescent cells that are unable to respond to growth factors. Healing of chronic wounds occurs as the molecular environment of the wound shifts to the environment of an acute wound. New therapies are designed to correct the molecular abnormalities of chronic wounds and correspond to the principles of wound bed preparation.

Self-Assessment Questions

1. Which of the following is NOT a reason why PCR as a diagnostic tool may be more desirable than standard swab cultures for measuring bacterial strains present in a biofilm?

   A. Results are obtained quicker than standard culture techniques

   B. It identifies more strains with greater accuracy

   C. The test can be done at the bedside like a rapid strep test

   D. It may be more cost effective

2. What does the M stand for in the TIME acronym approach to wound management?

   A. Manage nutrition

   B. Manage moisture

   C. Manage edema

   D. Manage infection

Answers: 1-C, 2-B

References

1.   Bennett NT, Schultz GS. Growth factors and wound healing: Part II. Role in normal and chronic wound healing. *Am J Surg.* 1993;166(1):74–81.

2.   Bennett NT, Schultz GS. Growth factors and wound healing: biochemical properties of growth factors and their receptors. *Am J Surg.* 1993;165(6):728–737.

3.   Lawrence WT. Physiology of the acute wound. *Clin Plast Surg.* 1998;25(3):321–340.

4.   Doughty DB, Sparks-DeFriese B. Wound-healing physiology. In: Bryant RA, Nix DP, eds. *Acute and Chronic Wounds.* 4th ed. St. Louis, MO: Elsevier Mosby; 2010:63–82.

5.   Wolcott RD, Rumbaugh KP, James G, et al. Biofilm maturity studies indicate sharp debridement opens a time-dependent therapeutic window. *J Wound Care.* 2010;19(8):320–328.

6.   Mast BA, Schultz GS. Interactions of cytokines, growth factors, and proteases in acute and chronic wounds. *Wound Repair Regen.* 1996;4(4):411–420.

7.   Harris IR, Yee KC, Walters CE, et al. Cytokine and protease levels in healing and non-healing chronic venous leg ulcers. *Exp Dermatol.* 1995;4(6):342–349.

8.   Trengove NJ, Bielefeldt-Ohmann H, Stacey MC. Mitogenic activity and cytokine levels in non-healing and healing chronic leg ulcers. *Wound Repair Regen.* 2000;8(1):13–25.

9.   Trengove NJ, Stacey MC, MacAuley S, et al. Analysis of the acute and chronic wound environments: the role of proteases and their inhibitors. *Wound Repair Regen.* 1999;7(6):442–452.

10.   Tarnuzzer RW, Schultz GS. Biochemical analysis of acute and chronic wound environments. *Wound Repair Regen.* 1996;4(3):321–325.

11.   Yager DR, Chen SM, Ward SI, Olutoye OO, Diegelmann RF, Cohen IK. Ability of chronic wound fluids to degrade peptide growth factors is associated with increased levels of elastase activity and diminished levels of proteinase inhibitors. *Wound Repair Regen.* 1997;5(1):23–32.

12.   Dowd SE, Wolcott RD, Sun Y, McKeehan T, Smith E, Rhoads D. Polymicrobial nature of chronic diabetic foot ulcer biofilm infections determined using bacterial tag encoded FLX amplicon pyrosequencing (bTEFAP). *PLoS One.* 2008;3(10):e3326.

13.   James GA, Swogger E, Wolcott R, et al. Biofilms in chronic wounds. *Wound Repair Regen.* 2008;16(1):37–44.

14.   Smith DM, Snow DE, Rees E, et al. Evaluation of the bacterial diversity of pressure ulcers using bTEFAP pyrosequencing. *BMC Med Genomics.* 2010;3:41.

15.   Cowan T. Biofilms and their management: from concept to clinical reality. Presented at the Second Annual Journal of Wound Care Lecture in Manchester Town Hall in Manchester, England, March 10, 2011.

16.   Schreml S, Szeimies R, Prantl L, Landthaler M, Babilas P. Wound healing in the 21st century. *J Am Acad Dermatol.* 2010;63(5):866–881.

17.   Yager DR, Nwomeh BC. The proteolytic environment of chronic wounds. *Wound Repair Regen.* 1999;7(6):433–441.

18.   Yager DR, Zhang LY, Liang HX, Diegelmann RF, Cohen IK. Wound fluids from human pressure ulcers contain elevated matrix metalloproteinase levels and activity compared to surgical wound fluids. *J Invest Dermatol.* 1996;107(5):743–748.

19.   Rogers AA, Burnett S, Moore JC, Shakespeare PG, Chen WY. Involvement of proteolytic enzymes—plasminogen activators and matrix metalloproteinases—in the pathophysiology of pressure ulcers. *Wound Repair Regen.* 1995;3(3):273–283.

20.   Bullen EC, Longaker MT, Updike DL, et al. Tissue inhibitor of metalloproteinases-1 is decreased and activated gelatinases are increased in chronic wounds. *J Invest Dermatol.* 1995;104(2):236–240.

21.   Ladwig GP, Robson MC, Liu R, Kuhn MA, Muir DF, Schultz GS. Ratios of activated matrix metalloproteinase-9 to tissue inhibitor of matrix metalloproteinase-1 in wound fluids are inversely correlated with healing of pressure ulcers. *Wound Repair Regen.* 2002;10(1):26–37.

22.   Wysocki AB, Staiano-Coico L, Grinnell F. Wound fluid from chronic leg ulcers contains elevated levels of metalloproteinases MMP-2 and MMP-9. *J Invest Dermatol.*

1993;101(1):64–68.

23. Grinnell F, Zhu M. Fibronectin degradation in chronic wounds depends on the relative levels of elastase, alpha1-proteinase inhibitor, and alpha2-macroglobulin. *J Invest Dermatol.* 1996;106(2):335–341.

24. Bucalo B, Eaglstein WH, Falanga V. Inhibition of cell proliferation by chronic wound fluid. *Wound Repair Regen.* 1993;1(3):181–186.

25. Katz MH, Alvarez AF, Kirsner RS, Eaglstein WH, Falanga V. Human wound fluid from acute wounds stimulates fibroblast and endothelial cell growth. *J Am Acad Dermatol.* 1991;25(6 Pt 1):1054–1058.

26. Agren MS, Eaglstein WH, Ferguson MW, et al. Causes and effects of the chronic inflammation in venous leg ulcers. *Acta Derm Venereol Suppl (Stockh).* 2000;210:3–17.

27. Trengove NJ, Langton SR, Stacey MC. Biochemical analysis of wound fluid from nonhealing and healing chronic leg ulcers. *Wound Repair Regen.* 1996;4(2):234–239.

28. Schultz GS, Sibbald RG, Falanga V, et al. Wound bed preparation: a systematic approach to wound management. *Wound Repair Regen.* 2003;11 Suppl 1:S1–S28.

29. Steed DL, Donohoe D, Webster MW, Lindsley L. Effect of extensive debridement and treatment on the healing of diabetic foot ulcers. Diabetic Ulcer Study Group. *J Am Coll Surg.* 1996;183(1):61–64.

30. Stojadinovic O, Brem H, Vouthounis C, et al. Molecular pathogenesis of chronic wounds: the role of beta-catenin and c-myc in the inhibition of epithelialization and wound healing. *Am J Pathol.* 2005;167(1):59–69.

31. Dowsett C, Ayello E. TIME principles of chronic wound bed preparation and treatment. *Br J Nurs.* 2004;13(15):S16–S23.

32. Cullen B, Smith R, McCulloch E, Silcock D, Morrison L. Mechanism of action of PROMOGRAN, a protease modulating matrix, for the treatment of diabetic foot ulcers. *Wound Repair Regen.* 2002;10(1):16–25.

33. Veves A, Sheehan P, Pham HT. A randomized, controlled trial of Promogran (a collagen/oxidized regenerated cellulose dressing) vs. standard treatment in the management of diabetic foot ulcers. *Arch Surg.* 2002;137(7):822–827.

34. Chin GA, Thigpin TG, Perrin KJ, Moldawer LL, Schultz GS. Treatment of chronic ulcers in diabetic patients with a topical metalloproteinase inhibitor, doxycycline. *WOUNDS.* 2003;15(10):315–323.

35. Stechmiller J, Cowan L, Schultz G. The role of doxycycline as a matrix metalloproteinase inhibitor for the treatment of chronic wounds. *Biol Res Nurs.* 2010;11(4):336–344.

36. Stechmiller JK, Kilpadi DV, Childress B, Schultz GS. Effect of Vacuum-Assisted Closure Therapy on the expression of cytokines and proteases in wound fluid of adults with pressure ulcers. *Wound Repair Regen.* 2006;14(3):371–374.

37. Edwards JV, Yager DR, Cohen IK, et al. Modified cotton gauze dressings that selectively absorb neutrophil elastase activity in solution. *Wound Repair Regen.* 2001;9(1):50–58.

38. Gibson D, Cowan LJ, Stechmiller JK, Schultz GS. Initial clinical assessment of a point of care device to rapidly measure MMP activities in wound fluid swab samples. Presented at the 25th Annual Conference of the Southern Nursing Research Society in Jacksonville, FL, February 16–19, 2011.

39. Steed DL. Clinical evaluation of recombinant human platelet-derived growth factor for the treatment of lower extremity diabetic ulcers. Diabetic Ulcer Study Group. *J Vasc Surg.* 1995;21(1):71–81.

40. Smiell JM, Wieman TJ, Steed DL, Perry BH, Sampson AR, Schwab BH. Efficacy and safety of becaplermin (recombinant human platelet-derived growth factor-BB) in patients with nonhealing, lower extremity diabetic ulcers: a combined analysis of four randomized studies. *Wound Repair Regen.* 1999;7(5):335–346.

41. Robson MC, Phillips TJ, Falanga V, et al. Randomized trial of topically applied repifermin (recombinant human keratinocyte growth factor-2) to accelerate wound healing in venous ulcers. *Wound Repair Regen.* 2001;9(5):347–352.

42. Robson MC, Phillip LG, Cooper DM, et al. Safety and effect of transforming growth factor-beta(2) for treatment of venous stasis ulcers. *Wound Repair Regen.* 1995;3(2):157–167.

43. Robson MC, Hill DP, Smith PD, et al. Sequential cytokine therapy for pressure ulcers: clinical and mechanistic response. *Ann Surg.* 2000;231(4):600–611.

44. Robson MC, Phillips LG, Lawrence WT, et al. The safety and effect of topically applied recombinant basic fibroblast growth factor on the healing of chronic pressure sores. *Ann Surg.* 1992;216(4):401–408.

45. Carson SN, Travis E, Overall K, Lee-Jahshan S. Using Becaplermin Gel with collagen products to potentiate healing in chronic leg wounds. *WOUNDS.* 2008.

46. Cowan L, Phillips P, Liesenfeld B, et al. Caution: when combining topical wound treatments, more is not always better. *Wound Practice & Research.* 2011;19(2):60–64.

47. Shi L, Ermis R, Kiedaisch B, Carson D. The effect of various wound dressings on the activity of debriding enzymes. *Adv Skin Wound Care.* 2010;23(10):456–462.

Effective Adult Education Principles to Improve Outcomes in Patients with Chronic Wounds

R. Gary Sibbald, BSc, MD, FRCPC(Med, Derm), MACP, FAAD, MEd, MAPWCA; **Afsaneh Alavi**, MD; **Matthew Sibbald**, BSc, MD; **Debra Sibbald**, B Pharm, PhD; **Laurie Goodman**, RN, BA, MHScN

Objectives

The reader will be challenged to:

- Describe the adult learning principles for effective educational planning and activities
- Integrate new educational scientific evidence (knowledge transfer) into day-to-day practice, including the need for interprofessional collaboration and communication skills
- Review practical ways of linking educational events to patient care outcomes
- Provide a learning culture to foster development of communities of practice and/or communities of learners.

Introduction

Traditionally, experts have delivered wound care education in didactic classroom settings. Facts and new knowledge have seldom been contextualized to the workplace or linked to healthcare professional performance and health outcomes.[1,2] Traditionally, medical and nursing instruction along with continuing education are taught in the classroom, but to increase the educational relevance, a shift needs to occur to the workplace. *Education should be related to patient care and everyday clinical, research, teaching, and administrative activities* (Figure 1).[3] For those individuals who are interested in becoming more knowledgeable, wound care societies have been created worldwide to examine current wound care topics in depth using large group lectures and occasional workshops. Many educators are concerned about the impact of the scientific content of these events on practice, because the content often does not focus on the educational process or on adult learning principles. In this chapter, we emphasize a need to go beyond content in wound care education to include the key elements of the educational process, including needs assessment, goals, objectives, interactive teaching methods, evaluation of healthcare professional performance, and patient outcomes.

Adult Learning Principles

Adult learning differs from learning for the first time. *Andragogy* centers on past experiences as the motivation and context for self-directed learning (SDL). As we collate

Sibbald RG, Alavi A, Sibbald M, Sibbald D, Goodman L. Effective adult education principles to improve outcomes in patients with chronic wounds. In: Krasner DL, Rodeheaver GT, Sibbald RG, Woo KY, eds. *Chronic Wound Care: A Clinical Source Book for Healthcare Professionals.* Vol 1. 5th ed. Malvern, PA: HMP Communications; 2012:37–54.

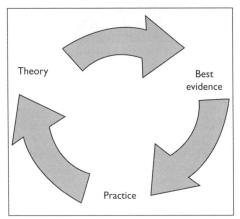

Figure 1. The circular pathway linking theory, best evidence, and practice.

and organize group experiences into a synthesized theory with reflection, our understanding deepens and brings meaning to our individual anecdotes (storytelling). Knowles[4] outlined this difference, coining the term andragogy, adult learning based on experience, as distinct from *pedagogy*, learning for the first time from an authoritative figure. Andragogy implies the need for individuals to be self-directed as they mature and to utilize experience as part of the learning process. Houle[5] divided learning styles into goal-, activity-, and learning-outcome-oriented types. Goal-oriented learners use education for accomplishing clear-cut objectives. Activity-oriented learners are course takers and group joiners. They enjoy the social contact almost to a greater degree than the learning activity. The learning-outcome-oriented individual is a knowledge seeker without reference to a specific goal.

Tough[6] highlighted the importance of pleasure and self-esteem as motivators for learning regardless of whether the activities are predominantly reading, listening, watching, or practicing. A certain amount of knowledge that is retained will be used for performing responsible actions at a higher level. The knowledge is then used as a skill base for understanding what is happening. This may lead to formalized recognition (certificate, diploma, and license). The public acknowledgment of this accomplishment often facilitates promotion, material rewards, or higher pay. The organizational culture of learning is the first step for a learning process and should be facilitated.[7]

The learning environment is important to effective teaching and must be optimized. Clinical practice environments may often act as barriers to translating this new knowledge into improved patient care. Successful healthcare professionals are usually independent and self-directed learners. They value learning that is relevant to them and integrate educational opportunities with the demands of everyday life. They are more motivated to learn by internal stimulation and are interested in a problem-centered approach. In adult learning theory, learners are their own richest resource. This learning must be integrated into interprofessional practice and systems to improve evidence-informed healthcare.

Learning is not a passive process but an active exercise constructed by the learner. In SDL models, students have control over their learning processes. Adult learners prefer to be independent and self-directed. They will find the ability to identify their learning gaps. By reflection on their performance outcome and learning processes, they will shift from superficial learning to deep learning. A learning contract is a valuable tool to conduct a curriculum that is learner-centered and self-directed. Learners need to be involved in their own learning. Mentorship is also a way to facilitate self-directed learning. A mentoring relationship plays an important role in individual personal growth of the healthcare professional.[8] In a mentoring relationship, the mentor and mentee work together to help the mentee's professional development at a particular point in his or her life.[8] An ultimate mentoring relationship is the development of a co-mentoring relationship between the mentor and mentee with both members learning from each other. The mentoring relationship enhances professional development that takes learning from the classroom to the workplace, facilitating learning from these experiences.

Schon[9] crystallized these ideas into a theory of adult learning (Figure 2). In the Schon model, we are confronted in daily clinical practice with "surprises" — situations that fail to fit into our accumulated knowledge rubric — a reflection *in action*. We manage the situation with an "experiment" that later requires retrospective reflection *on action* to complete the learning cycle. Failure to reflect on action and integrate the experiment

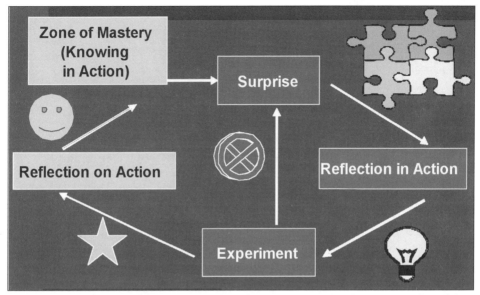

Figure 2. Schon Theory of Adult Learning. Modified and reprinted with permission from Schon DA. *The Reflective Practitioner.* Boston, MA: Basic Books; 1984.[9]

into our knowledge base strips us of the experiential lesson and leaves us surprised by the repeating situation. It is often this latter step that is missed in the busy current healthcare day-to-day activities. How many times have we as healthcare professionals been faced with surprises in clinical patient care situations or with challenging patients with whom we really were not sure what to do? Wound care practitioners encounter many clinical questions in patient care, but what compels us to follow up on some questions and not others? *If we do not complete the process of reflection on learning, we often encounter a similar problem with another surprise.*

Kolb's experiential learning theory is based on social psychology and educational philosophy.[10] The central principles include:
- Having experience (reflection in practice)
- Thinking about how it happened (reflection on practice)
- Integrating our own reflection (build over our previous knowledge)
- Making a change for future plans (conclusion).

The building of adult learning on past experience and the linking of education to patient care is the theme of this chapter.

Brundage[11] completed an extensive synthesis of the literature on adult education. His research demonstrated that:
- Learning involves a dynamic equilibrium between change and stability, structure and process, and content and activity
- Learning occurs over time and within societal contexts and relationships
- Adult learners have past experiences, present concerns, and roles relevant to work and family as well as to learning
- Adult learners bring not only their minds but also their physical bodies, emotional responses, and cherished values to learning
- Teachers are also adult learners.

Pine[12] and Horn were pioneers in the study of adult education. They studied a counseling training program for 120 community aides and, when they reviewed the data, were able to extract a number of adult learning principles and conditions for learning.

The following statements best exemplify adult learning principles:
1. Learning is an experience that occurs inside the learner and is activated by the learner
2. Learning is a discovery of the personal meaning and relevance of ideas
3. Learning is the consequence of experience

4. Learning is a cooperative and collaborative process
5. Learning is an evolutionary process
6. Learning can sometimes be a painful process
7. One of the richest resources for learning is the learner himself/herself
8. The process for learning is emotional as well as intellectual
9. The processes of problem solving and learning are highly unique and individual.

Learning is facilitated in an atmosphere that:
1. Encourages people to be active
2. Promotes and facilitates the individual's discovery of personal meaning
3. Emphasizes the uniquely personal and subjective nature of learning
4. Allows people to express their differences
5. Recognizes people's right to make mistakes
6. Tolerates ambiguity
7. Promotes evaluation as a cooperative process with an emphasis on self-evaluation.

Change in Professional Performance

How can we make a change in practice performance and link changes to education? Professionals move back and forth from practice to new evidence and try to apply and integrate new information. Davis et al[13] reviewed the education literature to determine educational strategies that were effective in changing physician performance and in improving healthcare outcomes. The researchers scanned a number of databases between 1975 and 1994 using continuing medical education (CME) and related terms as key words. The review identified 99 randomized controlled trials that contained 160 interventions linking educational strategies to objective physician performance measures and/or healthcare outcomes. Almost two-thirds of the continuing education (CE) interventions displayed improvement in at least one major outcome. Seventy percent of the interventions aimed at physician performance demonstrated a positive change, and 48% of the interventions aimed at healthcare outcomes also produced a positive change. This study concluded that commonly used delivery systems, such as conferences, had little direct impact on improving professional practice. An educational event is referred to as a primary strategy. Secondary strategies enable or reinforce practice (Table 1).

The most successful secondary strategies utilized in some of these interventions included reminders, patient-mediated interventions, outreach visits, opinion leaders, and multifaceted activities. Audit with feedback and educational materials were less effective. This study heightened our awareness of the importance of linking educational events to strategies that integrate new knowledge into practice.

Impact of Formal Continuing Interprofessional Education

In a follow-up review, Davis et al[32] analyzed 14 studies based on didactic primary educational events without any secondary strategies. The studies included in this analysis were randomized controlled trials of formal didactic and/or interactive CME interventions. These primary interventions included conferences, courses, rounds, meetings, symposia, and lectures. To qualify for this analysis, participants had to include 50% or more practicing physicians or residents. Sixty-four studies were initially identified, and 14 qualified for the analysis. The studies were analyzed to determine if they were didactic, interactive, or had a mixed format. Fourteen studies met the selection criteria and generated 17 interventions. Nine of the studies resulted in positive changes in professional practice, and 3 of the 4 interventions that measured healthcare outcomes showed an improvement in one or more measurement. Seven of these studies had sufficient data to calculate overall effect sizes. The data demonstrated that *didactic sessions alone did not appear to be effective in changing physician performance.* Some evidence suggested that interactive CE sessions that enhance participant activity or provide the opportunity to practice skills could effect change in professional practice and, on occasion, healthcare outcomes.

These conclusions are not surprising when we refer to the often-quoted educational principle that passive learning will result in little retained knowledge, perhaps as low as 10%. With interactivity, knowledge retention may be as high as 25%. These figures would relate to primary interventions in the reviewed analyses. It is not a foregone conclusion that new knowledge will be translated into everyday activities. This is where secondary strategies are necessary to in-

Table 1. Toolkit of secondary educational strategies	
Academic detailing[14,15]	Healthcare professional provides mini-educational session in the practice setting to provide new knowledge
Pharmacist (academic detailing)[16,17]	Usually relates to new drug or appropriate use of therapeutic agent(s)
Standardized patients[18]	Trained (standardized) patients respond to history, physical examination, and treatment plans; these patients are able to identify deficiencies in healthcare providers' knowledge, skills, and attitudes
Opinion leaders[19–21]	An influential healthcare professional educates other healthcare professionals, colleagues, and peers
Patient educational materials/patient reminders[22–27]	The patient becomes empowered to better understand the disease process and treatment
Physician reminders (22/26 studies showed positive change; 2 studies did not)[13]	Chart prompts, mailings, computer-generated reminders to monitor or diagnose physical findings or treatment
Audit and feedback (10 positive, 14 negative outcomes)[13]	A retrospective analysis of previous charts for diagnostic criteria and treatment; direct (active) chart review with the healthcare professional made this strategy more effective[28–31]

terpret learning for practice. With these bridging methodologies, knowledge retention may increase to as high as 75%. We need to overcome the barriers that may exist to adapt this knowledge into practice. Secondary strategies that facilitate a change are often referred to as enablers. Enablers may be as simple as a summary chart that clarifies a concept (eg, usual antibiotic sensitivity for common systemic antimicrobials that can help link the result from a bacterial swab to appropriate antimicrobial therapy in the absence of specific sensitivity testing). Other enablers may outline 4 or 5 critical diagnostic and treatment steps or a simplified clinical pathway for venous leg ulcers or pressure ulcers. *The first time that a healthcare professional integrates new knowledge into practice, the participant must reflect on action as he or she follows up patient care.* This is the second and most important part of the Schon model. When innovation is integrated into everyday activities, fine-tuning is often necessary. This is where the role of reinforcing activity becomes important. The reinforcing step can be facilitated by consulting with an opinion leader or a network of advanced practitioners to iron out the kinks in the new knowledge being integrated into patient care. Implementation of new knowledge into practice often requires more than one attempt before it improves patient care. One of the commonly used methods

of standardizing practice is to develop consensus statements, guidelines, or algorithms.

Translating Guidelines into Practice

Davis and Taylor-Vaisey[33] performed a systematic review of the adoption of clinical practice guidelines. *Many professional organizations spend a lot of time and energy producing guidelines, but little attention is paid to the implementation and process of ensuring that these guidelines become integrated into everyday practice.* Audit plus feedback is a moderately effective method, but this method is even more effective when targeted to specific providers and delivered by peers or opinion leaders. The best methods for successful guideline implementation include reminder systems, academic detailing, and the use of a toolkit of multiple interventions. Academic detailing may involve a key opinion leader imparting new knowledge to another healthcare setting for the purpose of changing practices. These methods illustrate the importance of subject expertise and other areas having a willingness to gain new knowledge for successful outcomes.

Guideline implementation is central to quality improvement, patient safety, and potential healthcare-system change.[34] In contrast, CE concepts are based on promoting and maintaining the clinical performance of healthcare professionals. Knowledge transfer is the bridge between these 2 concepts (Figure 3).[34]

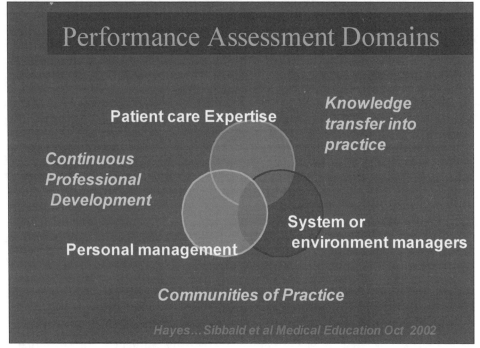

Figure 3. Relationship of knowledge, systems, and individual growth to patients.

Wound care learning often occurs in formal settings outside the workplace (such as conferences or lectures). This formal learning is complemented with the informal process of knowledge transfer within everyday practice. It is usually relevant and has a greater chance of improving patient care outcomes. A modified knowledge translation (implementation research, utilization research) definition from the Canadian Institutes of Health Research is:

...*the exchange, synthesis, and ethically sound application of knowledge — within a complex system of interactions among researchers and users — to accelerate the capture of the benefits of research for "citizens" (Canadians) through improved health, more effective services and products, and a strengthened healthcare system.*[35]

Many different methods for implementation of knowledge transfer have been proposed. Knowledge translation is a framework for healthcare professionals to integrate best scientific evidence into day-to-day practice. The different stages of awareness, agreement, adoption, and adherence are compatible with different educational strategies, such as lectures, enabling (patient education

and flow sheets), and reinforcing strategies, such as feedback and audit.[34]

The process of knowledge transfer starts with the appraisal of the best evidence and links these evidence summaries to clinical pathways for application to practice. Knowledge translation encompasses the multiple perspectives of the system, learner, and educational process, closing the gap between evidence and implementation in practice.[36,37] For all healthcare professionals, CME is the longest learning period (often over 30 years) compared to undergraduate and postgraduate training (each 2 to 5 or more years). ***Continuing professional development (CPD) is a combination of adult learning and personal growth[38] that shifts learning from the teacher (facilitator) in the classroom to the learner in the workplace.***

Continuing professional development is individualized and can allow personal autonomy within an interprofessional team. It is a dynamic process involving all healthcare professionals from physicians to nurses and allied healthcare professionals. Learners can modify their adult learning priorities to accommodate different interests and

Table 2. The difference between continuing education (CE), continuing professional development (CPD), knowledge translation (KT), and guideline implementation (GI) (adapted from Davis et al[34,38])

	Continuing Education	Continuous Professional Development	Knowledge Translation	Guideline Implementation
Setting	• Teaching settings	• Any learning situation	• Primary practice settings	• Primarily in a practice environment
Tools	• Primary educational methods (lectures, print materials)	• Wide variety of learning methods	• Methods of overcoming barriers to change emphasizing prompts, reminders, and patient-mediated methods	• Academic detailing • Reminders • Audited feedback • Policy changes
Targets	• Individual healthcare professionals • CE credits	• Healthcare professionals • Creation of learning portfolio or SDL	• Practitioners (clinicians, teams) • Payers (health systems) • Patients, population • Policy makers	• Healthcare organizations • Teams, with less emphasis on the individual learners • Patients and family members
Content	• Mostly clinical (healthcare expert)	• Clinical plus other practice-related areas	• As in CE and CPD, possible focus on evidence appraisal • Incorporates other professional competencies (communication, collaborations, manager functions)	• Mostly clinical • Knowledge transfer into practice • Practical healthcare system issues • Patient-education issues
Guiding models	• Primarily educational • CE credits and accreditation important	• SDL • May relate to professional performance	• Holistic: incorporates clinician-learner and educational delivery system • Evidence based from content of activity to testing of intervention (healthcare professional performance or patient outcomes)	• Improve health status • Quality improvement • Clinical accountability • Reduce medical error
Relevant disciplines	• Discipline-specific healthcare knowledge education • Educational psychology	As for CE, plus: • Organizational learning theory • Social psychology	As for CE and CPD, plus: • Systems management • Health services research • Social marketing • Patient education • Bioinformatics and others	• Professionals (healthcare) • Policy makers • Payers • Patients • Researchers • Educators

job requirements. Continuing professional development has been defined as "a process of lifelong learning for all individuals that also meets patient needs and delivers healthcare-system priorities."[39] Alternatively, guideline implementation is another way to integrate best evidence into practice

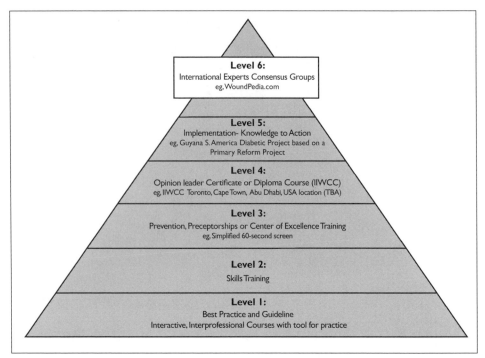

Figure 4. Pyramid of educational continuous professional development.

and change the healthcare system. Table 2 compares these 4 perspectives.

Chronic wound care is interprofessional. Short educational courses have been designed based on adult education theory with interactive teaching methods to increase the impact for practice (Level 1). See Figure 4. The Registered Nurses' Association of Ontario has developed guidelines for the prevention and treatment of most types of chronic wounds that have been implemented both locally and internationally. The methodological quality of a guideline can be checked with the Appraisal of Guidelines for Research and Evaluation (AGREE II) instrument, which can be located online at http://www.agreetrust. org. This instrument asks the rater to score 23 statements with one of the 4 anchors (strongly agree, somewhat agree, somewhat disagree, and strongly disagree), and there is a section for comments. The questions are divided into 6 subscales that include scope and purpose, stakeholders, rigor of evidence-based review, clarity, applicability, and editorial independence. The score should be tabulated in each of the 6 subscores but not

assigned an overall summative score. The tool should be completed by 2 or more assessors and discrepancies resolved. Assessors are then asked to indicate their preference for guideline implementation: strongly recommend, recommend, not recommend, or unsure of the guideline.

The knowledge-to-action cycle requires identifying the best guidelines through the AGREE II tool, then summarizing them for practice. The Canadian Association of Wound Care (CAWC; http://cawc.net/) has translated guidelines for practice by providing secondary enablers or templates to use at the bedside. These Quick Reference Guides include wound bed preparation, diabetic foot ulcers, venous leg ulcers, and pressure ulcers along with best practice articles that are posted on the website.

Figure 4 outlines the 6-level educational vision for successful integration of evidence-based literature into wound care practice. Each distinctive level from 1 to 6 engages the healthcare learner on a progressive level from novice to expert. This 6-level educational plan is "fluid" and ever-changing based on education and healthcare needs.

For example, in the foundation of the pyramid is the CAWC Level 1 series, which utilizes an interactive format with touch pads to familiarize attendees with the major principles of diagnosis and treatment of common chronic wounds. In the CAWC Level 2 course, attendees practice the skills of portable Doppler evaluation for ankle brachial pressure index (ABPI), compression bandaging, and debridement. This level involves skills training that builds on basic knowledge training from Level 1. The third level of education is designed around prevention, including a simplified 60-second tool for screening the high-risk diabetic foot to avoid ulcer formation. Successful team integration requires working in a reflective interprofessional practice. This exercise helps learners to become aware of healthcare system skills, including communication, collaboration, and manager activities. It also develops an awareness of health promotion and professionalism in addition to observing the expert clinician with the scholarly application of knowledge to patient care. The first 3 levels are part of the CAWC educational programs that go beyond the outdated paradigm of didactic non-interactive lectures at a meeting. The vision is that each level purposefully builds on the previous knowledge base. To add to this, a partnership with the CAWC and the University of Toronto has allowed the development of the Level 4 to 6 educational interventions.

A Level 4 activity trains the trainers to be key opinion leaders or champions. This is exemplified by the annual International Interprofessional Wound Care Course (IIWCC) that was established at the University of Toronto in 1999 and at the Stellenbosch University, Cape Town, South Africa, in 2010, and will be held in Abu Dhabi in 2012. It is well recognized that chronic wound care is interprofessional, and the care of these patients represents a substantial growing cost to the healthcare system. Usual wound care treatment is often not evidence based or anchored in best clinical practice.

The IIWCC objectives are to help learners:

- Assess and critically review wound care literature in key subject areas
- Integrate wound care principles using a self-directed learning program formulated with a learning contract
- Demonstrate applications of best practices by developing a selective related to the students' everyday activities
- Incorporate the components of clinical practice with small groups and patient problem solving.

This key opinion leader course is facilitated over two 4-day residential weekends with a 7- to 12-month period for self-study modules. In addition, a selective is required to encourage participants to complete a project linking the course material to their day-to-day activities. The residential weekends are interactive, and participants discuss the educational process as well as their wound care knowledge base. Each student's baseline knowledge is evaluated with interactive techniques, eg, touch pads. Patient demonstrations allow students to integrate wound care principles into patient care through working in assigned small group interprofessional teams. The self-study modules are based on sections of this textbook (*Chronic Wound Care: A Clinical Source Book for Healthcare Professionals*). Selected chapters in the text cover modules on education, local wound care, leg ulcers, foot ulcers, and pressure ulcers as compulsory modules. These chapters are supplemented with other key readings chosen by the faculty for some of the optional modules, including holistic patient care, wound care processes, infection, and chronic wounds in special populations. These optional modules were designed to encourage learners to match course curriculum to their clinical needs. To achieve this goal, a selection of readings is also included in the course for additional modules on acute postsurgical wounds, burns and trauma, ostomy and local skin care, lymphedema, and acute wound infections. The self-study modules have questions on each selected book chapter or articles related to specific content, interpretation of the material, or implications for practice.

The course selective process includes a presentation to classmates and faculty at the final residential weekend. The best presentations from small groups are peer-chosen and presented in a large group setting. This course issues a certificate of completion for individuals who complete 9 modules, attend the 2 residential weekends, and complete the selective.

The course predominantly attracts wound care

nurses along with a smaller number of doctors and allied healthcare professionals, including foot care specialists (chiropodists, podiatrists) and rehabilitation specialists (occupational, physical therapists). The student enrollment is also open to leaders in healthcare from industry who have at least 5 years of wound care experience. Enrollees from around the world, including the United States, Mexico, Belgium, Italy, Switzerland, Japan, Singapore, Australia, Iran, South America, and Africa, have participated in the Toronto course. The West Asian courses have been conducted in Iran, Saudi Arabia, and currently in Abu Dhabi with participants in the past from more than 10 gulf and hosting countries.

The collaboration in Cape Town, South Africa, established in 2010, has trained students from South Africa and 7 Sub-Saharan countries (Cameroon, Ghana, Kenya, Malawi, Nigeria, Tanzania, Uganda) representing key opinion leader training for a population of more than 400 million people.

The IIWCC is part of a certificate of completion at the University of Toronto and is one of 5 components of a flex-time applied professional masters in the Dalla Lana School of Public Health. Each course provides opportunities for networking with more than 80 classmates and faculty from around the world, creating potential communities of learning.

Collated course evaluations in the past have encompassed qualitative and quantitative methodologies. Qualitative survey answers highlight the benefits of the course, including networking, sharing and exchanging information with others, and obtaining expert opinion from the faculty. The 9 wound care modules (5 compulsory, 4 optional) have a wealth of current information, and participants are appreciative of the pre-selection of the articles from an expert faculty. The attendees choose their selective based on practice-related needs as well as personal requirements for educational growth and a desire to educate patients and staff within their facilities. The most positive overall aspects of the IIWCC are the learning of new information about current wound care practices, networking, and the knowledgeable and enthusiastic faculty. More than 90% of the course participants enjoyed working with colleagues, developing new relationships, and experiencing a sense of contagious enthusiasm. Stu-

dents claimed that the information gained from the IIWCC clearly influenced their practice. The students felt empowered, experienced increased self-confidence, and considered it worth all the hard work. In order to change wound care, more initiatives that take advantage of current educational literature need to be linked to practice.

The Level 5 professional masters program in wound prevention and care links the IIWCC with a 2-part educator course. The third component explores the basics and application of public health and the prevention of disease. The last 2 components are a practicum to learn new skills, including an elective to promote adult self-directed learning. The design of this masters program is centered on subject expertise (wound care key opinion leader training), systems training (public health courses), and personal development of educator skills (teaching and learning courses).

These 5 levels have been mirrored in a project abroad. Part of the knowledge-to-action cycle at this level has included the application of all these principles through a Canadian International Development Agency (CIDA) grant in Guyana, South America. Here, an interprofessional center of excellence has been established at the Georgetown Public Hospital Corporation (GPHC) with a 48% reduction in amputations between 2008 and 2010. This has been accomplished with:

• Basic training of doctors, nurses, and rehabilitation specialists in an interactive, interprofessional format
• Knowledge translation and skills training
• Modeling of interprofessional care and implementation of a simplified 60-second screening tool program to identify the high-risk foot, preventing ulcers and amputation
• Key opinion leader training of health professionals over 3 years at the IIWCC Toronto
• Systems support from a CIDA grant, the CEO and Chief of Staff of the GPHC, and the Ministry of Health, including 2 Health Ministers.

There is a need to bring local consensus documents and guidelines to international consensus forums. Level 6 of this educational framework provides a forum for experts around the world to evaluate the evidence base in wound care and to translate this for practice. The World Union of

Wound Healing Societies meeting in Toronto established the WoundPedia website (www.Wound-Pedia.com) to accomplish this task of gathering just-in-time wound care information for practice. The material is arranged in practical, relevant, and adaptable educational toolkits following the wound bed preparation paradigm (treat the cause, patient-centered concerns, local wound care — debridement, infection-inflammation control, moisture balance, and finally the edge effect for wounds that are healable but not progressing at the expected rate). The evidence-based summary should be adapted for local needs and based on local expertise and resources in developed, developing, and emerging healthcare systems.

This 6-level educational master plan is the vision for successful integration of the evidence-based literature into practice. Expert opinion and patient preference are embedded within this structure to facilitate improved and cost-effective utilization of valuable healthcare resources.

Strategies for Improving Educational Effectiveness

Well known primary strategies of large-group continuing education include conferences, meetings, symposia, and courses. More effective and interactive teaching methods that are woven through these course curriculums include the following:
- Pre-tests/post-tests
- Asking questions
- Using voting cards
- Utilizing touch pads or audience-response systems
- Reading abstracts or passages
- Buzz groups
- Mini-quizzes
- Progressive presentation of a patient problem with audience participation
- Discussion with panels or vignettes to get commentary
- Debates
- Patient-related interventions: have a patient present at a session or discuss a case
- Video vignettes
- Standardized patients: training patients or actors to teach students aspects of history and physical examination
- Phil Donahue or talk-show-host technique of taking the microphone and going out into the audience
- Question cards to filter questions with a moderator.

Secondary and ongoing educational strategies to promote interprofessional practice change include:
- Enablers or tabular summaries and charts for transfer into practice at the bedside
- Toolkits for implementation of new knowledge
- Communities of practice (COPs): informal networks of individuals with similar interests
- Mentorship
- Small learning groups
- Patient empowerment
- Educational outreach visits
- A combination of strategies.

Community of Practice as "An Informal Continuing Education" Methodology

In a successful wound care team, members may start with an informal network or interprofessional team. As the members become more integrated in practice, a common care plan is written, and this becomes truly interprofessional. Many teams even go a step further with a transprofessional perspective. The concept of a transprofessional team expands the expertise from individual members to all the team members. If a team member is absent, another professional can institute appropriate care within his or her scope. Healthcare professionals can learn from each other through group discussion. A team is a formalized structure that also may form an informal COP. Wenger[40] defines COPs as people who come together around common interests. These are self-directed and self-organized learning groups that have a common domain of interest, requiring a minimum level of knowledge of the domain and shared competence that differentiate members from other people.[41]

Highlighted in the wound care educational process are the needs assessment, interactive learning, knowledge transfer, evaluation, and continuous reevaluation/quality improvement. Our goal in every educational program is enhanced if it is linked to improved health outcomes. If we want to increase our odds of success to change healthcare professional performance, we need to embrace the concepts necessary for effective knowledge transfer, continuing professional development, and a COP. These groups often discuss the latest developments in the common field of interest and share difficult challenges in wound care practice. Members of the group may discuss novel ideas or work together on common agendas, such as a volunteer educational organization or a common political agenda. COPs often have a core voluntary membership but not formalized leadership. A COP has learning potential for expanding the members' core knowledge and through acquiring new knowledge from the periphery. A community of learners may be used interchangeably with a COP, but a community of learners may be focused on educational objectives without any practice to apply the knowledge to everyday activities.

Importance of Communities of Practice in Wound Care

Learning is a social process, and knowledge stems from our day-to-day practice. The COP originated from industry and its members' educational needs. The COP facilitates new knowledge production and translation.[36] Chronic wound care is often a relatively new concept, and a COP is a place for sharing experiences and receiving feedback about new approaches to care. A COP can involve wound care professionals who may or may not also be involved in a formalized institution or agency team. It will be more successful when members of the group are actively involved and mutual engagement is established. Every community needs a facilitator who also may play the role of group administrator (arrange meeting locations, remind participants of upcoming meetings, and circulate background material or literature).

Educators can facilitate networking through programs and Internet-based contacts and can identify unperceived gaps and needs. The educator may then help design educational interventions to improve practice. Communities of practice define themselves in 3 dimensions:

1. Common practice or educational needs, eg, the care of persons with diabetes and foot complications
2. Common social bond, eg, professional networking
3. Ability to increase capacity through resource sharing, eg, enablers for practice, recent survey, or research related to practice.

Communities of practice are different from task forces or committees because COPs are not task-centered and do not dissolve when the task is completed. Shared learning and interest of the group is the central reason for collaboration. Communities of practice are more active than a network and have a long-term and consistent collaborative association that helps identify members with their formal and tacit knowledge.

Knowledge-Building Communities

Most computer-learning models are passive and are simply a transfer of the lecture format to technology. However, technology can be used in innovative ways to optimize the students' interaction and develop a virtual facilitated collaboration in the community of learners.

Membership in COPs[42,43] and in *communities of practice networks*[44] makes development of expertise more likely.[45] By collaboration, the implicit is made explicit through participation and reification, using meta-cognitive focusing processes. Both must exist to ensure sufficient mutual understanding to reach common goals and anchor activities.

Scardamalia and Bereiter[46,47] describe an educational model called *knowledge-building communities (KBC)* based on knowledge construction and collaborative opportunistic approaches to learner and idea-centered reasoning.[48] The premise is that ideas are the real and malleable material of knowledge building. It asserts that the process to create knowledge remains the same regardless of how the purpose or outcomes differ across learning levels. It is defined as the production and continual improvement of ideas of value to a community: The community accomplishments are greater than the sum of individual contributions and are part of broader cultural efforts. Certain technologies and social structures facilitate growth and spreading of ideas, encouraging intentional learning, reflection, and communication. Knowledge-building communities provide a hospitable environment for crystallizing collaboration to improve ideas. The essence is cooperation to create understanding, working toward advancing individual knowledge and that of the group. Collective expertise produces higher order conceptual frameworks.[45,49]

The model involves learners investigating

problems over a sustained period of weeks or months. Ideas and research findings are entered as notes in a communal knowledge base. The intent is engaging learners in progressive knowledge building, continually developing their understanding through problem identification, research, and community discourse. The emphasis is progress toward collective goals of understanding, rather than individual learning and performance.

This process is clarified through 12 determinants developed by Scardamalia,[50] which link practices with technological supports for knowledge-building discourse. These guide activity in distributed networks of learners and articulate the process of expertise. When operationalized, they enable community members to emulate expert behavior regardless of individual or collective levels of ability. Some of these determinants in particular underlie the shift from learner-inquirers to members of a KBC.[51] They include knowledge advancement as a community rather than individual, idea improvement, knowledge of skills and abilities rather than content, discourse as collaborative problem solving, constructive use of authoritative information, and emergent understanding. Other determinants critical to knowledge building include epistemic agency (students themselves find knowledge and share through self-direction), idea diversity, embedded transformative assessment, and knowledge building that is symmetric, pervasive, and democratic.

Scardamalia and Bereiter[51] developed computer software called *Knowledge Forum*™ *(KF)*, which employs affordances for knowledge creation. As a platform for such communities, it provides the technical infrastructure necessary to support, document, and research knowledge building. It is a stable Internet application easily mastered by most people. The embedded analytic tools provide a useful and streamlined method for collecting and examining quantitative data, allowing users to customize their working spaces to provide multiple views and appropriate scaffolds.

A public forum writing space supports community sharing of ideas. Written permanence permits reflection, challenges, evidence citation, and improvements, enabling community creativity from dispersed locations in an asynchronous discussion. Scaffolds support student inquiry; address major steps; encourage theory articulation, question formulation, and identification of deeper learning needs; and lead to specialized expertise in particular domains. Build-ons allow students to discuss ideas or conflicts to clarify or develop new ideas and approach deeper understanding.

Quotation of notes can link back automatically to the original, fostering idea synthesis and reflection. Views organize notes. Students see related ideas from multiple perspectives, supporting deep understanding and synthesis. "Rise-above-it notes" allow consolidation and synthesis of ideas, enabling reflection, elimination, and integration of new ideas. Publication of the most important contributions can occur.

Importance of Online Technological and Social Supports for Wound Care Specialists

Wound care specialists, as an international, interprofessional group, represent a unique cohort that has specific needs for a knowledge-building community, particularly if clinicians work in isolation or at a distance from other experts in the field. Most are faced with significant time constraints on participating in continuing adult education while balancing the ongoing daily demands of their workplaces. Inexperience with retrieving online resources or limited connectivity may pose practical challenges to accessing current and prompt authoritative sources, particularly when dealing with an urgent and specific patient issue.

Knowledge-building theory would suggest that the individualist orientation of this specialty and limited enculturation is at odds with the community network values necessary to initiate and sustain knowledge work. The current mode that promotes knowledge acquisition through independent reading, participation in isolated or sporadic continuing education events, or completion of distance education lessons does not provide sufficient context for community knowledge, itself a vital facet of knowledge building. Creating a networking milieu through an online asynchronous, software-supported, knowledge-building environment would provide wound care professionals with a more robust learning setting and the opportunity to truly engage in the knowledge work necessary to sustain and advance wound care practice. It might establish a longitudinal enhancement for this community.

Quantitative/Qualitative Measures Applied Dixon's Model of Evaluation		
	Quantitative	Qualitative
1. Opinions	happiness index	structured interview focus group
2. Competence	pre-test/post-test	survey, interview
3. Clinical	prescribing data	explore barriers to change
4. Health outcomes	clinical endpoint	quality-of-life interviews
5. Economic	pharmaco-economic studies	costs from case studies
Adapted with permission from Davis D, Taylor-Vaisey A. Two decades of Dixon: the question(s) of evaluating continuing education in the health professions. J Contin Educ Health Prof. 1997;17(4):207–213.		

Figure 5. Fitzpatrick-Dixon levels of evaluation (modified).[44,45]

Importance of Communication Skills

Effective communication is essential for promoting adherence to treatment. *Adherence* (to follow through on a treatment or regime) is more patient-centered than the healthcare-provider-dominated term compliance (to obey an order or command). A healthcare professional's communication skills have a prominent effect on improving provider care and enhancing patient outcomes. Ineffective communication has been associated with an increased incidence of medical errors and malpractice claims. According to Keller and Carroll,[52] healthcare professionals must perform certain skills to increase their communication for improved patient care. This is known as the *4-E model*. The components are Engaging (a human connection with the patient creates an ethically sound and supportive relationship with patients and families), Empathizing (being present and with the patient, using patient language and not sympathy, using effective listening skills to facilitate a relationship), Educating (not just providing information but making information comprehensible for the patient and being sure of the patient's perception of the information), and finally Enlisting (increasing patient responsibility and competence to care by involving him or her in the decision making and encouraging adherence).[52,53]

Dixon[54] first proposed evaluation criteria for educational interventions in 1978. This proposal included 4 levels of outcome analysis, and each analysis could be approached using quantitative and qualitative measures. Twenty years later, in 1997, Davis and Taylor-Vaisey[55] reevaluated this

model, and for this discussion, we have added a fifth level, the economic analysis (Figure 5).

The first level of evaluation is based on participant opinion. Opinions come from evaluation forms after an educational event. This is an important process to obtain information as part of a *needs assessment* for future planning and to evaluate the various individuals and formats that are part of a primary educational intervention. Educators often jokingly refer to this as a "happiness index" because it does not measure whether the participants actually increased their knowledge as a result of attendance at the event that is being evaluated. Quantitative methodology refers to mathematical analysis and needs to be distinguished from qualitative research methods. *The quantitative results often tell us what the impact of an educational activity has been, but the qualitative result can answer the important question of why.* Qualitative research methods are useful in measuring attitudes as opposed to knowledge and skills. One of the best ways to sample attitudes of participants in a course is through structured interviews with a neutral facilitator or a small focus group. A group of 6 to 10 individuals will be asked questions about various aspects of the course they have just attended. It is important to have a neutral facilitator (and not one of the course faculty) to permit participants to be comfortable and honest in the focus group setting. The participants are probably best selected at random from educational activity attendees at the beginning of the activity. The focus group can sometimes be conducted during a lunch or afternoon break in a separate room from other attendees. Other methodologies for selecting focus group participants may include the selection of various professions from an inter-professional intervention, targeting a subset of attendees (eg, new graduates) or individuals working in the community versus those who work in a hospital setting.

The second level of evaluation measures *newly acquired knowledge or competencies*. Quantitative methodologies include a pre-test or post-test. Questionnaires, surveys, or interviews can accomplish the same objective in a qualitative way. With the first 2 levels of intervention, we still have not measured the integration of new knowledge into clinical practice.

At Level 3, the pharmaceutical industry has realized the importance of this data for years and has tracked physician prescribing data and the integration of new drugs into everyday practice. Qualitative methodologies can determine if the integration of new modalities into practice is due to a knowledge deficit or relates to various barriers for change. An example in wound care would be the 4-layer bandage. The 4-layer bandage is effective in achieving sustained compression for up to a week.[56] If the clinic setting does not have a nurse trained in the procedure, there may be a reluctance to change. The bandages may not be on the clinical formulary, or there may be no formula for reimbursement. All these barriers may prevent new innovations from being translated into everyday activities.

At Level 4, measuring healthcare outcomes and relating education to patient care are two of the strongest ways to evaluate best practices. In a quantitative way, this would reflect a clinical endpoint, such as the prevalence of pressure ulcers within an institution or home care setting. Alternatively, a prevalence study could be conducted on the number of patients with leg or foot ulcers that fail to heal over a 12-week period as a useful baseline determination prior to an educational intervention designed to improve practice and in the end linked to a repeat audit. Our final goal is to reduce patient suffering and disability. Our customer is in fact our patient and, often, little attention is paid to patient attitude and suffering. Quality-of-life tools[57-60] that are general (non-disease specific and relate to overall health) and disease specific (related to disability associated with leg ulcers, etc) have been developed. Validated quality-of-life tools have been used in the past as research instruments, but they also may have utility in everyday practice.

In the final analysis, our healthcare systems require economic accountability. The fifth level of evaluation measures economic analyses. Several formalized pharmacoeconomic models are used to create theoretical frameworks with mathematical models to analyze the cost of proposed new therapies.[61] It is important to show cost effectiveness (alternatively, cost minimization, cost efficacy, or cost utility) for new technologies before innovations will become widely accepted, often through treatment reimbursement. The hypothetical economic models require individual cases or case series to give insight into appropriate clinical use and possible confounding variables that may increase cost in the real clinical situation.

Professional Roles to Enhance the Clinical Expert

Just as clinical outcomes have become central to the assessment of learning, professional outcomes have become integral to learning objectives. A global shift in healthcare education has occurred. Instead of curricula being planned around content, new educational interventions are often centered on the varied roles of healthcare professionals. This movement began in 1999 with Holden's ideas that a reflective medical practitioner requires 3 cornerstones:

1. Technical intelligence: Medical knowledge and its application
2. Creative intelligence: The ethics and moral judgment required to approach medical practice
3. Personal intelligence: Consciousness of an individual role within a larger system.[62]

When the principal Canadian educational organization for specialists, the Royal College of Physicians and Surgeons of Canada, overhauled its evaluative framework of medical degrees and residency programs, it used a similar role-based format. The same roles apply to nursing, rehabilitation, and other healthcare professional education programs. The 3 domains were expanded into 7 key functions: medical (healthcare) expert, communicator, collaborator, manager, health advocate, scholar, and professional. Similarly, a collaborative group of undergraduate medical programs in Scotland, the Scottish Dean's Medical Curriculum Group, took the same idea of outcome-oriented education and itemized 12 domains: what the doctor is able to do (clinical skills, practical procedures, patient investigation and management, health promotion, communication, and informatics), how the doctor approaches practice (scholarship, attitudes, and decision-making skill), and professionalism.

The relevance of this domain/outcome-oriented approach reaches beyond undergraduate and postgraduate education. It reinforces the *broad spectrum of skills necessary to productive practice, not only for doctors but for all healthcare professionals.* These models highlight why education should go beyond healthcare, scholarly, medical, and nursing content. For improved patient outcomes, it is important to learn complementary managerial skills to optimize local resource utilization and overcome common communication barriers. Interprofessional collaboration can improve care, and health promotion along with advocacy within the community can improve the available resources and shift the focus of care from disease management to prevention. Success requires balanced learning in all domains, but many programs are not balanced. As adult self-directed learners, this requires planning. Similar to the Can MEDS objectives set out by the Royal College and the 12 domains itemized by the Scottish Dean's group, each learner from all professions must add context to the roles in his or her practice. A concerted effort must be made to construct learning objectives in each of these domains.

Of note, the original Can MEDS roles proposed by the Canadian College of Physicians and Surgeons included an eighth role — *a balanced lifestyle* — that was omitted from the final version. Perhaps this speaks tellingly about our attitude toward our medical roles and education. Nonetheless, it probably should not be so easily dismissed: balancing other interests outside of our professional roles undoubtedly is both healthy and important.

Acknowledgments

We would like to acknowledge Dr. Dave Davis and Darlyne Rath for their contributions to earlier versions of this chapter and Patricia Coutts, President, CAWC, for review of the content in this version.

Practice Pearls

- Wound care education needs to be linked to outcomes, including improved professional performance and patient healthcare outcomes.
- Educational process evidence base is just as important as the scientific content of the course (interactive, longitudinal, and link to practice, including enablers and reinforcers).
- Successful programs should be linked to the principles of:
  - Knowledge transfer for practice (implementation research)
  - Communities of practice or communities of learners
  - Professional performance domains other than the clinical expert in scientific evidence
  - Communication skills
  - Collaboration
  - Manager role
  - Health and patient advocacy
  - Professionalism
  - Scholarly activities.

Self-Assessment Questions

1. Continuing professional development is mostly focused on:
   A. Accreditation and CME credit
   B. Quality improvement
   C. Improved health status
   D. Improved professional performance

2. According to Keller and Carroll, all of the following are important communication skills for the healthcare professional EXCEPT:
   A. A human engagement with the patients and their families
   B. Sympathizing with the patient
   C. Educating the patient
   D. Enlistment to involve the patient in decision-making

3. All of the following attributes characterize a COP EXCEPT:

A. A formal group

B. Based on common interests

C. Not task-centered

D. Facilitates new knowledge production and translation

Answers: 1–D, 2–B, 3–A

References

1. Holmström IM, Rosenqvist U. Misunderstanding about illness and treatment among patients with type 2 diabetes. *J Adv Nurs*. 2005;49(2):146–154.

2. Sharp LK, Lipsky MS. Continuing medical education and attitudes of health care providers toward treating diabetes. *J Contin Educ Health Prof*. 2002;22(2):103–112.

3. D'Amour D, Oandasan I. Interprofessionality as the field of interprofessional practice and interprofessional education: an emerging concept. *J Interprof Care*. 2005;19 Suppl 1:8–20.

4. Knowles M. The emergence of a theory of adult learning: andragogy. In: *The Adult Learner: A Neglected Species*. 2nd ed. Houston, TX: Gulf Publishing Company; 1978:27–59.

5. Houle CO. *The Design of Education*. 2nd ed. San Francisco, CA: Jossey-Bass Higher and Adult Education Series; 1996.

6. Tough A. How adults learn and change. *Diabetes Educ*. 1985;11 Suppl:21–25.

7. Stinson L, Pearson D, Lucas B. Developing a learning culture: twelve tips for individuals, teams and organizations. *Med Teach*. 2006;28(4):309–312.

8. Belcher AE, Sibbald RG. Mentoring: the ultimate professional relationship. *Ostomy Wound Manage*. 1998;44(4):76–78.

9. Schon DA. *The Reflective Practitioner*. Boston, MA: Basic Books; 1984.

10. Mezirow J. A critical theory of self directed learning. In: Brookfield S, ed. *Self-Directed Learning: From Theory to Practice (Jossey Bass Higher and Adult Education Series)*. San Francisco, CA: Jossey-Bass; 1985;(25):17–29.

11. Brundage DH. *Adult Learning Principles and their Application to Program Planning*. Toronto, Ontario, Canada: Ontario Ministry of Education; 1980.

12. Pine GJ. *Operation Mainstream: A Report on Problem Solving and the Helping Relationship*. Durham, NH: New England Center for Continuing Education; 1968.

13. Davis DA, Thomson MA, Oxman AD, Haynes RB. Changing physician performance. A systematic review of the effect of continuing medical education strategies. *JAMA*. 1995;274(9):700–705.

14. Avorn J, Soumerai SB. Improving drug-therapy decisions through educational outreach. A randomized controlled trial of academically based "detailing." *N Engl J Med*. 1983;308(24):1457–1463.

15. Steele MA, Bess DT, Franse VL, Graber SE. Cost effectiveness of two interventions for reducing outpatient prescribing costs. *DICP*. 1989;23(6):497–500.

16. Avorn J, Soumerai SB, Everitt DE, et al. A randomized trial of a program to reduce the use of psychoactive drugs in nursing homes. *N Engl J Med*. 1992;327(3):168–173.

17. Raisch DW, Bootman JL, Larson LN, McGhan WF. Improving antiulcer agent prescribing in a health maintenance organization. *Am J Hosp Pharm*. 1990;47(8):1766–1773.

18. Rabin DL, Boekeloo BO, Marx ES, Bowman MA, Russell NK, Willis AG. Improving office-based physician's prevention practices for sexually transmitted diseases. *Ann Intern Med*. 1994;121(7):513–519.

19. Stross JK, Bole GG. Evaluation of a continuing education program in rheumatoid arthritis. *Arthritis Rheum*. 1980;23(7):846–849.

20. Stross JK, Bole GG. Evaluation of an educational program for primary care practitioners, on the management of osteoarthritis. *Arthritis Rheum*. 1985;28(1):108–111.

21. Stross JK, Hiss RG, Watts CM, Davis WK, Macdonald R. Continuing education in pulmonary disease for primary-care physicians. *Am Rev Respir Dis*. 1983;127(6):739–746.

22. Brimberry R. Vaccination of high-risk patients for influenza. A comparison of telephone and mail reminder methods. *J Fam Pract*. 1988;26(4):397–400.

23. Magruder-Habib K, Zung WW, Feussner JR. Improving physicians' recognition and treatment of depression in general medical care. Results from a randomized clinical trial. *Med Care*. 1990;28(3):239–250.

24. McPhee SJ, Bird JA, Fordham D, Rodnick JE, Osborn EH. Promoting cancer prevention activities by primary care physicians. Results of a randomized, controlled trial. *JAMA*. 1991;266(4):538–544.

25. Pierce M, Lundy S, Palanisamy A, Winning S, King J. Prospective randomised controlled trial of methods of call and recall for cervical cytology screening. *BMJ*. 1989;299(6692):160–162.

26. Rosser WW, McDowell I, Newell C. Use of reminders for preventive procedures in family medicine. *CMAJ*. 1991;145(7):807–814.

27. Vinicor F, Cohen SJ, Mazzuca SA, et al. DIABEDS: a randomized trial of the effects of physician and/or patient education on diabetes patient outcomes. *J Chronic Dis*. 1987;40(4):345–356.

28. Everett GD, deBlois CS, Chang PF, Holets T. Effect of cost education, cost audits, and faculty chart review on the use of laboratory services. *Arch Intern Med*. 1983;143(5):942–944.

29. Martin AR, Wolf MA, Thibodeau LA, Dzau V, Braunwald E. A trial of two strategies to modify the test-ordering behavior of medical residents. *N Engl J Med*. 1980;303(23):1330–1336.

30. Pinkerton RE, Tinanoff N, Willms JL, Tapp JT. Resident physician performance in a continuing education format. Does newly acquired knowledge improve patient care? *JAMA*. 1980;244(19):2183–2185.

31. Restuccia JD. The effect of concurrent feedback in reducing inappropriate hospital utilization. *Med Care*. 1982;20(1):46–62.

32. Davis D, O'Brien MA, Freemantle N, Wolf FM, Mazmanian P, Taylor-Vaisey A. Impact of formal continuing medical education: do conferences, workshops, rounds, and other traditional continuing education activities change physician behavior or health care outcomes? *JAMA*. 1999;282(9):867–874.

33. Davis DA, Taylor-Vaisey A. Translating guidelines into practice. A systematic review of theoretic concepts, practical experience and research evidence in

the adoption of clinical practice guidelines. *CMAJ.* 1997;157(4):408–416.

34. Davis D, Davis N. Selecting educational interventions for knowledge translation. *CMAJ.* 2010;182(2):E89–E93.

35. Tetroe J. Knowledge translation at the Canadian Institutes of Health Research: a primer. Available at: http://www.ncddr.org/kt/products/focus/focus18/. Accessed January 17, 2012.

36. Estabrooks CA, Thompson DS, Lovely JJ, Hofmeyer A. A guide to knowledge translation theory. *J Contin Educ Health Prof.* 2006;26(1):25–36.

37. Lockyer JM, Fidler H, Hogan DB, et al. Assessing outcomes through congruence of course objectives and reflective work. *J Contin Educ Health Prof.* 2005;25(2):76–86.

38. Davis D, Evans M, Jadad A, et al. The case for knowledge translation: shortening the journey from evidence to effect. *BMJ.* 2003;327(7405):33–35.

39. Mohanna K, Wall D, Chambers R. *Teaching Made Easy: A Manual for Health Professionals.* Oxford, UK: Radcliffe Medical Press; 2004:41–57.

40. Wenger E. Communities of practice: a brief introduction. Available at: www.ewenger.com/theory/index.htm. Accessed March 2007.

41. Pereles L, Lockyer J, Fidler H. Permanent small groups: group dynamics, learning, and change. *J Contin Educ Health Prof.* 2002;22(4):205–213.

42. Austin Z, Duncan-Hewitt W. Faculty, student, and practitioner development within a community of practice. *Am J Pharm Ed.* 2005;69(3):55.

43. Duncan-Hewitt W, Austin Z. Pharmacy schools as expert communities of practice? A proposal to radically restructure pharmacy education to optimize learning. *Am J Pharm Ed.* 2005;69(3):54.

44. Barab S, Duffy T. From practice fields to communities of practice. In: Jonassen D, Land S, eds. *Theoretical Foundations of Learning Environments.* Marwah, NJ: Lawrence Erlbaum Associates; 2000:25–55.

45. Bereiter C, Scardamalia M. *Surpassing Ourselves: An Inquiry into the Nature and Implications of Expertise.* Chicago, IL: Open Court Publishing Company; 1993.

46. Scardamalia M, Bereiter C. Engaging students in a knowledge society. In: *The Jossey-Bass Reader on Technology and Learning.* San Francisco, CA: Jossey-Bass Inc; 2000:312–319.

47. Scardamalia M, Bereiter C. Engaging students in a knowledge society. *Educational Leadership.* 1996;54(3):6–10.

48. Bereiter C. *Education and Mind in the Knowledge Age.* Mahwah, NJ: Lawrence Erlbaum Associates; 2002.

49. Choo CW. *The Knowing Organization: How Organizations Use Information to Construct Meaning, Create Knowledge, and Make Decisions.* New York, NY: Oxford University Press, Inc; 1998.

50. Scardamalia M. CSILE/Knowledge Forum®. In: Kovalchick A, Dawson K, eds. *Education and Technology: An Encyclopedia.* Santa Barbara, CA: ABC-CLIO; 2002.

51. Scardamalia M, Bereiter C. Knowledge building: theory, pedagogy, and technology. In: Sawyer RK, ed. *Cambridge Handbook of the Learning Sciences.* New York, NY: Cambridge University Press, Inc; 2006:97–118.

52. Keller VF, Carroll JG. A new model for physician-patient communication. *Patient Educ Couns.* 1994;23(2):131–140.

53. Rider EA, Keefer CH. Communication skills competencies: definitions and a teaching toolbox. *Med Educ.* 2006;40(7):624–629.

54. Dixon J. Evaluation criteria in studies of continuing education in the health professions: a critical review and a suggested strategy. *Eval Health Prof.* 1978;1(2):47–65.

55. Davis D, Taylor-Vaisey A. Two decades of Dixon: the question(s) of evaluating continuing education in the health professions. *J Contin Educ Health Prof.* 1997;17(4):207–213.

56. Sibbald RG, Coutts P, Paterson DM. Sustained vs. graduated compression in the management of leg ulcers. Presented at The Wound Healing Society Meeting in Toronto, Ontario, June 4–6, 2000.

57. Phillips T, Stanton B, Provan A, Lew R. A study of the impact of leg ulcers on quality of life: financial, social, and psychologic implications. *J Am Acad Dermatol.* 1994;31(1):49–53.

58. Price PE, Harding KG. Measuring health related quality of life in patients with chronic leg ulcers. *WOUNDS.* 1996;8(3):91–95.

59. Franks PJ, Moffatt CJ. Quality of life issues in patients with chronic wounds. *WOUNDS.* 1998;10(Suppl E):1E–9E.

60. Franks PJ, Moffatt CJ, Connolly M, et al. Community leg ulcer clinics: effect on quality of life. *Phlebology.* 1994;9(2):83–86.

61. Phillips TJ. Cost effectiveness in wound care. In: Krasner D, Kane D, eds. *Chronic Wound Care: A Clinical Source Book for Healthcare Professionals.* 2nd ed. Wayne, PA: Health Management Publications, Inc; 1997:369–372.

62. Holden J. How much informal education in general practice? *Educ Gen Pract.* 1999;10:83–84.

Teaching Wound Care to Patients, Families, and Healthcare Providers Around the Globe

Paula Erwin-Toth, MSN, RN, CWOCN, CNS, ET;
Brenda Stenger, MEd, RN, CWOCN, ET;
Linda Stricker, MSN/ED, RN, CWOCN;
James Merlino, MD, FACS, FASCRS

Objectives

The reader will be challenged to:

- Utilize wound management resources to provide support as well as financial and reimbursement information to healthcare providers, patients, and caregivers
- Analyze appropriate, culturally congruent, wound care education programs for healthcare providers, patients, and caregivers based on principles of adult education and nursing (healthcare) theory
- Critique methods to facilitate acquisition of wound care skills/techniques by healthcare providers, patients, and caregivers.

Introduction

Effective patient/caregiver education is an essential component of successful wound management no matter where the patient lives or where the healthcare provider practices. In order for successful learning to take place, healthcare personnel providing patient/caregiver education must possess knowledge and skills in wound care and adult education that is culturally congruent. Decreasing lengths of stay in the acute care setting have given further impetus to healthcare personnel to provide meaningful patient/caregiver education in a variety of settings. Interventions derived from research-based outcome criteria will further standardize care. In the United States, *The Joint Commission and the Agency for Healthcare Research and Quality (AHRQ) have identified patient/caregiver education as a critical component of clinical care in general and of wound care specifically.*[1-5]

Work redesign efforts directed at decreasing healthcare costs may result in licensed and unlicensed healthcare personnel participating in chronic wound management. All healthcare providers acting in this capacity must be well rounded in chronic wound management. Skills in patient/caregiver competency in chronic wound care are essential to the success of the management plan. The licensed healthcare professional takes the lead on assessing all aspects of the wound and plan of care. Assessment includes the wound condition, barriers to healing, psychosocial needs, support needs for direct wound care, and follow-up evaluation. When an unlicensed caregiver is participating in direct

Erwin-Toth P, Stenger B, Stricker L, Merlino J. Teaching wound care to patients, families, and healthcare providers around the globe. In: Krasner DL, Rodeheaver GT, Sibbald RG, Woo KY, eds. *Chronic Wound Care: A Clinical Source Book for Healthcare Professionals.* Vol 1. 5th ed. Malvern, PA: HMP Communications; 2012:55–62.

wound care, appropriate delegation is important for safe and effective delivery of that care. It is important to determine the learning needs and skills of the unlicensed person, provide the education and skill development for direct wound care, and follow up to ensure that learning has occurred and safe care was provided.[3,6,7]

Principles of Adult Learning

Adult learning theory. In 1984, Knowles, a major adult learning theorist, reflected, "Learning is an elusive phenomenon."[8] Educational activities are designed to initiate a change in behavior, knowledge, and skill. This process starts with the educator asking if learning has actually taken place. The key questions are:

• Has the learner truly demonstrated a change in behavior, knowledge, and skill?
• Will this change endure across time and place?
• How do you accurately assess and document these findings?
• How do you modify your educational plan if effective learning is not taking place?[3,7,8]
• Does the learner have past experiences that are relevant to the current learning need?

Andragogy is defined by Knowles as the "art and science of helping adults learn."[8] Knowles's andragogical model is based on *6 major assumptions*:

1. **The need to know:** Adults need to know why they must learn something before learning it.
2. **The learner's self-concept:** Adults have a self-concept of being responsible for their own lives. They resent and resist situations in which they feel others are imposing their wills upon them.
3. **The role of the learner's experience:** In a group of adults, there will be a wider range of individual differences than in a group of youths. A group of adults will be more heterogeneous in terms of background, learning style, motivation, needs, interests, and goals than a group of youths. Hence, the great emphasis in adult education is on individualization of teaching and learning strategies.
4. **Readiness to learn:** Adults become ready to learn those things that they need to know and to be able to do in order to cope effectively with their real-life situations.

5. **Orientation to learning:** Adults are life-centered (or task-centered or problem-centered) in their orientations to learning. Adults achieve new knowledge, understanding, skills, values, and attitudes most effectively when these items apply to real-life situations.
6. **Motivation:** While adults are responsive to some external motivations (eg, better jobs, promotions, higher salaries), the most potent motivators are internal pressures (eg, the desire for increased job satisfaction, self-esteem, quality of life).[8]

While andragogy is appropriate for most types of adult learning situations, Knowles recognized that occasionally *pedagogical strategies* used in teaching children may be selectively or temporarily applied to adult learners. In the pedagogical model, the teacher assumes "full responsibility for making all decisions about what is learned, how it will be learned, when it will be learned, and if it has been learned."[8,9] Learners that need to be taught by the pedagogical model characteristically are dependent, have no experience with the content area, do not perceive the relevance of the content, need to accomplish a required performance, or feel no internal need to learn the content. However, for learning to develop and endure, applying andragogical strategies once the initial learning has taken place is important.[8] In contrast, adults have knowledge from previous experience and can further their knowledge and learn new concepts through active experimentation and reflection on action.[10] Using an approach that combines *adult learning principles with a structured curriculum* provides the adult learner the opportunity to self-direct some of the learning based on previous knowledge and still have information crucial for self care.

Adult education. In a prospective study of pressure ulcer risk in patients with spinal cord injuries, researchers discussed the importance of discerning health beliefs and ongoing educational programs to reinforce learning related to pressure ulcer prevention.[11] They discovered that little or no education was provided following the initial acute care and rehabilitation phase for patients with spinal cord injuries. Despite the high prevalence of pressure ulcers in the 60 study participants (25% from the control group and 28%

from the experimental group), none of them requested additional information about skin care or to be reevaluated for pressure-related problems. Although the subjects recognized the importance of skin care and pressure ulcer prevention, they neither requested nor were provided information.

When planning an adult educational program, the following components should be included:[8,12,13]

1. **Needs and priorities assessment:** What does the learner perceive to be important?
   - **Learning style assessment:** How does the individual learn best, eg, through audio, visual, or kinesthetic methods?
   - **Cultural assessment:** Are there specific cultural influences to perception of illness?
   - **Literacy assessment:** Are there barriers to learning that must be included in the teaching plan?
2. **Content analysis:** What does the content mean to the overall or long-term plan?
3. **Objectives:** What is the content? How will it be presented?
4. **Evaluation:** How will the learner's knowledge be assessed? How will he or she evaluate the education?
5. **Related arrangements:** Where will the teaching take place? What audiovisual aids or materials will be used?
6. **Organizational considerations:** Where does the burden of cost for direct wound care lie? How does the culture of the organization impact flow of care from start of care to delivery of care to community resources? Does the interdisciplinary team interact together or individually? Where can networking skills increase referrals?

Brookfield identified the following 6 principles of adult education:
1. Participation is voluntary
2. Respect for self-worth is fostered
3. Adult learning is collaborative
4. Ongoing evaluation is critical for the endeavor's success
5. Adult education fosters a spirit of critical reflection
6. The aim of adult education is the nurturing of self-directed, empowered adults.[14]

Other factors to consider are *family and cultural influences* that are important in adult learning. Current and past interactions of families and significant others with the patient will influence the effectiveness of education. Knowledge of the learner's ethnic and cultural background can provide valuable insight into identifying learning needs and developing effective teaching strategies. However, one must be cautious to avoid stereotyping learners based on family relationships and ethnic background.[15–18]

The educator should consider the **chronological ages and developmental stages** of the patient and caregivers when creating the teaching plan. For example, older adults are capable of learning new information and new skills, but the educator must consider the effects of concomitant medical and social conditions that can influence the patient's/caregiver's ability to learn.[6,8,19]

Attention to *pain management* should be addressed along with self-care activities. Patients who are in pain may not be capable of learning new behaviors. Caregivers may be reluctant to participate in activities that they perceive as being hurtful to their patients. Not only can the effect of pain differ culturally, it can also influence readiness to participate in learning activities.[1,17,18] Coping with complex chronic illnesses, such as diabetes, adds to the burden of compliance. Learning to incorporate self-care into a new lifestyle is a process that takes time, and each person adjusts individually. When anxiety and depression manifest as a person is learning, barriers occur and the healthcare provider will see behaviors inconsistent with compliance. Assessing the person based on individual problems provides clues to when and how to intervene.

Body image in patients with chronic wounds is not well researched. Since positive self-esteem has been identified as an important component of adult learning, it is logical to assume that a negative body image may contribute to low self-esteem and may have a negative impact on learning. Patients with chronic or disfiguring wounds should be encouraged to maintain good physical hygiene and an optimal physical appearance. People who feel good about themselves are more likely to feel motivated in their own care.[20]

When developing a *patient-circle of care teaching plan*, the educator should consider the literacy of the patient/caregiver. The educator must be sensitive during this portion of the assessment. Asking for an individual's highest level of education is rarely sufficient. There are several standardized tests available to determine reading level; however, use of these instruments is rarely practical in a clinical setting. Yasenchak and Bridle[21] recommended asking patients/caregivers the question, "Do you like to read?" instead of the more threatening, "How well do you read?" Before beginning to teach, have the patient/caregiver read a section of the written instructions aloud. Reading ability and comprehension can then be assessed. In a literature review, Boyd reported that a majority of the people in the United States has a reading level at or below the eighth grade. However, 60%–92% of patient education materials require a reading level of eighth grade or higher. The use of clear and plain language that focuses on the important concepts provides opportunity for understanding and assessment of learning. Developing focus groups of potential patients from varied backgrounds, age groups, and cultural and economic backgrounds provides data that reflect the specific needs of the communities served by the organization or healthcare professional.[18,21,22]

Learning styles and activities. Developing a teaching plan based on assessment of health literacy, learning readiness, and cultural influences is a critical phase in the planning process. Taking the added step of determining learning style preferences provides the learner with an optimal learning approach. Identifying learning preferences can be as simple as asking the patient how he or she prefers to learn, or by asking the question, "The last time you learned a new hobby, what did you use to help you master the skill?" This question will help set the tone for what type of learning activities should be set up to guide the patient to learning appropriate wound care skills. Utilizing an *interactive and multimedia approach* through the use of printed material, video clips, computer modules, and return demonstration with the products offers reinforcement to all learning styles. Using *teach–back methods*, where the patient teaches the new skill back to the clinician, provides an opportunity to assess mastery of the necessary components of care.[13] Documentation of individual learning is an important part of learning assessment. Developing forms or electronic systems that incorporate learning objectives and specific learning needs combined with learning assessment parameters provides evidence of what learning occurred.

Numerous nursing models and theories can be applied to enhance patient/family education. *Orem's Self Care Deficit Theory*[22] and *Roy's Adaptation Model*[23] can provide theoretical frameworks to assist nurses in developing effective teaching plans. Dorthea Orem held the assumption that people are individuals who should be self-reliant and responsible for their own care and that self-care is a learned behavior. Roy's adaptation model considers individual self-awareness and how individual decisions are based in relationships and the environment. Incorporating these 2 models into the assessment process includes where the person is with self-care adaptation and abilities and where to individualize specific teaching interventions.

Reimbursement Issues and the Interprofessional Team Approach

In this era of cost containment and shrinking healthcare dollars, there may be pressure to reduce educational activities no matter what part of the world one is in. In the 1960s and 1970s, the fee-for-service system expanded to include education and other services, because costs could be directly or indirectly absorbed into an institution's or agency's operating budget.

These changes have left many patients, families, providers, and insurers scrambling to form a new healthcare paradigm. It is vital for wound care providers to be aware of the financial issues at stake and promote the role of *education as a key to reducing healthcare costs*. More recently, financial sanctions reducing or eliminating reimbursement for nosocomial wounds has further challenged the healthcare system.[1,24,25]

Educating patients, families, caregivers, and healthcare providers is the key to *a proactive program of prevention* and timely, appropriate interventions. This approach will improve the quality of life for clients, and it will improve outcomes. It also will reduce the amount of healthcare resources spent for wound care.[1–3,5,6,8,9,16,18,26] The best educational programs are linked to patient care outcomes and modified when these outcomes do not meet goals or current standards.

An *interprofessional team* best serves this approach. The goal should be to provide seamless care to the client regardless of the setting. Often, a case manager or social worker can coordinate this continuum of care. Ideally, in this system, the care is patient-focused. All interprofessional team members are focused on improving outcomes for clients. At times, *case mapping or critical pathways* can facilitate this process. Variance analysis can reveal where clients are not following the expected pattern, and the team can modify the plan of care to address these variances. The key to success in this approach and all educational activities is the active role played by the client/family and the interprofessional, interdepartmental, and interagency cooperation evidenced by the healthcare team.[6,8]

Teaching Healthcare Providers

Education of licensed and unlicensed healthcare providers should be an ongoing process. Although educational preparation and responsibilities among healthcare providers may vary, optimal wound management is dependent upon knowledge of, and compliance with, the wound care plan.[6,8]

A *needs assessment* should be conducted before planning wound care education programs. Needs assessments take several forms including questionnaires, surveys, focus groups with a neutral facilitator, or examination of data (prevalence rates, medical and nursing errors, adverse events, recurrence rates, etc.). Most healthcare providers — licensed and unlicensed — are motivated by the desire to provide quality care. The activity and volume of patient assignments may result in the healthcare provider feeling overwhelmed and underappreciated.[3,6,9] Focusing on methods of wound prevention and management techniques that can be completed effectively and efficiently will enhance the educational experience of the healthcare providers.[5,6,8,17,18]

The content of an educational program depends on the learner. A nursing assistant may need to know the rationale and the techniques for proper positioning, turning, and skin care. He or she needs to know how to identify changes in the patient's skin and overall condition. Knowledge of basic nutrition and hydration is important as well. Just telling unlicensed personnel what to do is not enough; they are adult learners, and they need to know why something is important.[8] Ed-

ucational programs should be directed at building on and developing wound care knowledge. This approach will help facilitate the nursing assistant's internal motivation to learn and to perform the learned activities.[6,8,9,12]

Licensed healthcare personnel should be provided with the *scientific rationale* for wound prevention and management techniques based on their scopes of practice. Educational programs relating to anatomy and physiology, nutrition, topical therapies, positioning techniques and support surfaces, psychosocial issues, and patient/caregiver education are only a few of the areas that licensed personnel may require to provide optimal care. As with unlicensed healthcare providers, licensed individuals need to have educational programs based on information and techniques that will directly affect their practices.[6,8,9,12]

Educational programming should be scheduled at regular intervals with updated needs assessment surveys at all healthcare provider levels. The location, duration, and timing of educational programs will vary. Clinicians practicing at the bedside may benefit from *situational educational experiences* with formats including patient simulation, workshops, and/or practice component demonstrations. Before effective patient/caregiver education can take place, all levels of healthcare providers need to be well versed in chronic wound management.[6,8,9,12] Using ongoing learning needs assessment and evaluation criteria provides information for future educational activities. Needs assessment through changes in healthcare regulations and monitoring quality management data complements learner satisfaction and provides important data in planning education to improve care and minimize errors in the delivery of care.

Teaching the Patient/Caregiver

A *patient/caregiver needs assessment* should be performed and documented. Baseline information relating to knowledge, beliefs, and health practices, as well as the learner's perceived educational needs, should be obtained. Information pertaining to psychosocial and cultural variables should also be utilized in program design, as these issues may influence teaching strategies.[16] Unperceived needs, often based on healthcare provider knowledge gaps, scientific evidence, and patient preferences, will form part of the curriculum as well. Finally, the healthcare provider needs to determine whether the patient and caregiver are ready to learn.[3,7,8,18,19]

The healthcare provider also needs to identify *barriers to learning*. These barriers may be environmental, physiological, or psychological. Lack of privacy, limited space, poor lighting, and frequent interruptions can all negatively impact learning. For example, finding a private room or at least pulling the curtain, turning off the television, providing adequate lighting, and turning off pagers can enhance the learning environment.[3,6–8,16,18] In an environment where reimbursement resources are scarce, education becomes a lower priority on an administrative level, and healthcare professionals are challenged to demonstrate its importance. Focusing on current elements of regulatory standards, such as the Hospital Consumer Assessment of Healthcare Providers and Systems (HCAHPS), provides important data and documentation to gain administrative support. HCAHPS is a survey used to assess quality of patient care from a patient perspective. Elements of this survey include care from nurses, education clarity, care from doctors, and the hospital environment.

Efforts should be made to optimize the patient's physical condition. Pain is a barrier to learning. Effective pain management through pharmacological treatments, electrical stimulation, positioning, and/or biofeedback techniques may be beneficial to both the patient and caregiver. Timing of these interventions should be done to elicit maximal relief with minimal effect on cognitive abilities.[1,17,26]

Identification of psychological, social, and cultural barriers is an important part of a comprehensive assessment. Techniques to promote effective coping skills and to facilitate *open communication* and efforts to acknowledge and work within cultural and religious values should be undertaken by the healthcare provider. Economic barriers to effective wound management should be considered as well. The inability to purchase proper food or nutritional supplements, medications, topical therapies, and/or assistive devices will have a negative impact on health. If any of these barriers are present, consultation with a social worker may benefit the patient/caregiver.[6,9,15,16]

In the acute care environment, healthcare pro-

viders may need to focus on *survival issues* (eg, need-to-know versus nice-to-know). Reinforcement of teaching and expansion of the breadth and depth of patient/caregiver education can be conducted at an extended care facility, at home, or in an ambulatory care setting. The goal is for the patient/caregiver to achieve independence and mastery of care.[6–8,12,14]

Each component of *patient teaching should be transparent*. Healthcare providers should collaborate with the patient/caregiver to identify the overall general learning goal and specific learning objectives. They should clearly describe the teaching method, timing, and venue. They should also conduct an evaluation of the effectiveness of patient/caregiver learning. Healthcare providers should list specific outcome-based criteria and note whether the patient/caregiver successfully demonstrated understanding and competence. If learning has been ineffective, the healthcare provider should reassess and revise the teaching plan.[8,12,14]

Ongoing assessment, reinforcement of previous instruction, and the addition of new material should continue during wound healing and after wound healing has occurred. Finally, patients/caregivers should have the opportunity to evaluate the quantity and quality of the education they have received.[8,12,14]

Linking Communication to Patient Satisfaction

Communication is an important measure of both provider and patient satisfaction. When physicians, nurses, and other healthcare providers communicate effectively to patients and their caregivers, the patients are more likely to be adherent with their plan of care and medications, experience less anxiety, and have improved health outcomes.[27]

Improving patient-provider communications is essential to providing an excellent patient experience. Effective communication also impacts patient safety and quality of care, and, most importantly, it is the right thing to do.

Measuring Patient Satisfaction

Patient surveys are key to addressing patient-centered concerns and increasing patient satisfaction. In the United States, there are several *survey instruments* and processes that measure patient satisfaction at different touch points. Examples include surveys sent to patients after care has been provided by home care providers (HH-CAHPS or Home Health Consumer Assessment of Healthcare Providers and Systems) and after inpatient visits (HCAHPS). US hospitals routinely conduct surveys of other patient care areas, including emergency department visits and ambulatory surgery procedures.[27] These surveys can be accessed at www.healthstream.com/HCAHPS.

Currently, in the United States, only inpatient (HCAHPS) and home healthcare (HH-CAHPS) surveys are mandated by the Centers for Medicare & Medicaid Services (CMS). In other countries, patient satisfaction is becoming an important benchmark of healthcare and can determine resource allocation in some settings. Patient surveys are intended to increase transparency and to help consumers in their health provider and hospital decisions. Every hospital in the United States that treats Medicare patients is required to administer these surveys or will face decreased reimbursement.[27]

HCAHPS provides a standardized methodology that allows objective and meaningful comparisons among hospitals on topics that are important to patients. Eight critical aspects of care, referred to as the HCAHPS domains, are covered in the survey questions, including communication with doctors and communication with nurses.[27] These domains include communication with doctors, communication with nurses, communication about medications, staff responsiveness, pain management, quality of discharge instructions, cleanliness of environment, and quiet of hospital environment.

In the United States, CMS only reports the "Top Box" scores, or the percentage of patients who respond in the most positive manner ("Always" response) to each question. Therefore, average is not acceptable: service must always be exceptional in order to note changes on HCAHPS scores.[27]

Considering the patient's point of view will help providers bring genuine, empathetic care to the bedside to transform the patient experience. As a healthcare provider, you can better appreciate what it is like to be in the patient's place when you recall a time when you have been a patient yourself.

Conclusion

Culturally congruent education is an essential component of successful chronic wound management. Knowledgeable healthcare providers will be better prepared to facilitate learning by patients/caregivers. Across the globe, principles of adult learning, adult education, and nursing and other healthcare professional theories can be applied to enhance the effectiveness of educational endeavors. Adult learning and learning principles are constant and used to guide curriculum plans in developing education programs. Identification of collaborating wound care professionals and educators, general learning goals, specific objectives, needs assessments, variable learning methods, and evaluation will help to create an effective wound management education plan.[3,6,8,12,14]

Practice Pearls

- Effective patient/caregiver education is an essential component of successful wound management.
- Older adults are capable of learning new information and new skills, but the educator must consider the effects of concomitant medical and social conditions that can influence the patient's/caregiver's ability to learn. The education must be culturally congruent.
- It is vital for wound care providers to be aware of the key financial issues and to promote the role of education as a key to wound prevention and reducing healthcare costs.
- Healthcare providers should collaborate with the patient/caregiver to identify the overall general learning goal and specific learning objectives.

Self-Assessment Questions

1. A 62-year-old woman with a venous insufficiency ulcer would most likely need what type of education?

    A. Admission to an acute care facility to provide intensive self-care education

    B. A learning needs assessment and education

care plan based on patient-specific data

C. Identification of a family member willing to provide totally compensatory care

D. Daily skilled home care visits until re-epithelization of the wound occurs

2. Which strategies are most effective in teaching adults wound management skills?

A. Build on previous knowledge, identify the learner's desire and ability to master care, and ensure teaching is task focused

B. Provide a lengthy theoretical overview of the principles of wound healing, always schedule instruction early in the day, and emphasize the need for a specific number of education sessions

C. Ensure the learner is given a pre- and post-test to evaluate acquisition of wound management knowledge

D. Implement a computer-based education program as the sole source of delivery of wound management instruction

Answers: 1-B, 2-A

References

1. Joint Commission on the Accreditation of Hospitals. *Hospital Accreditation Standards, 2006: Accreditation Policies Standards Elements of Performance Scoring.* Chicago, IL: JCAHO; 2005.

2. Panel for the Prediction and Prevention of Pressure Ulcers in Adults. *Clinical Practice Guideline Number 3: Pressure Ulcers in Adults: Prediction and Prevention.* Rockville, MD: US Department of Health and Human Services. Agency for Health Care Policy and Research; 1992. AHCPR publication 92-0047.

3. Stotts NA, Hopf HW. Facilitating positive outcomes in older adults with wounds. *Nurs Clin North Am.* 2005;40(2):267–279.

4. Sibbald RG, Williamson D, Orsted HL, et al. Preparing the wound bed — debridement, bacterial balance, and moisture balance. *Ostomy Wound Manage.* 2000;46(11):14–22,24–28.

5. Bonham PA. Assessment and management of patients with venous, arterial, and diabetic/neuropathic lower extremity wounds. *AACN Clin Issues.* 2003;14(4):442–456,548–550.

6. Sunderhaus C. Wound care. Wound care education: educational barriers for patients and case managers. *Care Management.* 2006;12(1):36–39.

7. Tomaselli NL. Teaching the patient with a chronic wound. *Adv Skin Wound Care.* 2005;18(7):379–390.

8. Knowles M. *The Adult Learner: A Neglected Species.* Houston, TX: Gulf Publishing Co; 1984.

9. Popoola MM. Complementary therapy in chronic wound management: a holistic caring case study and praxis model. *Holist Nurs Pract.* 2003;17(3):152–158.

10. Schon DA. *Educating the Reflective Practitioner: Toward a New Design for Teaching and Learning in the Professions.* San Francisco, CA: Jossey-Bass Inc., Publishers; 1987.

11. Rodriguez GP, Garber SL. Prospective study of pressure ulcer risk in spinal cord injury patients. *Paraplegia.* 1994;32(3):150–158.

12. Knox AB. *Helping Adults Learn.* San Francisco, CA: Jossey-Bass; 1987.

13. Chang M, Kelly AE. Patient education: addressing cultural diversity and health literacy issues. *Urol Nurs.* 2007;27(5):411–417.

14. Brookfield S. *Understanding and Facilitating Adult Learning.* San Francisco, Calif: Jossey-Bass; 1986.

15. Leahy M, Wright L. *Families and Psychosocial Problems.* Springhouse, PA: Springhouse Corporation; 1987.

16. Pieper B. Wound management in vulnerable populations. *Rehabil Nurs.* 2005;30(3):100–105.

17. Krasner D. The chronic wound pain experience: a conceptual model. *Ostomy Wound Manage.* 1995;41(3):20–25.

18. Gibson MC, Keast D, Woodbury MG, et al. Educational intervention in the management of acute procedure-related wound pain: a pilot study. *J Wound Care.* 2004;13(5):187–190.

19. Boyd MD. A guide to writing effective patient education materials. *Nurs Manage.* 1987;18(7):56–57.

20. Willis J. *Beautiful Again: Restoring Your Image and Enhancing Body Changes.* Santa Fe, NM: Health Press; 1994.

21. Yasenchak PA, Bridle MJ. A low-literacy skin care manual for spinal cord injury patients. *Patient Educ Couns.* 1993;22(1):1–5.

22. Orem D. *Nursing: Concepts of Practice.* 2nd ed. New York, NY: McGraw-Hill; 1980.

23. Roy C. Adaptation: a basis for nursing practice. *Nurs Outlook.* 1971;19(4):254–257.

24. Coleman J. MCO trends. *Case Manager.* 1986;7(3):44–47.

25. Ranja J. Ethics: conflicts of interest and the health provider's role as a "fiduciary." *Case Manager.* 1996;7(3):40–43.

26. Meaume S, Teot L, Lazareth I, Martini J, Bohbot S. The importance of pain reduction through dressing selection in routine wound management: the MAPP study. *J Wound Care.* 2004;13(10):409–413.

27. Hardee JT, Kasper IK. A clinical communication strategy to enhance effectiveness and CAHPS scores: the ALERT model. *Perm J.* 2008;12(3):70–74.

Addressing Concerns of People with Chronic Wounds and Their Circle(s) of Care

Strategies for Optimal Patient-Centered Care

Elizabeth A. Ayello, PhD, RN, ACNS-BC, CWON, ETN, MAPWCA, FAAN;
Nicole Courchene, MSW;
R. Gary Sibbald, BSc, MD, FRCPC(Med, Derm), MACP, FAAD, MEd, MAPWCA

Objectives

The reader will be challenged to:

- Describe practical approaches to developing patient-centered care strategies for skin and wound care practice
- Identify motivational interviewing skills and techniques to use in communicating to enhance patient adherence/coherence to the wound care plans of care
- Explore methods to improve medication/treatment adherence.

Introduction

Patient- and family-centered care has been defined as "an approach to the planning, delivery, and evaluation of healthcare that is grounded in mutually beneficial partnerships among patients, families, and healthcare practitioners."[1] This approach is "respectful and responsive to the preferences, needs, and values of patients"[2] and has been linked to quality of care. Key principles of patient-centered approaches can be found in Table 1. Within the specialty of wound care, patient-centered concerns are part of the *wound bed preparation (WBP)* framework (see Chapter 4.15 in *Chronic Wound Care: A Clinical Source Book for Healthcare Professionals*, Volume 1, 5th edition), a model that is a widely used framework for assessing, diagnosing, and treating wounds.[3] Besides treating the cause and local wound care comprised of **D** (debridement), **I** (infection/inflammation), and **M** (moisture) before **E** (edge), patient-centered concerns are an important component of WBP.[3] Sibbald and colleagues have discussed 2 broad issues regarding patient-centered concerns elsewhere.[3] They are:

1. Assess and support individualized concerns including quality of life, pain, activities of daily living, psychosocial well-being, smoking, access to care, and financial limitations
2. Provide education and support to the person and his or her circle of care (including referral) to increase adherence (coherence) to the treatment plan.[3]

In this chapter, we will address some of the strategies professionals can use to deliver patient-centered care to persons

Ayello EA, Courchene N, Sibbald RG. Strategies for optimal patient-centered care. In: Krasner DL, Rodeheaver GT, Sibbald RG, Woo KY, eds. *Chronic Wound Care: A Clinical Source Book for Healthcare Professionals.* Vol 1. 5th ed. Malvern, PA: HMP Communications; 2012:65–76.

Table 1. Key principles of patient-centered approaches[2]

- Treating patients, consumers, carers, and families with dignity and respect
- Encouraging and supporting participation in decision-making by patients, consumers, carers, and families
- Communicating and sharing information with patients, consumers, carers, and families
- Fostering collaboration with patients, consumers, carers, families, and healthcare professionals in program and policy development and in health service design, delivery, and evaluation

with wounds as well as how to more effectively partner with these individuals when the plan of care calls for changes in patient behavior.

Building a Patient-Centered Culture

Patient-centered care, sometimes also known as patient-focused care, needs to be addressed at either a systems or institutional level as well as at the patient/professional level. Both of these approaches are necessary if the individual professional working within the healthcare institution desires to provide care that places the needs of the patient as paramount. When healthcare institutions and professionals truly partner with patients and their families, this means not only involving them in decisions about their care but also gaining their insights and the benefit of their help to better plan and deliver care.[1] By coordinating care, improved patient outcomes, improved healthcare system resource utilization value for all patients, and increased staff satisfaction can be achieved.[1] First, we will describe some approaches to designing patient-centered models that require institutional buy-in. This will be followed by a discussion of motivational interviewing as a useful approach to engaging clients in the process of health behavior change. Then we will apply these principles for patient-clinician communication to improve treatment adherence.

Institutional Level Approaches

Several guides to developing patient-centered care models are available on the Internet. Inherent in most of them is the notion that patient-centered care is a partnership between the patient and the staff. In Australia, several resources

describe how to focus on and support both the partner and the patient in patient-centered care. These resources include the Australian Safety and Quality Framework for Health Care, the Australian Charter of Healthcare Rights, and the National Safety and Quality Health Service Standards.[2] The Australian report includes 22 recommendations to help promote patient-centered care.[2] The American Hospital Association (AHA) has partnered with the Institute for Family-Centered Care and Planetree (a global catalyst and leader with a vision to promote the development and implementation of innovative models of healthcare that focus on healing and nurturing body, mind, and spirit). This tripartite collaboration developed a toolkit, Strategies for Leadership, and a video, Patient- and Family-Centered Care: Partnerships for Quality and Safety.[1] The video (run time 13:50), available for download on their website, describes core concepts of patient- and family-centered care and provides illustrative stories/case studies from patients, families, and hospital leaders.[1] According to the Picker Institute,[4] most important to patients is how staff interacts with them, and communication is critical. There is a difference between communicating *to* patients and their families and communicating *with* them. Some hospitals have developed scripting tools to help staff communicate more effectively. The Cleveland Clinic uses the acronym **HEART** to help staff respond to patients and families. The HEART mnemonic represents the following components:

- **H**ear the story
- **E**mpathize
- **A**pologize
- **R**espond to the problem
- **T**hank them.[4]

Another strategy to help patients and their families is to provide communication boards that are conveniently located so that staff can write information and families can provide messages to the patient.[4] TVs can provide educational videos that can be accessed whenever it is convenient for patients and their families.[4] Since hospitalized patients might forget questions that they want to ask their healthcare providers, having a pad of paper or booklet handy for the patient/family to write down their questions is helpful.[4] Since scripting tools are effective in a patient-centered

Table 2. Core components and barriers to implementing patient-centered care for underserved populatons[8]

Core Components of Patient-Centered Care in Underserved Populations

- **Welcoming environment:** provide a physical space and an initial personal interaction that is welcoming, familiar, and not intimidating.
- **Respect for patients' values and expressed needs:** obtain information about patient's care preferences and priorities; inform and involve patient and family/caregivers in decision-making; tailor care to the individual; promote a mutually respectful, consistent patient-provider relationship.
- **Patient empowerment or "activation":** educate and encourage patients to expand their role in decision-making, health-related behaviors, and self-management.
- **Sociocultural competence:** understand and consider cultural, economic, and educational status; health literacy level; family patterns/situation; and traditions (including alternative/folk remedies). Communicate in a language and at a level that the patient understands.
- **Coordination and integration of care:** assess the need for formal and informal services that will have an impact on health or treatment, provide team-based care and care management, advocate for the patient and family, make appropriate referrals, and ensure smooth transitions between different providers and phases of care.
- **Comfort and support:** emphasize physical comfort, privacy, emotional support, and involvement of family and friends.
- **Access and navigation skills:** provide what patients can consider a "medical home," keep waiting times to a minimum, provide convenient service hours, promote access and patient flow, and help patient attain skills to better navigate the healthcare system.
- **Community outreach:** make demonstrable, proactive efforts to understand and reach out to the local community.

Barriers to Patient-Centered Care

- Difficulty recruiting and retaining underrepresented minority physicians
- Lack of defined "boundaries" for outreach staff who may be overwhelmed dealing with interrelated health, social, cultural, and economic issues of patients
- Strict hiring requirements that pose obstacles to hiring neighborhood residents
- Lack of tools to gauge and reward patient-centered care performance
- Financial constraints
- Traditional attitudes among staff unwilling to change the "old school" provider/patient relationship or acknowledge and address cultural and socio-economic issues
- Fatigue and competing priorities

approach to communicating with patients and families, how can they be incorporated into skin and wound care practice?

SBAR is a standardized communication technique that healthcare professionals can use to efficiently and accurately share patient information and set expectations. The SBAR mnemonic represents **S**ituation, **B**ackground, **A**ssessment, and **R**ecommendation.[5] An example of using SBAR for communicating pressure ulcer information among healthcare professionals can provide a template for effective transdisciplinary communication.[6] Other strategies for transforming institutions to more patient-centered care in the Veterans Administration (VA) system are outlined on the Internet.[7]

A report that addresses the special needs of patient-centered care for underserved populations was prepared for the WK Kellogg Foundation and is available from the Economic and Social Research Institute.[8] Core components and barriers to implementing patient-centered care can be found in Table 2.[8] A strategy used by one of the chapter authors for clinic patients is to include a note about something personal about the patient in the medical record, so the next time the patient comes for the healthcare appointment, the healthcare professional can make a follow-up comment that is unique and individual to that patient. For example, on a visit to the wound clinic, the patient with an ulcer remarked that he is excited and hoping that the pain can be controlled so that he can attend his child's wedding. The healthcare professional put a reminder that the patient's child was getting married on a removable "sticky" note on the front of the patient's chart as a prompt to ask how he enjoyed the wedding at the next appointment.

Changing Patient Behaviors

Changing and improving the care of a patient may be a complex and challenging undertaking. Having a wound may require a person to change his or her typical routines and life practices. For example, the smell and exudate of a venous ulcer that will be repulsive to other family members may cause the affected individual to eat alone. Compression therapy is part of the typical care for a person with a venous leg ulcer, and when the wound has healed, compression stockings need to be worn for life in the absence of significant arterial disease. Sometimes, using less compression initially or a different type of bandage might help the patient tolerate the compression. Alternately, a person with diabetes mellitus needs to wear an appropriate shoe that accommodates his or her foot size, and during ulcer healing, adequate offloading of pressure is part of the treatment plan.

Among persons with lower leg and foot disease, smoking adversely impacts wound healing.[9] Smith and Smith reported that "smoking a single cigarette creates a vasoconstrictive effect for up to 90 minutes, while smoking a pack results in tissue hypoxia that lasts an entire day."[10] Individuals who smoke 1 pack a day have 3 times the risk of tissue necrosis and those who smoke 2 packs a day have 6 times the risk of those who do not smoke.[10] For individuals who stop smoking, 85% who have intermittent claudication will improve their walking distance by 50%–75%.[11] Despite these and other well known detrimental effects of smoking on the arterial endothelial function and wound healing, persons with wounds may continue to smoke. Success of intervention strategies varies, but most agree that multicomponent strategic approaches that involve behavioral intervention are effective.[9] More education about the effects of smoking on the vasculature is not enough to reduce or to stop smoking behaviors. This can be frustrating to a clinician when education alone is not effective. Sometimes we find ourselves attempting to sway patients' behaviors by:

Table 3. Motivational interviewing
• Resistance
• Change talk
• OARS
o **O**pen-ended questions
o **A**ffirmations
o **R**eflective listening
o **S**ummarization
• Importance and confidence

- Lecturing
- Using scare tactics
- Arguing
- Bargaining
- Bullying
- Begging.

An alternative approach that can help to inspire behavior change is ***motivational interviewing***.

Motivational Interviewing

Motivational interviewing (MI) has been used in clinical conditions (eg, smoking, dietary adherence, substance abuse) as a method of helping patients through the process of change. Miller and Rollnick[12] have defined MI as "a directive, patient-centered counseling style for enhancing intrinsic motivation by helping patients explore and resolve ambivalence."

Components of MI can be found in Table 3. Additionally, several presentations and tip sheets are downloadable on the Internet.[13,14]

The general principles of MI start with empathy and acceptance. MI requires clinicians to use active and reflective listening skills as much, if not more, than information sharing and education. MI is used to help the patient identify discrepancies between their current health behaviors, the goals of treatment, and important personal goals or values. As clinicians, we may have a long list of reasons why the patient should adopt new behaviors — for example, a patient with venous ulcers should stop smoking — but in MI, the patient identifies his or her own individual argument for change. When a behavior comes into conflict with a deeply held value or goal, behaviors are more likely to change. Drawing the patient's attention to the discrepancies can be much more effective than other tactics, such as lecturing, that may cause the patient to defend his or her behaviors. It is important to avoid arguing for change.

When patients show resistance, it is best not to directly oppose or confront them. Resistance is a signal to respond differently.

Engaging in Change Talk

You can use a scale of 0 to 10 to begin a discussion about the patient's willingness to change, with 0 representing not at all willing and 10 representing extremely willing.

Following are several example discussion questions:
- "How important is it for you to _____?"
- "If you did decide to change _____, how confident are you that you can do it?"
- "How *motivated* are you to change _____?"
- "How *important* is it for you right now to change _____?"

You should follow each question above with more probing, such as:
- "Why did you pick that number and not a 0 or a 10?"
- "What would need to happen for you to get from X to Y?"

For example, for a person with a venous ulcer, you might ask, "What would need to happen for you to get from smoking to not smoking?" Alternatively, you might ask, "What would need to change for you to wear your compression stockings?"

You may find that the patient is ambivalent about making a behavior change. Following is a tool you can use to help a patient weigh the pros and cons and to help him or her verbalize motivators. It is likely that the patient will have a multitude of reasons not to change. Of course, we want to help the patient shift his or her decisional balance (Table 4 and Table 5) toward changing. It is best not to *give* reasons to change. Rather, it is better to *elicit* reasons to change from the patient.

Once you have discussed importance, confidence, and motivation, you should have a good idea of the patient's willingness to continue the discussion and move through the change process.

The *transtheoretical model of behavior change* evaluates the patient's readiness to act on a new, healthier behavior. Numerous resources and guides for evaluating readiness are available on the Internet. Knowing the patient's stage of change is helpful, but it is only one element contribut-

Table 4. Benefits and costs of staying the same or changing

	Staying the Same: NOT wearing a compression garment	Changing: Wearing a compression garment
Benefits of:	• Easier than changing • Takes no effort • The ulcer may not heal	• Health could get better/not get worse • May help healing occur
Cost of:	• Same or more health complications • Negative QOL due to an unhealed ulcer (pain, odor, etc)	• I might feel uncomfortable • It might be warm • I could feel embarrassed

ing to why and how patients move through the change process. Patients change because their values support the change; they think the change is important; they believe they can change; they work through their ambivalence; they are ready; and they have a well structured plan with adequate support.[15]

What is OARS?

Open questions, Affirmation, Reflective listening, and Summary reflections (OARS)[16] are the basic interaction techniques that should be used when employing the MI approach.

Open-ended questions cannot be answered with a yes or no. Most conversations should start with an open-ended question; this invites the patient to speak openly. Some examples include the following:
- "So can you tell me about _____?"
- "What does that mean to you?"
- "What information do you have/need about that?"

Affirmations are the best and fastest ways of building rapport with a patient. They convey to the patient verbal support. Some examples of affirmations include the following:
- "Thanks for sharing that with me."
- "It seems like you know a lot about your condition."

Table 5. Decisional balance

Why should I change?

When we think about making changes in our lives, most of us do not really consider all aspects of the decision process. Instead, we often do what is immediately gratifying, or we avoid doing the things that we see as difficult or uncomfortable. Sometimes we are just so confused or overwhelmed that we give up thinking about it at all.

Thinking through the pros and cons of your choices is one way to help you be sure that you have fully considered all the possibilities. Take a look at the examples listed below.

	Continue Smoking	Quit
Pros	I like it Last vice I have Reward system/take a break Avoid discomfort Fun/cool Social norm (friends, family smoke) Wakes me up Stress relief/calms me down Linked to lifestyle	Freedom Better health/breathe easier Longer life Look better Save money Hair and clothes smell better Taste food better Family will be proud Set better example
Cons	Health consequences/life expectancy Smoking is expensive Smelly clothes, house, and car Causes wrinkles and yellow teeth Slave to nicotine Cannot smoke at work Habit is looked down upon Family worries about health Not setting good example	Withdrawal symptoms Physical or emotional discomfort Cravings Feeling deprived Quitting means I am "old" Weight gain concerns Affects friendships/social life Stress management difficulties Failed before

• "That is very insightful."

Reflective listening is a critical skill to acquire when using MI. Reflections are short summaries reflecting back what the patient has told you in a meaningful way. Consider some of the following examples:

   • "It sounds like you are…"
   • "It sounds like you are concerned about…"
   • "It sounds like you are ambivalent about…"

Reflections can be statements or questions. To elicit how difficult a component of the treatment plan has been for a patient, you might use one of the reflective listening techniques as either a question or a statement:

   • Question: "How difficult was that for you?"
   Statement: "That must have been difficult."

   • Question: "What did you do in the past regarding your _____ habits? What has worked?"
   Statement: "It sounds like you continue to try to make changes despite some setbacks."

Once you have built rapport with the patient and understand his or her current situation, you can continue to use questions to transition the conversation into taking action. Here are some examples of questions that you might use in your practice:

   • "So what options are you considering?"
   • "Where do we go from here?"
   • "What do you think has to change?"
   • "What strategies work best for you?"
   • "What are your dreams for the future?"

Table 5. Decisional balance *continued*

**Now try it yourself. Fill out the table below with your own responses.
You need to really think about this, so take your time.**

	Continue Smoking	Quit
Pros	_____ _____ _____	_____ _____ _____
Cons	_____ _____ _____	_____ _____ _____

So, out of all the pros and cons you have written, which are the most significant to you?

_____

_____

Are any of the reasons you have given for not changing more important than the reasons that you have given for changing? Why?

_____

_____

What would it mean for you to change now?

_____

_____

Imagine your ideal future. What are the discrepancies between your current behaviors and your vision of the future?

_____

_____

_____ 1. On a scale from 0–10 with 0 being not at all important and 10 being extremely important, how important is it for you to quit smoking?

_____ 2. On a scale from 0–10 with 0 being not at all confident and 10 being extremely confident, how confident are you that you could quit smoking?

© Courchene 2010
This is the original work of Courchene based on the concept of Decisional Balance Grid from Prochaska JO, Norcross JC, DiClemente CC. How you change. In: *Changing for Good.* New York: Avon Books; 1995.

At this point you can use all the information the patient has provided to work together and negotiate a plan you can both feel good about. You can address the patient's perception of his or her unhealthy behavior and provide more information regarding risk factors and consequences if you feel the patient is open to it. You can reiterate the positive change talk the patient volunteered earlier and discuss the rewards of making the change. Remember that resistance is part of the process and you must roll with resistance.

If the person is especially resistant, ask for permission to give information, such as, "I'd like to share some information with you…" or offer as a general suggestion, "Some people have found ____ to be helpful." Always reinforce that small steps are all that are necessary by asking questions, such as, "What is the first small step you want to take?"

Formulating a plan is the next step in the process. Table 6 provides an example of a plan template. You can find many other helpful goal setting documents on the Internet. The goal you work together to create should align with the patient's treatment plan and should be *SMART.* SMART stands for *Specific, Measurable, Attainable, Realistic,* and *Tangible/Time Framed.*

Summation is the final step in the MI process and should include a quick review of the patient's reason for change and reinforcement of his or her positive motivators. As the clinician, you should summarize the specific changes and reiterate how the plans relate to improving the patient's health. Finally, you should formally close the deal with a verbalized agreement. Ask a final question like, "Is this what you want to do?" If not, what is the patient willing to do? Commitment and accountability can be the missing pieces that finally compel the patient to take action.

Always remember that small steps toward change lead to small successes…

Which lead to confidence…

Which leads to self-efficacy…

Which leads to progress…

Which leads to rewards (health improvement and, for wound patients, prevention of a wound developing or that the wound heals)…

Which lead to sustainable, permanent changes…

That equates to positive, big results!

Adherence to Medication/Other Treatments

Patient-centered care is also reflected in excellent patient communication and good relationships with the interprofessional team. Osterberg and Blaschke reviewed the issue of adherence to treatment.[17] The term *adherence* is more patient-centered than compliance based on obeying a healthcare provider order. In chronic conditions (including chronic wounds), adherence rates are only 43%–73%.[18-20] Wound care patients often have multiple comorbidities and may require multiple medications for treatment of their underlying diseases. Indirectly, adherence can be measured by self-reporting or direct observation (eg, blood test of drug concentration/biological marker, pill count). Pill counts can be complicated by patients switching pill containers or discarding medication. Rates of prescription refills are another direct measure utilized by healthcare systems.

There are 6 patterns of medication taking:[21,22]
• Perfect adherence
• Nearly all doses taken, timing irregularities
• Miss the occasional daily doses, timing irregularities
• Drug holidays — 3–4 times per year occasional dose omissions
• Drug holidays — monthly or more often, frequent omitted doses
• Few or no doses often with appearance of good adherence

Patient Communication and Barriers to Adherence

Nonadherence to medication and treatment is often the greatest reason for treatment failure. It is important to be non-judgmental about missed treatments. The following statement is modified from Osterberg and Blaschke:[17] "I know it must be difficult to wear your support stockings regularly. How often do you miss wearing them?"

Several patient barriers include forgetfulness, other priorities, decisions to omit doses, and lack of information. Claxton and colleagues[20] determined that it is best to make prescribing regimes simple with once-daily treatment having higher adherence rates than multiple dosing regimens. Prescribing must be patient-centered, considering lifestyle, medication or treatment side effects,

Table 6. Wellness Plan for You

Step 1. Select a Behavior to Change

A. Behavior you wish to change:

 1._____

Step 2. Identify the Benefits of Changing this Behavior

A. The benefit(s) of the behavior change:

 1._____

 2._____

 3._____

Step 3. Identify Your Goals

A. List short-term goal(s):

 1._____

 2._____

 3._____

B. Long-term goal:

 1._____

Step 4. Take the Target Behavior Test

A. Target Behavior Test

1. Changing this specific behavior is important to me.	❑ Yes	❑ No
2. I am optimistic about my ability to successfully change this behavior with support.	❑ Yes	❑ No
3. I am likely to live in a healthier environment if I change this behavior.	❑ Yes	❑ No
4. If necessary, I am able and willing to spend the money to assist in changing this behavior.	❑ Yes	❑ No
5. I am willing to make time to change this behavior.	❑ Yes	❑ No
6. I have chosen a target behavior that I can measure, observe, and evaluate.	❑ Yes	❑ No
7. I have selected an achievable goal (eg, "I will exercise three times a week for 30 minutes each session" is probably a realistic goal. "I will lose 10 pounds each month" is an unrealistic goal and is unsafe).	❑ Yes	❑ No
8. I have or will obtain support from others to change this behavior.	❑ Yes	❑ No

Step 5. Identify Strategies for Accomplishing Your Goal

A. List any strategies for achieving your goal(s):

 1._____

 2._____

 3._____

B. List possible obstacles to achieving your goal(s) and solutions for overcoming those obstacles:

 1._____

 2._____

Table 6. Wellness Plan for You *continued*

Step 6. Determining Your Support System

A. Your support network will consist of?

    1. _____

    2. _____

    3. _____

B. Enlist the support of a few friends. Try using the following Behavior Change Contract.

Behavior Change Contract

I, _____, pledge to meet the following goal: _____

I will use the following tools to monitor my progress toward reaching my goal(s).

    1. _____

    2. _____

I sign this contract as an indication of my personal commitment to reach my goal. I have also recruited a helper who will witness my contract and support me throughout this process.

_____   _____

Your Signature   Date   Signature of Friend   Date

Step 7. Reward Yourself

A. List rewards for accomplishing your goal(s):

    1. _____

    2. _____

    3. _____

Step 8. Implement your Strategies and Record Your Progress

As a brief review for behavioral change:

    1. Consider the benefits of your behavior change (thoughts and feelings).
    2. Be clear and realistic about your goal(s).
    3. Use behavior change strategies that you believe will work for you.
    4. Plan to encounter and overcome obstacles—"go around," "over and under."
    5. Adapt your environment to support your lifestyle changes.
    6. Reward yourself for positive behavioral change.
    7. Enjoy yourself —balance work and play.

Step 9. Make Adjustments

If you realize that your success is not happening as you had planned, review your goal(s), barriers, and support system and then make appropriate adjustments. Remember, goals should be realistic and attainable to continually build success and self confidence.

_____

_____

_____

Source: National Wellness Institute. http://www.nationalwellness.org

and cost. A poor therapeutic relationship will decrease adherence. To test your therapeutic relationship with a patient, use the 4 E-components of the Keller and Carroll communication tool:[23]

- Engage
- Empathy
- Educate
- Enlist

Score one point for fulfilling the criteria and a half point for partial or suboptimal achievement of criteria. For engagement, do you know something about a patient/client other than the reason for the visit (eg, family wedding, birth, death)? Express true concern or empathy for the patient's condition — this should be different than sympathy. Determine patients' current beliefs or explanation for their illness as a needs assessment to educate them about their condition and its treatment. Did you negotiate a treatment that also considers their choices (coherence)? Did you actively enlist the patient to be part of the treatment process (pain diary, adherence chart for plantar pressure redistribution device, etc)? Most successful patient visits should have a score of 3 or 4 out of a possible 4 points.

Conclusion

Patient adherence to skin and wound care regimens can be challenging. Engaging and motivating the patient to change healthcare behaviors using motivational interviewing techniques can be effective. Open-ended questions provide the opportunity to learn what it will take to move the patient to embrace strategies that prevent or treat his or her skin problems and/or wounds.

Self-Assessment Questions

1. What factor(s) will increase patient adherence to treatment?
   A. A good therapeutic relationship with the clinician
   B. Easy accessibility to healthcare providers to answer questions
   C. Regularly scheduled follow-up appointments
   D. All of the above

2. Which one of the following is a component of motivational interviewing (MI)?
   A. Bargaining

Practice Pearls

Patient-centered care involves optimizing organizational and clinician communication to improve the therapeutic relationship, including adherence to treatment:

- Organizational communications: think **HEART** (**H**ear the story, **E**mpathize, **A**pologize, **R**espond to the problem, **T**hank them)
- Healthcare professional communication: **E**ngage, **E**mpathize, **E**ducate, and **E**nlist
- Make patients central to treatment decisions (choices) and give them an active part in the treatment program (eg, diary or monitoring function).

   B. Lecturing
   C. Affirmations
   D. Begging

3. Which of the following is an example of an open-ended question?
   A. Did you wear your compression stockings all the time?
   B. What is your hemoglobin A1C level?
   C. Have you ever had a pressure ulcer on your heel before?
   D. What information about having an instant contact cast do you need?

Answers: 1–D, 2–C, 3–D

References

1. American Hospital Association. Quality and patient safety. Available at: http://www.aha.org/advocacy-issues/quality/index.shtml. Accessed November 13, 2011.
2. Australian Commission on Safety and Quality in Health Care. Patient and consumer centred care. Available at: http://www.safetyandquality.gov.au/internet/safety/publishing.nsf/Content/PCCC. Accessed November 13, 2011.
3. Sibbald RG, Goodman L, Woo KY, et al. Special considerations in wound bed preparation 2011: an update©. Adv Skin Wound Care. 2011;24(9):415–436, quiz 437–438.
4. Picker Institute. Patient-centered care is quality care. Available at: http://pickerinstitute.org/patient-centered-care-is-quality-care/. Accessed November 13, 2011.
5. Safer Healthcare. What is SBAR and what is SBAR communication? Available at: http://www.saferhealthcare.com/sbar/what-is-sbar/. Accessed November 26, 2011.
6. Sibbald RG, Ayello EA. From the experts. SBAR for wound care communication: 20-second enablers for

practice. *Adv Skin Wound Care.* 2007;20(3):135–136.

7.   Perlin JB, Kolodner RM, Roswell RH. The Veterans Health Administration: Quality, value, accountability, and information as transforming strategies for patient-centered care. *Am J Manag Care.* 2004;10(part 2):828–836. Available at: http://www.ajmc.com/media/pdf/AJMCnovPrt2Perlin828to836.pdf. Accessed January 15, 2012.

8.   Silow-Carroll S, Alteras T, Stepnick L. *Patient-Centered Care for Underserved Populations: Definition and Best Practices.* Washington, DC: Economic and Social Research Institute; 2006.

9.   Rayner R. Effects of cigarette smoking on cutaneous wound healing. *Primary Intention.* 2006;14(3):100–102,104.

10.   Smith JB, Smith SB. Cutaneous manifestations of smoking. Available at: http://emedicine.medscape.com/article/1075039-overview. Accessed March 19, 2012.

11.   Tierney B, Fennessy F, Hayes DB. ABC of arterial and vascular disease. Secondary prevention of peripheral vascular disease. *BMJ.* 2000;320(7244):1262–1265.

12.   Miller WR, Rollnick S. *Motivational Interviewing. Preparing People for Change.* 2nd ed. New York: The Guilford Press; 2002.

13.   Motivational interviewing: preparing people to change health behaviors. Available at: http://www.yourhonor.com/dwi/motivation/MIapr07.pdf. Accessed December 27, 2011.

14.   Motivational interviewing: preparing people to change health behaviors. Tip sheet. Available at: http://www. yourhonor.com/dwi/motivation/tipsheet.pdf. Accessed December 27, 2011.

15.   Prochaska JO, Velicer WF. The transtheoretical model of health behavior change. *Am J Health Promot.* 1997;12(1):38–48.

16.   Rollnick S, Miller WR, Butler CC. *Motivational Interviewing in Health Care: Helping Patients Change Behavior.* New York: The Guilford Press; 2007.

17.   Osterberg L, Blaschke T. Adherence to medication. *N Engl J Med.* 2005;353(5):487–497.

18.   Cramer J, Rosenheck R, Kirk G, Krol W, Krystal J; VA Naltrexone Study Group 425. Medication compliance feedback and monitoring in a clinical trial: predictors and outcomes. *Value Health.* 2003;6(5):566–573.

19.   Waeber B, Leonetti G, Kolloch R, McInnes GT. Compliance with aspirin or placebo in the Hypertension Optimal Treatment (HOT) study. *J Hypertens.* 1999;17(7):1041–1045.

20.   Claxton AJ, Cramer J, Pierce C. A systematic review of the associations between dose regimens and medication compliance. *Clin Ther.* 2001;23(8):1296–1310.

21.   Urquhart J. The electronic medication event monitor. Lessons for pharmacotherapy. *Clin Pharmacokinet.* 1997;32(5):345–356.

22.   Urquhart J. The odds of the three nons when an aptly prescribed medicine isn't working: non-compliance, non-absorption, non-response. *Br J Clin Pharmacol.* 2002;54(2):212–220.

23.   Keller VF, Carroll JG. A new model for physician-patient communication. *Patient Educ Couns.* 1994;23(2):131–140.

Health-Related Quality of Life and Chronic Wounds: Evidence and Implications for Practice

Patricia Price, BA(Hons), PhD, AFBPsS, CPsychol, FHEA;
Diane L. Krasner, PhD, RN, CWCN, CWS, MAPWCA, FAAN

Objectives

The reader will be challenged to:

- Distinguish between the concepts of health-related quality of life (HRQoL) and life quality
- Discuss the benefits of HRQoL for clinical practice, research, and audit/quality improvement
- Identify the limitations associated with measuring HRQoL using generic and condition-specific tools, such as pain and wound assessment tools
- Value quality-of-life issues for people with wounds and incorporate this assessment into clinical practice.

Introduction

There is growing awareness that an individual's perspective on health and illness represents an important aspect of total healthcare. Increasingly, the person's experience plays a significant role in helping professionals adapt their care to the needs of the individual. Healthcare providers are increasingly formalizing the way in which this information is reported using *patient-reported outcome measures (PROMs)*.[1] These measures provide a way in which professionals can gain insight into how patients perceive their conditions and the impact their conditions have on the quality of their lives, as well as monitor the impact of different treatments on life quality. This information will help the clinicians of the future deliver individualized care that focuses not only on healing the wound, but also on optimizing the quality of life of the person with a wound and his or her circle of care.

There have been substantial changes in this field over the past 10–15 years as researchers and clinicians have worked together to build on earlier work that described patient experiences while living with acute or chronic wounds. This fundamental work has led to the increased availability of tools for use in research and clinical contexts that allow us to measure improvements in this area. For example, in the United States, the Centers for Medicare & Medicaid Services (CMS) now require that residents in long-term care facilities be interviewed about their quality of life as part of the Minimum Data Set (MDS) 3.0 regulatory process. Every facility is required to capture person-centered concerns on an ongoing basis and to connect them to the care planning process. Few clinicians

Price P, Krasner DL. Health-related quality of life and chronic wounds: evidence and implications for practice. In: Krasner DL, Rodeheaver GT, Sibbald RG, Woo KY, eds. *Chronic Wound Care: A Clinical Source Book for Healthcare Professionals*. Vol 1. 5th ed. Malvern, PA: HMP Communications; 2012:77–84.

would disagree that the presence of a wound has a great impact on the individual. This chapter will outline key considerations in defining **health-related quality of life** and using robust tools to measure this outcome and outline the importance of qualitative work in reviewing the life quality of patients with nonhealing wounds. We will provide examples of ways in which consideration for quality-of-life issues for the person with a wound and his or her circle of care can be built into routine clinical care.

What is Quality of Life?

The term *quality of life* first appeared in the United States in the 1950s as a slogan to represent "the good life" and was featured during the next decade in European political discussions. More recently, however, it has become part of a holistic view of the individual within healthcare systems. Quality of life is a broad concept that reflects an individual's perspective on the level of life satisfaction experienced in a variety of situations, including housing, recreation, and environmental conditions. In this way, it is a subjective measure that is affected by factors well beyond health status.

Consequently, most authors since the 1980s have restricted their definitions to **health-related quality of life (HRQoL)** outcomes, referring to the impact of health and illness on physical and social functioning and psychological well-being. In the 1990s, HRQoL assessments were further refined and aimed to capture data on both objective functioning and subjective well-being. This approach tackles the controversy over the relative importance of these two aspects of this concept while acknowledging the patient's experience of disease and treatment as a central component of healthcare and healthcare research.[2,3]

HRQoL is a complex multidimensional concept that reflects the total impact of health and illness on the individual. However, many studies infer improvements in HRQoL from change in a single clinical parameter, usually pain. While all those involved in wound care would acknowledge the profound impact pain can have on an individual, it is important to note that pain and HRQoL are not equivalent concepts. Just as a clinician will require information on a range of physiological parameters before making a diagnosis, so, too, is information on a range of dimensions needed before statements can be made about the HRQoL status of an individual.[4]

PROMs include a range of validated tools that are designed to measure either a person's perception of his or her general health or in relation to a specific disease or conditions (eg, pain, chronic wound). HRQoL tools come into this category: HRQoL is measured using robust, validated questionnaires where people rate their health in response to individual items. These tools may be a **generic measure** of HRQoL when the questions are related to general health, allowing for HRQoL comparisons to be made across a range of health states, or **condition-specific measures**, where tools have been developed to assess the impact of a particular condition or illness. Condition-specific tools are often more sensitive to change in a person's condition over time (eg, improvement toward healing) as the individual items included in the questionnaire have been developed from the experiences of people who have lived with that particular condition. However, **generic HRQoL tools** allow the health state of a person with a chronic wound to be compared with any other health state, for example, a person with a fractured femur — such comparative data can be important when planning resource allocation and the provision of services.

However, important qualitative approaches also are used to ensure that the rich data that emerges from this approach can capture the detail of the everyday life experiences of people with chronic wounds, such as the social stigma, guilt, and shame associated with living with a malignant wound.[5,6] Work in this area has shown that an improvement in daily life quality is an important health outcome that may, in the short term, affect a person's motivation to continue with treatment in the long term and so improve clinical outcomes.[7] Research into the life quality of people with wounds using qualitative approaches is just as important as quantitative research in informing our clinical practice so that wound care outcomes can be optimized.

Why Measure HRQoL?

Improved HRQoL for people has become increasingly recognized as an important outcome measure for a range of interventions and particularly important for people with chronic conditions or those receiving palliative care. The importance of the measure can be grouped under 3 headings: *clinical practice, research,* and *audit/quality improvement-quality assurance.*

Clinical practice. During routine clinical practice, healthcare professionals intuitively take into account life quality issues when making clinical decisions. Robust quality data in this area will help formalize some of these decisions. HRQoL data may be particularly relevant when expensive or hazardous options need to be considered for those patients not healing using conventional treatment. With the increasing costs associated with patient care, HRQoL may be a useful measure for allocating finances to patient care. There is, as yet, no "gold standard" to measure cost effectiveness or to analyze costs, but at some point in the development of appropriate formulae, the "human" cost needs to be considered. On the individual level, considerations about treatment options may be influenced by those aspects of living with a wound that have the greatest impact on the person, while at the population level, HRQoL data are generally considered as valid indicators of service needs and intervention outcomes.

Research. HRQoL data may prove to be useful as an additional outcome measure for research in wound care, as an alternative to "days to healing" (particularly for those patients where healing is not a realistic option), or as an additional measure of efficacy of the clinical treatment plan. In some areas, HRQoL has become an accepted endpoint in clinical trials, particularly when comparing treatments with similar or no impact on disease progression or survival.[8] The development of new therapies, particularly those using new technologies, should include HRQoL data: enormous amounts of time could be devoted to the development of a new technique only to find that it is not acceptable to patients (eg, because of side effects like burning or stinging).

Audit/quality improvement-quality assurance. HRQoL data may be extremely useful within audits or quality improvement or quality assurance programs to demonstrate effectiveness and as a means of measuring change. Certainly, the work within this area could eventually allow us to provide a patient-based view of the service and treatment provided. Measuring HRQoL can help identify the burden of disease and disabilities and help countries monitor health objectives (eg, iden-

tify subgroups with poor perceived health in order to guide service interventions).[9] HRQoL data may be particularly important for planning services for the elderly in an era when life expectancy is increasing, given the expectation for improving both the number and quality of life years despite the consequences of the normal aging process.[9]

Quality of Life and Pressure Ulcers

Compared to other wound types, there is limited empirical evidence for the impact of pressure ulcers on HRQoL, although a systematic review[10] in 2009 included 31 studies with 2,463 patients. These studies included 10 qualitative studies (described as "good quality" studies) on life quality and 21 quantitative studies (described as "poor quality" studies) across a range of patients, including frail elderly and those with spinal-cord injury. Collectively, these studies cover 11 key themes that cover a range of issues from physical restrictions, social isolation, the impact of wound symptoms, body image, and self-concept, as well as the importance of the relationship between the patient and the healthcare provider. The major issues raised related to *severe wound pain* and the concern that healthcare providers did not listen to patient concerns, particularly in relation to responding to early warning symptoms of deterioration.

The age range of patients included in this review and the range of conditions included make it difficult to assess whether the issues raised by those with spinal-cord injury are the same as those who are elderly. Many of those who develop pressure ulcers are elderly and frail with profound mobility problems and a wide range of additional concomitant disorders. Such patients are often unable to complete self-ratings of HRQoL due to impairment in cognitive functioning, so qualitative studies are more likely to capture the extent of their experiences, while high-quality, large scale studies using validated tools are still urgently needed.

While the sociological and psychological histories of the patient are deemed important aspects of patients' assessment, it is clear that the majority of work in this area focuses on symptom control (eg, pain at dressing change) or overall patient discomfort.[11,12] The need for detailed research work in this area is paramount, and clinicians and researchers must tackle and address the methodological difficulties inherent in conducting research in this area.

Clinical Application

Using HRQoL measures to drive the wound care plan of care. Many of the issues raised by those with pressure ulcers can be approached with good communication between the patient and healthcare provider. Activities, such as attentive listening, responding to the patient's needs for information, and reacting proactively to patient concerns, can help to build a strong relationship around managing wound symptoms in a way that the patient feels supported and a partner in his or her own care.

HRQoL measures that can drive the pressure ulcer plan of care include:

- *Attention to the person's pressure ulcer-related concerns/complaints, especially wound pain*
- *Timely assessment of changes in pressure ulcer status/deterioration*
- *Appreciation for the person's psychosocial concerns*
- *Attention to the individual's mobility problems and other comorbidities.*

Quality of Life and Diabetic Foot Ulceration

While the literature contains many references to the devastating effects of diabetic foot wounds for the person with diabetes, the literature specifically on HRQoL has taken longer to emerge. However, recent studies have shown that the emotional status of the person at the time when the first diabetic ulcer appears can have long-term consequences for the individual, as a 5-year follow-up study has shown a 2-fold increase in mortality for those with depressive symptoms at initial presentation.[13]

Research work using generic questionnaires to measure HRQoL have indicated that **people with diabetic foot ulcers have a significantly poorer quality of life** than those with diabetes but no foot ulcers. For example, in a cross-sectional study in Norway[14] with 127 adults with diabetic foot ulcers compared with 221 patients with diabetes but no ulcers and 5,903 controls from the general population, Ribu and colleagues demonstrated that those with foot ulcers had statistically significantly poorer HRQoL when measured using the Short Form 36 (SF-36) — with particular restrictions in physical functioning that limited their abilities in activities of daily living. These findings were confirmed in a longitudinal study from the same group who followed these patients for 1 year. HRQoL scores improved significantly for those patients whose ulcers went on to heal.[15] Data from Spain[16] also

support the finding that having a diabetic foot ulcer reduces HRQoL; a study of 258 people with diabetes but no foot ulceration compared with 163 people with diabetes-related foot ulcers indicated a statistically poorer HRQoL when an ulcer is present using the SF-36. The study also showed that **neuropathy, amputation history, and poor metabolic control were all associated with poorer quality of life**. Data from Brazil also indicate this pattern of poorer HRQoL in those with active ulceration, although the study showed no difference in self-esteem scores.[17]

The impact of wound healing on quality of life was confirmed by an American study (N = 253) that showed a 5- to 6-point deterioration in the mental component of the SF-36 for those whose diabetic foot ulcers did not heal over an 18-month period.[18] Similar patterns were observed in a Swedish study (N = 75) that showed mental health summary scores, social functioning, and limits on daily living through physical and emotional limitations were significantly higher in those who went on to heal over a 12-month period, again using SF-36.[19] However, a British multicenter study of 317 patients[20] with diabetic foot ulcers found no statistical differences between those who had healed ulcers and those with ongoing ulceration/withdrawn at either 12 or 24 weeks using the SF-36. The researchers were able to demonstrate a statistically significant difference in physical functioning and well-being in those who were healed at both 12 and 24 weeks and a difference also in social functioning at 24 weeks alone when a condition-specific tool, the *Cardiff Wound Impact Schedule* or *CWIS*, was used.

The CWIS has been shown to be a valid and reliable condition-specific tool for chronic wounds on the lower limb. This tool has been recommended as a research outcome measure when evaluated for use in people with diabetic foot ulcers.[21] This is just one of a number of condition-specific tools that can be used to assess HRQoL in this group. A review of all the available tools is outside the scope of this chapter, but those interested in finding out more about the range of tools available should refer to a systematic review by Hogg et al.[22]

Studies on the life quality of people with diabetic foot ulceration have emphasized that this is a life of fear, mainly of amputation but also infection, with wound pain being an underestimated problem in this group.[23,24] Qualitative studies have shown that the presence of a diabetic foot ulcer is "inconvenient" and "burdensome," with the fear of amputation precipitating anxiety and stress.[25] For people with diabetes, ongoing experiences of pain affected the ability to sleep and impacted mobility and social life. These people also described feelings of depression, isolation, and loss of independence.[26] Patients with unhealed ulcers were frustrated with healing and had anxiety about the wound, reported problems with a range of activities of daily living, had problems with footwear, and complained of a limited social life.[27] One qualitative study indicated that both the ulcer and the treatment for the ulcer restricted mobility and independence, leading to feelings of anger, fear, depression, helplessness, and boredom, and also showed that podiatrists were aware of the negative impact of ulceration on their patients' lives but felt they lacked the skills necessary to deal with their patients' emotional needs.[28]

Nearly 20 years ago, Williams[29] noted the severity of a situation in which we did not have quantitative information on the impact of foot disorders on quality-of-life dimensions and stated, "The lack of such information must rank as the most serious deficiency in our current knowledge of the impact of these disorders." Considerable steps were taken during that time to address the situation, with both qualitative data on life quality and quantitative data on HRQoL collected from a range of countries using a range of methods, all indicating the profound impact that diabetic foot ulceration has on patients. A greater understanding of these issues should help us tailor clinical practice to assist patients while they live with ulceration and work to adopt positive foot self-care as a preventive measure against further deterioration.

Clinical Application

Be aware of the potential for unrecognized pain in this group and consider the frustrations that patients may experience during the long road to healing and the lifetime of changes that will be needed to prevent recurrence. Using an holistic approach will help to pick up on the anxieties and stress that patients may feel and consider approaches, such as motivational interviewing, to assist in behavior change.[30]

HRQoL measures that can drive the diabetic foot ulcer plan of care include:

- *Attention to the person's diabetic foot ulcer-related concerns, including pain*
- *Empathy for the person's change in mobility and functioning (activities of daily living), sleep, and social functioning*
- *Appreciation of any signs and symptoms of anxiety, stress, or depression*
- *Assessment of concerns related to amputation and infection.*

Quality of Life and Chronic Leg Ulceration

There is probably more data on quality-of-life issues and patients with leg ulceration than any other wound type due to the qualitative and quantitative work undertaken in the early 1990s. A synthesis analysis[31] in 2007 included 12 qualitative studies from the United States, Australia, Sweden, and the United Kingdom that identified **5 common themes: physical effects of leg ulceration, describing the leg ulcer journey, patient-professional relationships, cost of a leg ulcer, and psychological impact**. Using software designed for the synthesis of qualitative research by the Joanna Briggs Institute,[32] the synthesis[31] clearly demonstrated that living with the physical symptoms associated with an open, chronic wound dominated the data from all 12 studies. These physical symptoms included pain, odor, itch, leakage, and infection. The synthesis also demonstrated how many patients had initially been guided by their own health beliefs and aided by family members before accepting that the wound was not a "simple scratch" and that professional help was needed. The relationship with the professional was described in both positive and negative ways. Positive themes associated with the relationship focused on therapeutic value, providing continuity of care, providing strategies to cope with a chronic condition, and — whenever possible — aiding patients in regaining control of their lives. The negative comments from the data included disputes between patients and their health professionals and patients being given conflicting advice. Across a number of studies (n = 8), patients perceived a lack of time, trust, empathy, and understanding — **patients felt they were not listened to, and dissatisfaction with treatment was highlighted**.

Although not all studies included in the synthesis[31] focused on psychological problems, many patients reported feelings of embarrassment associated with the leg ulcer, the negative impact on body image, fear of amputation, negative self-esteem, anger, depression (in some cases linked to suicidal thoughts), and a general sense of identity loss (as the wound dominated their lives).

The authors concluded that many professionals work to a code of practice whereby the *emphasis is on the route to healing*, with the assumption that a healed wound will improve quality of life. However, they also noted that aiming for healing may not be the most appropriate route for those with large, hard-to-heal wounds or those whose wound duration is extensive, as this may "initiate a spiral of hopelessness."

A more recent review that only included 8 qualitative studies[33] (focusing on venous leg ulceration) confirmed that *physical symptoms, especially pain, dominate everyday living with mobility, sleep disruption, exudate, and odor all causing significant problems.* The authors also commended qualitative studies for their ability to provide insight into the lives of people with chronic wounds.

Integrative reviews that included both qualitative and quantitative studies[34,35] looking at quality-of-life issues for people with venous leg ulceration also have concluded that the impact of living with a chronic ulcer is profound, with individuals reporting more pain, more restrictions on their physical and social lives, and poorer sense of well-being compared to controls. Together, these data suggest that regardless of methodology, theoretical philosophy, or study location, the findings are increasingly confirmative that the impact on people is extensive, and we, as health professionals, now have to investigate ways in which we can deliver care that addresses these concerns.

Two recent reviews focused on the different tools that have been used to conduct quantitative studies of HRQoL,[35,36] including both generic and condition-specific questionnaires. The reviews demonstrated that many researchers still question the relevance of using generic tools (those designed to be used with any health condition), as the resulting data make it difficult to attribute HRQoL scores to leg ulceration rather than any other comorbidity that may be present. Both reviews also described the growing number of condition-specific tools that are available and have been developed based on the experiences of

people with chronic wounds. These reviews concluded that many tools have been able to demonstrate acceptable levels of reliability, validity, and discrimination between healed and active ulceration. Some are available in several languages, and some are still in the early stages of development. Researchers have concluded that at this stage in the development of these relatively new tools, it may be wise to use both a generic and condition-specific tool in clinical trials.[37] HRQoL work with condition-specific tools may still be in its infancy, but we must endeavor to investigate the specific impact of wounds on the individual if we are to truly understand the condition from the perspective of the person. Those interested in finding out more about specific tools will find relevant details in these reviews.[35,36]

Clinical Application

The data strongly suggest that patients' experiences of living with wounds are dominated by symptom management, with all studies showing that the wound and its treatment have a profound effect on quality of life. Nurses predominate in the care of these patients, and where that relationship works well, the benefits to the patients are substantial. Unfortunately, not all relationships work so well, indicating a need for more training and education around quality-of-life issues as the patient's needs go far beyond the routine treatment of wounds. The data suggest that a holistic approach to assessment is important and that patients and professionals need to build relationships based on mutual trust and respect if the patient's overall experience is to improve.

HRQoL measures that can drive the venous ulcer plan of care include:

- *Attention to the person's venous ulcer-related concerns, including symptoms, body image changes, and other psychosocial concerns*
- *Appreciation for the person's change in mobility and functioning (activities of daily living), sleep, and social functioning*
- *Regular review of patient concerns through active listening.*

Conclusion

Formal HRQoL assessment in patients with chronic wounds is relatively new, with investigators using a range of methodologies and measures with this patient population. Many of the studies are cross-sectional in design and descriptive in nature, indicating that there is still a large amount of basic theoretical and empirical work yet to be completed despite the huge progress that has been made in recent years. Compared to trials in other patient populations (eg, cancers, AIDS, asthma), relatively few randomized, controlled, chronic wound trials have included HRQoL data, although some studies are now including such measures as secondary outcomes.[8] Yet, anyone who spends even a short amount of time with a frail elderly patient who is house-bound with large wounds on both legs cannot help but be moved to appreciate the impact of living with that condition on everyday life. Attention to and appreciation for a person's HRQoL concerns should drive the individual's wound care plan of care.

The challenge for the future is to ensure that we pay as much attention to HRQoL and life quality as we do to other important clinical parameters and start to build new ways of delivering care that ensure that we keep patients' well-being as our central focus. The data are now consistently showing us that the quality of life of patients with chronic wounds is very poor — regardless of where the study has been conducted, whether qualitative or quantitative approaches have been used, or the sector within which the healthcare was provided. We now need to go beyond describing the situation and consider ways in which we can work in partnership to ensure we provide optimal care and work for the best possible outcomes for people with wounds, including an improvement in their sense of well-being.[38]

Self-Assessment Questions

1. Why is assessing HRQoL important?
   A. Patients like to talk to us about their lives
   B. Government tells us to assess everything
   C. Clinical, research, audit/quality reasons exist that can lead to improved outcomes
   D. Clinicians do it routinely, so there is no need to assess HRQoL

2. What sort of tool would you use to assess HRQoL in a way that you could compare it for different groups of patients?
   A. Condition-specific tools
   B. Generic tools
   C. Qualitative methods
   D. Ask the clinician

3. If you wanted to find out more about the life quality of your patients, which approach would you take?
   A. Condition-specific tools
   B. Generic tools
   C. Qualitative methods
   D. Ask the clinician

Answers: 1–C, 2–B, 3–C

Practice Pearls

- HRQoL measures will help the clinicians of the future deliver individualized care that focuses not only on healing the wound but also on optimizing the quality of life of the person with a wound and his or her circle of care.
- HRQoL is a complex multidimensional concept that reflects the total impact of health and illness on the individual.
- HRQoL measures should help guide clinical practice, research, and audit/quality improvement-quality assurance initiatives.
- HRQoL data suggest that a holistic approach to assessment is important and that patients and professionals need to build relationships based on mutual trust and respect if the patient's overall experience is to improve.

References

1. Dawson J, Doll H, Fitzpatrick R, Jenkinson C, Carr AJ. The routine use of patient reported outcome measures in healthcare settings. *BMJ*. 2010;340:c186.
2. Muldoon MF, Barger SD, Flory JD, Manuck SB. What are quality of life measurements measuring? *BMJ*. 1998;316(7130):542–545.
3. Gandek B, Sinclair SJ, Kosinski M, Ware JE Jr. Psychometric evaluation of the SF-36 health survey in Medicare managed care. *Health Care Financ Rev*. 2004;25(4):5–25.
4. Price P. An holistic approach to wound pain in patients with chronic wounds. *WOUNDS*. 2005;17(3):55–57.
5. Dolbeault S, Flahault C, Baffie A, Fromantin I. Psychological profile of patients with neglected malignant wounds: a qualitative exploratory study. *J Wound Care*. 2010;19(12):513–521.
6. Piggin C, Jones V. Malignant fungating wounds: an analysis of the lived experience. *J Wound Care*. 2009;18(2):57–64.
7. Speight J, Reaney MD, Barnard KD. Not all roads lead to Rome — a review of quality of life measurement in adults with diabetes. *Diabet Med*. 2009;26(4):315–327.
8. Gottrup F, Apelqvist J, Price P; European Wound Man-

agement Association Patient Outcome Group. Outcomes in controlled and comparative studies on non-healing wounds: recommendations to improve the quality of evidence in wound management. *J Wound Care.* 2010;19(6):237–268.

9. Centers for Disease Control and Prevention. Health-Related Quality of Life (HRQOL). Available at: http://www.cdc.gov/hrqol/concept.htm. Accessed January 3, 2012.

10. Gorecki C, Brown JM, Nelson EA, et al; European Quality of Life Pressure Ulcer Project group. Impact of pressure ulcers on quality of life in older patients: a systematic review. *J Am Geriatr Soc.* 2009;57(7):1175–1183.

11. Benbow M. Quality of life and pressure ulcers. *J Community Nursing.* 2009;23(12):14–18.

12. Rastinehad D. Pressure ulcer pain. *J Wound Ostomy Continence Nurs.* 2006;33(3):252–257.

13. Winkley K, Sallis H, Kariyawasam D, et al. Five-year follow-up of a cohort of people with their first diabetic foot ulcer: the persistent effect of depression on mortality. *Diabetologia.* 2012;55(2):303–310.

14. Ribu L, Hanestad BR, Moum T, Birkeland K, Rustoen T. A comparison of the health-related quality of life in patients with diabetic foot ulcers, with a diabetes group and a nondiabetes group from the general population. *Qual Life Res.* 2007;16(2):179–189.

15. Ribu L, Birkeland K, Hanestad BR, Moum T, Rustoen T. A longitudinal study of patients with diabetes and foot ulcers and their health-related quality of life: wound healing and quality-of-life changes. *J Diabetes Complications.* 2008;22(6):400–407.

16. Garcia-Morales E, Lázaro-Martínez JL, Martínez-Hernández D, Aragón-Sánchez J, Beneit-Montesinos JV, Gonzàlez-Jurado MA. Impact of diabetic foot related complications on the Health Related Quality of life (HRQol) of patients — a regional study in Spain. *Int J Low Extrem Wounds.* 2011;10(1):6–11.

17. de Meneses LC, Blanes L, Francescato Veiga D, Carvalho Gomes H, Masako Ferreira L. Health-related quality of life and self-esteem in patients with diabetic foot ulcers: results of a cross-sectional comparative study. *Ostomy Wound Manage.* 2011;57(3):36–43.

18. Winkley K, Stahl D, Chalder T, Edmonds ME, Ismail K. Quality of life in people with their first diabetic foot ulcer: a prospective cohort study. *J Am Podiatr Med Assoc.* 2009;99(5):406–414.

19. Löndahl M, Landin-Olsson M, Katzman P. Hyperbaric oxygen therapy improves health-related quality of life in patients with diabetes and chronic foot ulcer. *Diabet Med.* 2011;28(2):186–190.

20. Jeffcoate WJ, Price PE, Phillips CJ, et al. Randomised controlled trial of the use of three dressing preparations in the management of chronic ulceration of the foot in diabetes. *Health Technol Assess.* 2009;13(54):1–86.

21. Jaksa PJ, Mahoney JL. Quality of life in patients with diabetic foot ulcers: validation of the Cardiff Wound

Impact Schedule in a Canadian population. *Int Wound J.* 2010;7(6):502–507.

22. Hogg FRA, Peach G, Price P, Thompson MM, Hinchliffe RJ. Measures of health-related quality of life in diabetes-related foot disease: a systematic review. *Diabetologica.* 2012;55(3):552–565.

23. Ribu L, Rustoen T, Birkeland K, Hanestad BR, Paul SM, Miaskowski C. The prevalence and occurrence of diabetic foot ulcer pain and its impact on health-related quality of life. *J Pain.* 2006;7(4):290–299.

24. Bengtsson L, Jonsson M, Apelqvist J. Wound-related pain is underestimated in patients with diabetic foot ulcers. *J Wound Care.* 2008;17(10):433–435.

25. Watson-Miller S. Living with a diabetic foot ulcer: a phenomenological study. *J Clin Nurs.* 2006;15(10):1336–1337.

26. Bradbury S, Price PE. Diabetic foot ulcer pain (part 2): the hidden burden. *EWMA J.* 2011;11(2):25–37.

27. Goodridge D, Trepman E, Sloan J, et al. Quality of life of adults with unhealed and healed diabetic foot ulcers. *Foot Ankle Int.* 2004;27(4):274–280.

28. Searle A, Campbell R, Tallon D, Fitzgerald A, Vedhera K. A qualitative approach to understanding the experience of ulceration and healing in the diabetic foot: patient and podiatrist perspectives. *WOUNDS.* 2005;17(1):16–26.

29. Williams DRR. The size of the problem: epidemiological and economic aspects of foot problems in diabetes. In: Boulton AJ, Connor H, eds. *The Foot in Diabetes.* 2nd ed. Chichester, UK: Wiley & Sons; 1994.

30. Gabbay RA, Kaul S, Ulbrecht J, Scheffler NM, Armstrong DG. Motivational interviewing by podiatric physicians: a method for improving patient self-care of the diabetic foot. *J Am Podiatr Med Assoc.* 2011;101(1):78–84.

31. Briggs M, Flemming K. Living with leg ulceration: a synthesis of qualitative research. *J Adv Nurs.* 2007;59(4):319–328.

32. Pearson A. Balancing the evidence: incorporating the synthesis of qualitative data into systematic reviews. *JBI Reports.* 2004;2(2):45–64.

33. Green J, Jester R. Health-related quality of life and chronic venous leg ulceration: part 1. *Br J Community Nurs.* 2009;14(12):S12–S17.

34. Herber OR, Schnepp W, Rieger MA. A systematic review on the impact of leg ulceration on patients' quality of life. *Health Qual Life Outcomes.* 2007;5:44.

35. González-Consuegra RV, Verdú J. Quality of life in people with venous leg ulcers: an integrative review. *J Adv Nurs.* 2011;67(5):926–944.

36. Green J, Jester R. Health-related quality of life and chronic venous leg ulceration: part 2. *Br J Community Nurs.* 2010;15(3):S4–S14.

37. Palfreyman S. Assessing the impact of venous ulceration on quality of life. *Nurs Times.* 2008;104(41):34–37.

38. Gray D, Boyd J, Carville K, et al. Effective wound management and wellbeing: guidance for clinicians, organizations and industry. *Wounds UK.* 2011;7(1):86–90.

Pain in People with Chronic Wounds: Clinical Strategies for Decreasing Pain and Improving Quality of Life

Kevin Y. Woo, PhD, RN, FAPWCA;

Diane L. Krasner, PhD, RN, CWCN, CWS, MAPWCA, FAAN;

R. Gary Sibbald, BSc, MD, FRCPC(Med, Derm), MACP, FAAD, MEd, MAPWCA

Objectives

The reader will be challenged to:

- Synthesize the complexity and pathophysiology of wound-associated pain
- Describe a systematized approach to address wound pain by examining the wound-related factors, procedure-related triggers, and modulating factors (cognitive, emotional, personal, sensory, and contextual)
- Identify methods to evaluate pain
- Appraise various pharmacological and non-pharmacological strategies to reduce pain.

Introduction

Pain is a common experience in people with chronic wounds. Pain impacts all aspects of everyday life, including physical activity, sleep, and social functioning, and erodes individuals' quality of life.[1-3] Even long after the ulcers are healed, some people continue to provide vivid descriptions of the pain experiences.[4] While wound-associated pain often is caused by intrinsic wound pathology and exacerbated by local manipulation that is part of routine wound management, the intensity of pain is subjected to influences of many personal and social factors. The complexity of pain necessitates a systematized approach to obtain a thorough pain history, evaluate aggravating and alleviating factors, assess the wound and surrounding tissue, and monitor outcomes. Optimal pain management must be incorporated as an integral part of comprehensive wound care/caring in order to improve quality of life.

Prevalence of Pain in People with Chronic Wounds

Studies of patients with various chronic wound types validate the enormity and pervasiveness of pain. Szor and Bourguignon[5] reported that as many as 88% of people with pressure ulcers in their study expressed pressure ulcer pain at dressing change and 84% experienced pain even at rest. Of people with venous leg ulcers, the majority experienced moderate to severe levels of pain described as aching, stabbing, sharp, tender, and tiring.[6] Pain has been documented

Woo KY, Krasner DL, Sibbald RG. Pain in people with chronic wounds: clinical strategies for decreasing pain and improving quality of life. In: Krasner DL, Rodeheaver GT, Sibbald RG, Woo KY, eds. *Chronic Wound Care: A Clinical Source Book for Healthcare Professionals*. Vol 1. 5th ed. Malvern, PA: HMP Communications; 2012:85–96.

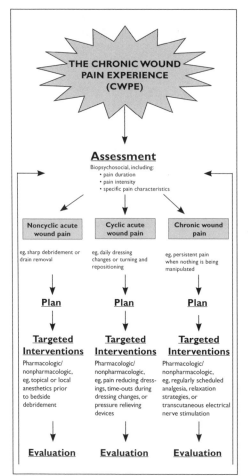

Figure 1. Proposed model of the chronic wound pain experience (CWPE). © 1995 Krasner.

jor stressor among people with chronic wounds.[3] Stress-induced cytokine and neuroendocrine activity can activate sympathetic outflow, leading to vasoconstriction and subsequent compromised tissue oxygenation levels.[2] As part of the cascade of stress response, the overproduction of cortisol and catecholamines can have a significant impact, delaying wound healing due to alteration in the immune system.[9] Numerous studies have validated the deleterious impact of stress (and emotional distress) on wound healing.[9] Time to achieve complete wound closure is significantly prolonged for high-stress individuals. Woo and Sibbald[10] followed 111 home care clients with either leg or foot ulcers prospectively for 4 weeks to determine the effectiveness of comprehensive wound assessment and management. Wound-related pain was addressed by education, careful selection of wound dressings, application of topical analgesics during dressing changes, and use of systemic analgesics. The average pain intensity score was reduced from 6.3 at baseline to 2.8 at Week 4 ($P < .001$). To examine the relationship between pain and wound healing, pain intensity scores were compared among those who achieved wound closure by the end of data collection to those who did not. The mean pain intensity score was 1.67 for subjects who achieved wound closure as compared to an average score of 3.21 among those who did not achieve complete wound closure ($P < .041$). The result lends credence to the importance of pain management to promote wound healing.

Conceptualizations of Wound-Related Pain

According to a conceptual framework developed by Krasner,[11] wound-related pain is complex and dynamic, integrating the experience of noncyclic acute wound pain, cyclic acute wound pain, and chronic wound pain (Figure 1).

Chronic or persistent wound pain is described as the background symptom that is often associated with intrinsic wound-related factors often connected with the cause or aggravating factors of the wound. In contrast, acute wound pain (cyclic due to dressing change procedures and non-cyclic often associated with debridement) is conceptualized as episodic and triggered by wound-related procedures that are performed by healthcare providers (Figure 1).

to persist up to at least 3 months after wound closure.[6,7] Contrary to the commonly held belief that most patients with diabetic foot ulcers do not experience pain due to loss of protective sensation, up to 50% of patients experience varying degrees of predominantly neuropathic spontaneous painful symptoms at rest and approximately 40% experience moderate to extreme pain climbing stairs or walking on uneven surfaces, according to Evans and Pinzur.[8]

Consequences of Wound-Associated Pain

Pain has been described as the worst part of living with chronic wounds and constitutes a ma-

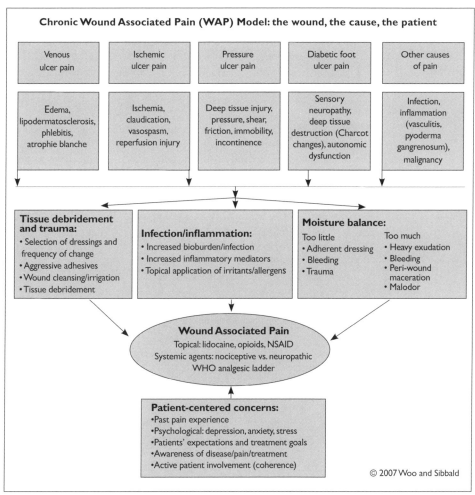

Figure 2. Chronic wound-associated pain model.

Another conceptualization proposed by Woo and Sibbald[12] provides further detail, linking various wound etiological causes, local wound factors, and patient-centered concerns to wound-associated pain (Figure 2).

Mechanisms of Wound-Related Pain

Wound-related triggers. Underlying mechanisms that lead to tissue breakdown also are implicated in the emergence of painful symptoms. According to Woo and Sibbald,[12] pressure ulcer pain stems from ischemic damages due to unrelieved pressure, shear, and friction. Proinflammatory mediators, such as bradykinin, histamine, serotonin, and prostaglandins, are released,

rendering peripheral nociceptors to be hyperactive. Venous ulcer pain is linked to venous abnormalities, including local leakage of fibrin that can become inflamed, precipitating acute lipodermatosclerosis; inflammation of the venous vessel wall and clotting, leading to thrombophlebitis; and venous hypertension with edema from leaky capillaries. Even in the absence of an ulcer, pain has been found in up to 43% of people with lipodermatosclerosis (due to acute inflammation of the dermal tissue).[13] Intermittent claudication (pain in the lower extremities that is precipitated by exercise) is a common yet extremely painful condition in people with peripheral arterial vascular disease. As arterial insufficiency progresses, ischemia rest pain may predominate.[14] Among persons with diabetes and coexisting neuropathy, spontaneous pain is thought to be caused by nerve damage (often accompanied with reddened and mottled skin, abnormal sensation to touch, and feelings of burning and electrical shocks) as a result of microvascular (vasa nervorum) and metabolic aberrations.[15]

Changes to the usual pattern of wound-associated pain can be a warning signal. The consensus among clinical experts is that the presence of unexpected pain/tenderness along with other criteria is indicative of infection in chronic wounds.[16,17] According to study results reported by Gardner et al,[18] pain as an indicator of infection has a specificity value of 100%; subjects did not experience any painful symptoms if wound infection was not detected based on bacteriology assessment. As a word of caution, there were only 31 subjects in this evaluation. The mechanism that explains how pain is connected to infection remains elusive. It may potentially involve *Toll-like receptors (TLRs)*, a family of pattern recognition receptors that mediate innate immune responses from pathogens or endogenous signals.[3] Following repeated insult, excessive and prolonged inflammation can lead to spontaneous "wind-up" pain or exaggerated or prolonged painful responses to normally painful stimuli (*hyperalgesia*) and even non-painful stimuli (*allodynia*).[19] The wind-up mechanism is complex, involving the remodelling of synaptic contacts between the neurons in the spinal dorsal horn circuitry (neuronal plasticity) and the increased activity of inflammatory substance P and glutamate on receptors for neurokinin 1 (NK1) and N-methyl-D-aspartic acid (NMDA).[20] Several types of exquisitely painful inflammatory skin lesions (eg, pyoderma gangrenosum, cutaneous vasculitis) are caused by sustained inflammatory response associated with autoimmune dysfunction. *Wound-associated pain may extend beyond the wound margins to periwound skin.* Unprotected skin in periwound regions is susceptible to irritation by enzyme-rich wound fluid. In a crossover, randomized, controlled trial,[21] patients with wound margin maceration and skin damage were prone to experience increased pain.

Practice tips to reduce wound-associated pain include the following:
• Identify and correct the wound cause
• Treat infection and inflammation
• Protect periwound skin from wound fluid.

Procedure-related triggers. Despite obvious therapeutic values and primary intentions to optimize wound healing, many wound management procedures are painful. Most obvious, debridement using a sharp surgical instrument can cause a considerable amount of pain.[22] A toolkit of various analgesic agents (topical or systemic), alternative debridement methods, and emerging technologies should be considered to minimize discomfort. Next to debridement, dressing removal has been documented to cause pain in several observational studies.[3] It has also been noticed that dressing materials often adhere to the fragile wound surface due to the glue-like nature of dehydrated or crusted exudate. Each time the dressing is removed, potential local trauma may evoke pain. In addition, the granulation tissue and capillary loops may grow into the product matrix — especially gauze dressings and with the use of negative pressure wound therapies — potentiating the likelihood of trauma and bleeding with dressing removal. According to a review of dressings and topical agents for secondary intention healing of post-surgical wounds, patients experienced significantly more pain with gauze than with other types of dressings.[23] *Wound care providers practicing evidence-based wound care should avoid the use of gauze products in painful wounds.* To ensure dressing securement, strong dressing adhesives or tapes are often used. However, repeated application and removal of adhesive tapes and dressings strip the stratum corneum from the skin epithelial cell surface, damaging the skin. In severe cases, contact irritant dermatitis results in local erythema, edema, and blistering of the wound margins.[24]

Next to dressing removal, *wound cleansing also is likely to cause pain* during dressing changes. In one study,[25] Woo asked 96 patients with chronic wounds to rate their levels of pain before dressing changes, at dressing removal, at wound cleansing, and after dressing reapplication. Wound cleansing was rated as most painful, indicating that *the routine practice of using abrasive materials and gauze to scrub the wound surface should be discouraged*. Clinicians must be mindful of the fact that pain can be caused by pressure-relieving equipment and treatment-

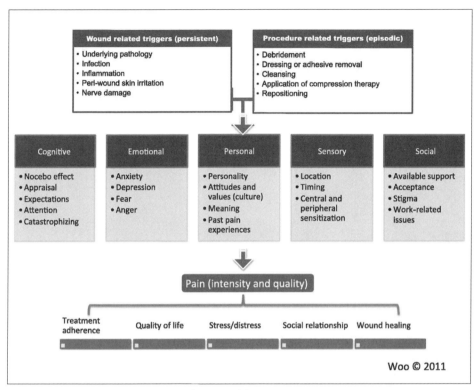

Figure 3. Integrated wound-associated pain model.

related activities, such as repositioning, especially among patients who have significant contractures, increased muscle spasticity, and spasms. Some patients consider compression therapy treatment of venous stasis to be uncomfortable. Briggs and Closs[26] indicated that only 56% of patients in their study were able to tolerate full compression bandaging, with pain being the most common reason for nonadherence. *Elastic compression systems exert high pressure at rest and may not be tolerated until adequate pain control has been achieved.* Nonelastic systems exert their main effect with high pressure only with muscle contraction (during movement), and they may be tolerated at rest where there is a lower pressure against a fixed resistance.

Practical tips for procedural pain include the following:
- Use atraumatic dressings
- Avoid frequent removal or the use of strong adhesives (consider silicone adhesive alternatives)
- Avoid aggressive scrubbing of the wound base
- Provide information and support for patients and their circle of care.

Pain and its Dimensions

Pain is a complex biopsychosocial phenomenon. Melzack[27] introduced the term **neuromatrix** to connote the intricate interactions among a number of modulating factors. Despite seemingly comparable levels of pain intensity, persons with pain experience varying degrees of physical limitations, emotional distress, and suffering. The integrated wound-associated pain model in Figure 3 posits the multidimensionality of pain in response to wound- and procedure-related triggers. Understanding that emotions, cognitive process, social environment, and attitudes can influence how people feel, the various separate dimensions are created merely for heuristic purpose.

For instance, **nocebo effect** or **negative placebo effect** delineates pain amplification by expectation of pain and heightened anxiety. Colloca and Benedetti[28] identified cholecystokinin (CCK) as a physiological mediator that augments nocebo hyperalgesia. Neuroimaging studies revealed that the link between anxiety and hyperalgesia may be located in the central nervous system (entorhinal area of the hippocampal formation, anterior cingulate cortex, amygdala, and insula).[29] The result is a vicious cycle of pain, stress/anxiety, and worsening of pain. In a study of 96 patients with chronic wounds, Woo[25] reported that patients who experienced high levels of anxiety also reported high levels of anticipatory pain, leading to high levels of pain at dressing change. Certain personalities may be more vulnerable to noxious stimuli in light of their propensity to experience anxiety and catastrophize their experience. *Comprehensive wound pain management should incorporate an assessment of the person's anxiety level, stress, expectation, and social environment.*

How to Assess Pain

Pain assessments should be well documented to facilitate the continuity of patient care and to benchmark the effectiveness of management strategies. Many methods of pain assessment have been developed, ranging from subjective self-reports to objective behavioral checklists. Pain is a subjective experience. An individual's self-report of pain is the most reliable method to evaluate pain. Other assessment methodologies include physiological indicators, behavioral manifestations, functional assessments, and diagnostic tests. Categorical scales, numerical rating scales, pain thermometers, visual analogue scales, faces scales, and verbal categorical scales are one-dimensional tools commonly used to quantify pain in terms of intensity, quality (characteristics), pain unpleasantness, and pain relief.[30] To obtain a comprehensive assessment of pain, multidimensional measurements are available to evaluate the many facets of pain and its impact on daily functioning, mood, social functioning, and other aspects of quality of life. The key questions to ask about pain can be remembered by *PQRSTU*:[31,32]

- **P — Provoking and palliating factors:** What makes your pain worse? What makes your pain better (eg, warm weather, walking, certain types of cleansing solutions or dressings)?

- **Q — Quality of pain:** What does your pain feel like? Descriptors (eg, burning, electrical shocks, pricking, tingling pins) may help to differentiate the 2 types of pain: nociceptive and neuropathic.

- **R — Regions and radiation:** Where is the pain and does the pain move anywhere (eg, in and around the wound, the wound region, unrelated)?

- **S — Severity or intensity:** How much does it hurt on a scale of 0–10 with 0 representing no pain and 10 representing pain as bad as it could possibly be?

- **T — Timing or history:** When did the pain start? Is it present all the time? A pain diary may help to map out the temporal pattern of pain, eg, the pain worsens at night.

- **U — Understanding:** What is important to you for pain relief? How would you like to get better?

As an alternative, studies have shown that the observation of nonverbal indicators encompassing a wide range of vocalized signals and bodily movements may provide a means of assessing pain in patients (eg, neonates or cognitively impaired) who are not able to verbalize their pain. Several tools are available, including the following:

- Abbey Pain Scale Assessment of Discomfort in Dementia (ADD) Protocol
- Checklist of Nonverbal Pain Indicators (CNPI)
- Discomfort Scale-Dementia of the Alzheimer's Type (DS-DAT)
- Face, Legs, Activity, Cry, and Consolability (FLACC) Pain Assessment Tool
- Pain Assessment in Advanced Dementia (PAINAD) Scale
- Pain Assessment Scale for Seniors with Severe Dementia (PACSLAC)

Despite the robust psychometric properties of these measurement tools, it is important to remember behaviors (eg, facial expression, body movements, crying) that signal pain may vary significantly among individuals, and there is no evidence that any single behavior or number of behaviors is more reliable to measure the presence or intensity of pain.[30,33] Pain measurement tools may include word descriptors to qualify pain and allow clinicians to differentiate *nociceptive* from *neuropathic pain.* Nociceptive pain is incurred by

Table 1. Patient-oriented and multifaceted approach to pain management

Strategy	Objectives

Education	• Web-based learning
	• Face-to-face education:
	  o Explain mechanism of pain
	  o Dispel misconceptions about pain
	  o Address concerns about addiction
	  o Emphasize the availability of multiple strategies

Pharmacological	• Topical:
	  o Topical ibuprofen (dressing not available in the United States)
	  o Morphine
	  o Topical lidocaine
	• Systemic:
	  o Nociceptive pain: ASA, NSAIDs, acetaminophen for mild to moderate pain
	  o Opioids for moderate to intense pain
	  o Neuropathic pain: SNRI, anticonvulsants

Local Wound Care	• Atraumatic interface (silicone) • Sequester: remove inflammatory mediators • Protect periwound skin • Treat infections
Physical Therapies	• Heat/cold compress • Massage • Exercise
Anxiety Reduction	• Relaxation • Imagery • Distractions • Education • Music therapy • Support groups
Cognitive Therapy	• Cognitive behavior therapy • Problem-solving skills • Positive thinking
Therapeutic Alliance	• Communication techniques, eg, reflective listening • Goal setting • Align expectations • Demonstrate sympathy
Empowerment	• Allow individual to call "time out" • Respect individual's choices • Maximize autonomy: active participation • Functional focused therapy

© Woo 2011

tissue damage stimulating pain receptors in the muscle, bone, joints, and ligaments (somatic pain) or in the viscera and peritoneum (visceral pain). Nociceptive pain is often described as sharp, dull, aching, throbbing, or gnawing. In contrast, neuropathic pain is caused by injury and sensitization of the peripheral or central nervous system. Neuropathic pain is mostly described as burning, electrical shocks, pricking, tingling pins, and in-creased sensitivity to touch. Specific assessment protocols are developed to evaluate neuropathic pain.[34] All in all, no one tool has been deemed universal and useful for all patients. The selection of a specific pain scale must take into account the patient's age, language, educational level, sensory impairment, developmental stage, and cognitive status. *Once chosen, the same measurement scale should be used for subsequent assessments for on-*

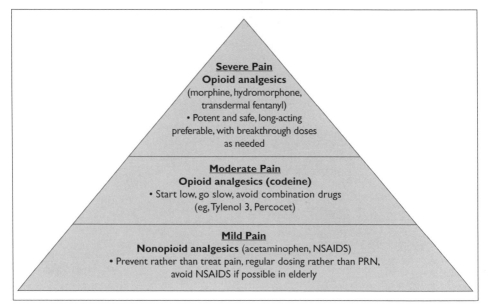

Figure 4. The World Health Organization (WHO) Analgesic Ladder.

Table 2. Neuropathic pain		
Type	**Symptom**	**Treatment**
Nerve irritation	Burning/stinging	Tricyclics — amitriptyline, nortriptyline, etc
Nerve damage	Shooting/stabbing	Anti-epileptics — gabapentin, carbamazepine

going comparison. Changes in pain levels may indicate a need to reassess the choice and timing of analgesics and/or other interventions used in pain management.

How to Manage Wound-Associated Pain

A patient-oriented and multifaceted approach (Table 1) is recommended for the management of wound-associated pain with the objectives to address pain relief, increase function, and restore overall quality of life. Pharmacotherapy continues to be the mainstay for pain management. Appropriate agents are selected based on severity and specific types of pain. The World Health Organization's analgesic ladder[35] proposes that treatment of mild (1–4 out of 10) to moderate (5–6 out of 10) nociceptive pain should begin with a non-opioid medication, such as acetaminophen and nonsteroidal anti-inflammatory drugs (Figure 4 and Table 2).

For controlling more severe (7–10 out of 10) and refractory pain, opioid analgesics should be considered. Management of neuropathic pain or associated symptoms (eg, anxiety and depression) may include the possibility of adding adjuvant treatments. Three classes of medications are recommended as first-line treatments for neuropathic pain (Table 3): antidepressants with both norepinephrine and serotonin reuptake inhibition (TCAs and selective serotonin and norepinephrine reuptake inhibitors [SSNRIs]), calcium channel $\alpha_2\delta$ ligands (gabapentin and pregabalin), and topical lidocaine (lidocaine patch 5%).[19] In addition to the severity and pain types, selection of appropriate pharmaceuticals should always take into account the characteristics of the drug (onset, duration, available routes of administration, dosing intervals, side effects) (Table 3) and individual factors (age, coexisting diseases, and other over-the-counter or herbal medications).[19]

Table 3. Analgesics: mode of action, dosage, and side effects

Medication	Mode of Action	Dosage	Side Effects
Non-Opioid			
Acetaminophen	Affects nitric oxide cycle, antipyretic property	325–650 mg q 4 h up to a maximum of 4 g/d in healthy people	Do not exceed 4 g/d to avoid liver toxicity
Acetylsalicylic acid (ASA)	Inhibits the enzyme cyclooxygenase (COX)	325–650 mg q 4–6 h up to 4 g/d	Gastritis, gastrointestinal bleeding, acute renal failure, may interact with anticoagulants
NSAIDs and COX-2 selective NSAIDs	Inhibit COX	Common NSAIDs: Ibuprofen 200–400 mg q 4–6 h Ketoprofen 25–50 mg q 6–8 h Naproxen 250 mg q 6 h Common COX-2 NSAIDs: Celecoxib 200–400 mg od Rofecoxib 25–50 mg od Meloxicam 7.5–15 mg od	Similar as ASA, less side effects with COX-2 NSAIDs
Co-analgesic (Adjuvant)			
Tricyclic antidepressant (TCA)	Inhibit serotonin and NE reuptake; block sodium channels	Common TCAs: Amitriptyline, doxepin, nortriptyline 10–25 mg q hs titrate up to 150–200 mg/d	Dry mouth, drowsiness, orthostatic hypotension
Anticonvulsants	Most agents block sodium channels; unknown for gabapentin	Common anticonvulsants: Carbamazepine 100 mg od to maximum dose 1200 mg/d, gabapentin 100 mg TID titrate up to 3000 mg/d	Drowsiness, dizziness, fatigue
Opioids (CR/SR)			
Morphine	Gold standard mu agonist	For patients who are opioid naive, start on morphine 2.5–10 mg po q 4 h with 10% of total daily dose (TDD) q 1 h as needed	Constipation, delirium, sedation, nausea, vomiting, urinary retention
Codeine	Weak mu agonist; 0.125 as potent as morphine; convert to active analgesic by enzyme CYP2D6	Codeine 100 mg = morphine 10 mg (~10:1)	
Oxycodone (may be combined with ASA or acetaminophen)	Mu and kappa agonist; 2x as potent as morphine	Oxycodone 5 mg or Percocet 1 tab (5/325) = morphine 10 mg (1:2)	
Hydromorphone	5–7.5x as potent as morphine	Hydromorphone 2 mg = morphine 10 mg (1:5)	
Methadone	Mu and delta agonist; blocks NMDA; 10x more potent than morphine	Variable	

©Woo 2011
Legend: h = hour; d = day; q = every; od = daily; hs = evening; TID = 3 times a day; NSAID = nonsteroidal anti-inflammatory drug; NE = norepinephrine; po = by mouth

How to Use Analgesics

As a general rule of thumb, analgesics should be taken at regular intervals until pain is adequately relieved. Whenever possible, the oral route of medication administration is preferred. After a titration period with short-acting preparations (it takes 5 half-lives of an analgesic agent to reach a steady state) to estimate the required dosing for managing continuous stable pain, controlled release medications should be considered to facilitate around-the-clock dosing, especially at night. Nonetheless, short-acting medications should still be made available for occasional breakthrough pain. In some cases, it may be necessary to consider the use of 2 or more drugs from different classes. Their complementary mechanisms of action may provide greater pain relief with less toxicity and lower doses of each drug. *For the elderly population, it is advisable to "start low and go slow"[36] in order to circumvent untoward adverse effects* (see common side effects of analgesics in Table 3). Common side effects, such as constipation, nausea, confusion, and drowsiness, should be monitored and managed appropriately. However, if the pain is (anticipated to be) severe pain, conscious sedation, combining sedatives and potent narcotic analgesics, such as sublingual fentanyl or sufentanil (approximately 100 times more potent than morphine) and ketamine, can be used with success.[19] In resistant cases, options may include general anesthesia, local neural blockade, spinal analgesia, or the use of mixed nitrous oxide and oxygen.

Topical agents play a critical role in alleviating wound-related pain. Slow-release ibuprofen foam dressings (available in Canada and Europe but not in the United States) have demonstrated reduction in persistent wound pain between dressing changes and temporary pain on dressing removal.[37] The topical use of morphine, tricyclic, nonsteroidal anti-inflammatory drugs (NSAIDs), capsaicin, and lidocaine/prilocaine (EMLA® or Eutectic Mixture of Local Anesthetics including lidocaine and prilocaine, AstraZeneca, Wilmington, Delaware) has demonstrated effectiveness for pain relief.[3,12,38] However, the lack of pharmacokinetic data precludes the routine clinical use of these compounds at this time. There are many advantages to using local rather than systemic treatment. Any active agent is delivered directly to the affected area, bypassing the systemic circulation, and the dose needed for pain reduction is lower, minimizing the risk of side effects.

How to Reduce Procedural Pain

In addition to pharmacotherapy, careful selection of *dressings with atraumatic and nonadherent interfaces, such as silicone, has been documented to limit skin damage/trauma with dressing removal and to minimize pain at dressing changes.*[39] Silicone coatings do not adhere to moist wound beds and have a low surface tension due to their unique structure, which consists of chains of hydrophobic polymers with alternate molecules of silicone and oxygen.

Numerous sealants, barriers, and protectants, such as wipes, sprays, gels, and liquid roll-ons, are designed to protect the periwound skin from trauma induced by adhesives.[40] Wound cleansing should involve less abrasive techniques, such as compressing and irrigating usually with normal saline or water. Topical antimicrobial dressings and related products should be considered when surface compartment critical colonization is indicated by increased pain.

Education is a key strategy to empower patients with wounds and individuals within their circle of care and to improve wound-related pain control. Patients and individuals within their circle of care should be informed of various treatment options and be empowered to be active participants in care. Being an active participant involves taking part in the decision-making for the most appropriate treatment, monitoring response to treatment, and communicating concerns to healthcare providers. Common misconceptions about pain management should be addressed.[2]

Fear of addiction and adverse effects has prevented patients from taking regular analgesics. In a pilot study,[41] chronic wound patients described dressing change pain as being more manageable after receiving educational information. Pain-related education is a necessary step in effecting change in pain management by debunking common misconceptions and myths that may obstruct effective pain management. *Cognitive therapy that aims at altering anxiety by modifying attitudes, beliefs, and expectations by exploring the meaning and interpretation of pain concerns* has been successful in the management of pain.[25] This may involve distraction techniques, imagery, relaxation, or altering the significance of the pain to an individual. Patients can learn to envision pain as less threatening and unpleasant through positive imagery by imagining pain disappearing or by conjuring a mental picture of a place that evokes feelings and memories of comfort, safety, and relaxation. In addition to pain, clinicians should pay attention to other sources of anxiety that may be associated with stalled wound healing, fear of amputation, body disfigurement, repulsive odor, social isolation, debility, and disruption of daily activities.[2]

Relaxation exercises can help to reduce anxiety-related tension in the muscle that contributes to pain.

Conclusion

Pain is a common concern and affects quality of life in people with chronic wounds. It is imperative to approach wound-associated pain by first identifying the triggers (related to wound pathologies or procedures), followed by evaluating the number of neurobiopsychosocial factors that may affect the pain experience. A variety of approaches drawing on expertise from interprofessional teams is crucial to optimize pain management.

Practice Pearls

- Wound-associated pain is complex: comprehensive assessment should entail how pain is affected by wound etiologies, procedure-related triggers, and biopsychosocial factors.
- Wound-associated pain assessment should be comprehensive. Remember PQRSTU.
- Selected pharmacological agents for the treatment of wound-associated pain should be based on the WHO recommendations, taking into account pain severity and types of pain (nociceptive versus neuropathic pain).
- A non-pharmacological approach to pain management should include the use of atraumatic dressings, education, empowerment, and anxiety reduction.

Self-Assessment Questions

1. Mrs. Lebert experiences severe pain due to her leg ulcers. The wound care clinician should assess which of the following?
   A. Lipodermatosclerosis
   B. Other signs of infection
   C. Anxiety due to cleansing of the wound
   D. All of the above

2. Mrs. Lebert rated her pain as 10 out of 10 on a numerical rating scale. Which of following pain management strategies is most appropriate for Mrs. Lebert?
   A. Give short-acting morphine 5 mg once daily
   B. Give acetaminophen every 6 hours
   C. Consider changing gauze dressings to silicone dressings
   D. Inform Mrs. Lebert that pain is a good indicator of healing

Answers: 1–D, 2–C

References

1. Krasner D. *Carrying on Despite the Pain: Living with Painful Venous Ulcers. A Heideggerian Hermeneutic Analysis* [dissertation]. Ann Arbor, MI: UMI; 1997.
2. Woo KY. Meeting the challenges of wound-associated pain: anticipatory pain, anxiety, stress, and wound healing. *Ostomy Wound Manage.* 2008;54(9):10–12.
3. Woo K, Sibbald G, Fogh K, et al. Assessment and management of persistent (chronic) and total wound pain. *Int Wound J.* 2008;5(2):205–215.
4. Flaherty E. The views of patients living with healed venous leg ulcers. *Nurs Stand.* 2005;19(45):78,80,82–83.
5. Szor JK, Bourguignon C. Description of pressure ulcer pain at rest and at dressing change. *J Wound Ostomy Continence Nurs.* 1999;26(3):115–120.
6. Nemeth KA, Harrison MB, Graham ID, Burke S. Understanding venous leg ulcer pain: results of a longitudinal study. *Ostomy Wound Manage.* 2004;50(1):34–36.
7. Pieper B, Szczepaniak K, Templin T. Psychosocial adjustment, coping, and quality of life in persons with venous ulcers and a history of intravenous drug use. *J Wound Ostomy Continence Nurs.* 2000;27(4):227–237.
8. Evans AR, Pinzur MS. Health-related quality of life of patients with diabetes and foot ulcers. *Foot Ankle Int.* 2005;26(1):32–37.
9. Kiecolt-Glaser JK, Marucha PT, Malarkey WB, Mercado AM, Glaser R. Slowing of wound healing by psychological stress. *Lancet.* 1995;346(8984):1194–1196.
10. Woo KY, Sibbald RG. The improvement of wound-associated pain and healing trajectory with a comprehensive foot and leg ulcer care model. *J Wound Ostomy Continence Nurs.* 2009;36(2):184–191.
11. Krasner D. The chronic wound pain experience: a con-

ceptual model. *Ostomy Wound Manage.* 1995;41(3):20–25.

12. Woo KY, Sibbald RG. Chronic wound pain: a conceptual model. *Adv Skin Wound Care.* 2008;21(4):175–190.

13. Bruce AJ, Bennett DD, Lohse CM, Rooke TW, Davis MD. Lipodermatosclerosis: review of cases evaluated at Mayo Clinic. *J Am Acad Dermatol.* 2002;46(2):187–192.

14. Aquino R, Johnnides C, Makaroun M, et al. Natural history of claudication: long-term serial follow-up study of 1244 claudicants. *J Vasc Surg.* 2001;34(6):962–970.

15. Grey JE, Harding KG, Enoch S. Venous and arterial leg ulcers. *BMJ.* 2006;332(7537):347–350.

16. Cutting KF, White RJ. Criteria for identifying wound infection--revisited. *Ostomy Wound Manage.* 2005;51(1):28–34.

17. Moore Z, Cowman S. Effective wound management: identifying criteria for infection. *Nurs Stand.* 2007;21(24):68,70,72.

18. Gardner SE, Frantz RA, Doebbeling BN. The validity of the clinical signs and symptoms used to identify localized chronic wound infection. *Wound Repair Regen.* 2001;9(3):178–186.

19. Jovey RD, ed. *Managing Pain: The Canadian Healthcare Professional's Reference.* Toronto, Ontario, Canada: Healthcare & Financial Publishing, Rogers Media; 2002.

20. Ji RR, Woolf CJ. Neuronal plasticity and signal transduction in nociceptive neurons: implications for the initiation and maintenance of pathological pain. *Neurobiol Dis.* 2001;8(1):1–10.

21. Woo KY, Coutts PM, Price P, Harding K, Sibbald RG. A randomized crossover investigation of pain at dressing change comparing 2 foam dressings. *Adv Skin Wound Care.* 2009;22(7):304–310.

22. Sibbald RG, Goodman L, Woo KY, et al. Special considerations in wound bed preparation 2011: an update©. *Adv Skin Wound Care.* 2011;24(9):415–436.

23. Ubbink DT, Vermeulen H, Goossens A, Kelner RB, Schreuder SM, Lubbers MJ. Occlusive vs gauze dressings for local wound care in surgical patients: a randomized clinical trial. *Arch Surg.* 2008;143(10):950–955.

24. Thomas S. Atraumatic dressings. Available at: www.worldwidewounds.com/2003/january/Thomas/Atraumatic-Dressings.html. Accessed February 7, 2008.

25. Woo KY. *Wound Related Pain and Attachment in the Older Adults.* LAP Lambert Academic Publishing; 2011.

26. Briggs M, Closs SJ. Patients' perceptions of the impact of treatments and products on their experience of leg ulcer pain. *J Wound Care.* 2006;15(8):333–337.

27. Melzack R. From the gate to the neuromatrix. *Pain.* 1999;Suppl 6:S121–S126.

28. Colloca L, Benedetti F. Nocebo hyperalgesia: how anxiety is turned into pain. *Curr Opin Anaesthesiol.* 2007;20(5):435–439.

29. Tracey I. Neuroimaging of pain mechanisms. *Curr Opin Support Palliat Care.* 2007;1(2):109–116.

30. Powell RA, Downing J, Ddungu H, Mwangi-Powell FN. Pain history and pain assessment. Available at: http://www.iasp-pain.org/AM/Template.cfm?Section=Home&Template=/CM/ContentDisplay.cfm&ContentID=12173. Accessed January 14, 2012.

31. RNAO. Assessment of pain: questions to consider during assessment of pain (PQRST). Available at: http://pda.rnao.ca/content/assessment-pain-questions-consider-during-assessment-pain-pqrst. Accessed December 28, 2011.

32. Herr K, Coyne PJ, McCaffery M, Manworren R, Merkel S. Pain assessment in the patient unable to self-report: position statement with clinical practice recommendations. *Pain Manag Nurs.* 2011;12(4):230–250.

33. City of Hope Pain & Palliative Care Resource Center. Pain and symptom management. Available at: http://prc.coh.org/pain_assessment.asp. Accessed December 28, 2011.

34. Arnstein P. Assessment of nociceptive versus neuropathic pain in older adults. Available at: http://consultgerirn.org/uploads/File/trythis/try_this_sp1.pdf. Accessed December 28, 2011.

35. World Health Organization. WHO's pain ladder. Available at: http://www.who.int/cancer/palliative/painladder/en/. Accessed December 28, 2011.

36. The AGS Foundation for Health in Aging. *Medications for Persistent Pain. An Older Adult's Guide to Safe Use of Pain Medications.* Available at: http://www.healthinaging.org/public_education/pain/know_your_pain_medications.pdf. Accessed December 28, 2011.

37. Romanelli M, Dini V, Polignano R, Bonadeo P, Maggio G. Ibuprofen slow-release foam dressing reduces wound pain in painful exuding wounds: preliminary findings from an international real-life study. *J Dermatolog Treat.* 2009;20(1):19–26.

38. Briggs M, Nelson EA. Topical agents or dressings for pain in venous leg ulcers. *Cochrane Database Syst Rev.* 2010;(4):CD001177.

39. Woo KY, Harding K, Price P, Sibbald G. Minimising wound-related pain at dressing change: evidence-informed practice. *Int Wound J.* 2008;5(2):144–157.

40. Woo KY, Sibbald RG. The ABCs of skin care for wound care clinicians: dermatitis and eczema. *Adv Skin Wound Care.* 2009;22(5):230–238.

41. Gibson MC, Keast D, Woodbury MG, et al. Educational intervention in the management of acute procedure-related wound pain: a pilot study. *J Wound Care.* 2004;13(5):187–190.

Creating Wound Care Processes — From Assessment to Healthcare Delivery Systems

Wound Assessment and Documentation

Lia van Rijswijk, RN, MSN, CWCN;
Morty Eisenberg, MD, MScCH, CCFP, FCFP

Objectives

The reader will be challenged to:
- Evaluate commonly assessed wound characteristics
- Explain the rationale for assessing different wound characteristics
- Analyze the purpose of wound assessment in clinical practice.

Introduction

Appreciation of the wound healing process, factors that may affect it, and the number of products available to manage wounds has increased dramatically during recent years. However, a significant portion of wound healing knowledge is based on the results of laboratory studies, while knowledge about the efficacy and clinical effectiveness of many wound care interventions remains limited or even nonexistent. As a result, clinicians not only must remain up-to-date about newly available evidence-based guidelines of care, they also must carefully monitor the outcome of all interventions.[1] Optimal patient and wound assessment practices not only guide all decisions of care, they also are crucial to assessing clinical outcomes.[2-4] At the same time, general education on the topic remains limited; many commonly used wound assessment terms remain poorly defined; and confusion about assessment and staging is common. This may explain why many clinicians continue to feel insecure about the process itself.[5]

Fortunately, we know which indices of wound healing are most appropriate to monitor outcome in clinical practice. Generally, it is better to regularly assess using the same possibly less-than-perfect tool than not to assess at all. Every plan of care and intervention, as well as the clinician's ability to determine the effectiveness of care, is based on a complete patient history, assessment, and regular follow-up assessments.[6]

This chapter will focus on the practical application of available research as it pertains to the clinical assessment and documentation of nonsutured, mostly chronic wounds. The

van Rijswijk L, Eisenberg M. Wound assessment and documentation. In: Krasner DL, Rodeheaver GT, Sibbald RG, Woo KY, eds. *Chronic Wound Care: A Clinical Source Book for Healthcare Professionals.* Vol 1. 5th ed. Malvern, PA: HMP Communications; 2012:99–115.

assessment of wound pain is reviewed in Chapter 2.8. The assessment of pressure ulcers will be reviewed in Volume III of *Chronic Wound Care: A Clinical Source Book for Healthcare Professionals.*

Assessment:
What it is and What it is Not

Verbs commonly used to describe the process of follow-up care include *assess*, *evaluate*, *monitor*, or *inspect*. It is important not to use them interchangeably, because their use affects the level of knowledge required to implement the process. To monitor or inspect means to watch, keep track of, or check, usually for a special purpose.[7] To evaluate — to determine the significance of an observation through appraisal and study — requires specific skills and knowledge. Similarly, to collect, verify, organize, and determine the importance of data (eg, to assess) is impossible without specific skills and an understanding of the condition involved.[6,7] For example, the plan of care for a home-bound patient may include 2 visits per week; once a week, the home health aide will change the dressing and monitor the patient and wound for signs of improvement, infection, or deterioration, and once a week, the registered nurse will change the dressing and complete a wound assessment to quantify progress. In the United States, for nurses, the type of assessment a nurse can perform is determined by statutory law (State Nurse Practice Acts): in most cases, registered nurses assess and evaluate; licensed practical nurses or licensed vocational nurses monitor and inspect.

Clinical Wound Assessment Rationale

Goals of care and wound care plans of care. The *patient history* and *wound assessment findings* are the foundation for developing the individual's goals of care and wound care plan of care, which will guide treatment. For example, a patient history will help determine if healing or palliation should be the goal of care, and a wound history can provide important insights about the need for further diagnostic testing. If pressure redistribution is needed, a patient history and assessment will determine if frequent turning is appropriate and feasible. Subsequent follow-up assessments designed to monitor and evaluate outcome(s) will determine whether the wound is moving in the direction of the ultimate outcome, the *goal of care*.[2-4]

Developing a realistic and clearly defined goal of care is particularly important when managing patients with chronic wounds because these patients often have a number of concomitant conditions that may affect the healing process or the wound care plan. A chronic wound presents a considerable burden to patients, caregivers, and, frequently, healthcare professionals.[8] If the goals of care are not realistic or not clearly defined, patients and caregivers may become discouraged. Research suggests that it is important for clinicians to communicate and provide information about wound healing expectations with patients.[9] Defining short-term as well as long-term goals of care may help. For example, the overall goal of care for a full-thickness wound with necrotic tissue may be complete healing, but the short-term goal of care could be to reduce pain and obtain a healthy granulating wound bed. In addition to developing realistic long-term and short-term goals of care, it helps to remember that even seemingly unstable patterns may result in a desired outcome, providing one does not lose sight of it.

Outcome and treatment effectiveness. In recent years, considerable efforts have been made to discover and test *physical, chemical, and biological markers of normal or abnormal healing*. Many studies have shown a correlation between molecular and cellular abnormalities in wound fluid and nonhealing.[10,11] If future research shows that these chemical abnormalities are the cause, not the effect, of nonhealing, tests may be developed to help clinicians diagnose chronic wounds and offer alternative approaches to treatment. No cause-and-effect relationship has been established thus far, and laboratory tests that yield valid, reliable, and clinically useful information to assess healing are not available. Decades of research have shown that regular clinical assessments can help clinicians determine whether the wound is moving in the direction of the goal of care or desired outcome. The effectiveness of interventions — that is, their ability to produce the decided, decisive, or desired effect — cannot be ascertained unless baseline assessment data are compared to follow-up data. By extension, the cost to obtain the desired effect — the cost-effectiveness of care — also cannot be calculated without comparing

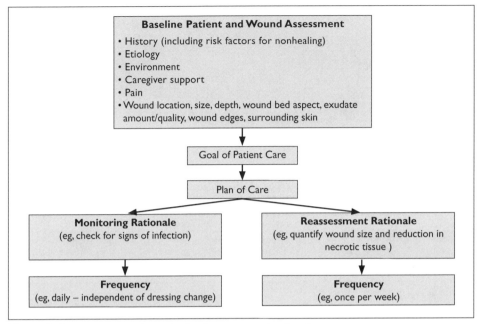

Figure 1. Reassessment and monitoring frequency and rationale.

standardized assessment data. In addition to monitoring the effectiveness of the plan of care, regular reassessments may help motivate patients and caregivers. Systematically gathered assessment and reassessment data will also help clinicians develop a treatment outcome database. The gathered data can be reviewed, analyzed, and compared to outcomes reported in the literature to develop or modify wound care guidelines and individual wound care plans of care. Because experiential outcome data is limited, this type of information is crucial when trying to develop care plans and pathways.[12,13] In summary, wound assessment and reassessment guidelines are a necessary and integral part of the individual patient's wound care plan of care as well as a tool to accumulate much needed outcome data on chronic wound care.[13,14]

Clinical Wound Assessment Frequency

After gathering baseline or admission assessment data, clinicians have to decide *how often and why the wound should be reassessed*. The latter seems obvious, but in some patient care settings, it is not unusual to encounter orders for twice daily wound assessments without any rationale for doing so. *Overall patient condition*,

wound severity, *patient care environment*, *goal*, and *overall plan of care* affect the reassessment and monitoring frequency and rationale (Figure 1). For example, when a patient has a systemic condition that may increase the risk of infection, the wound may require more frequent monitoring and assessments. Dressing/treatment selection also may be affected by reassessment frequency. For example, if a wound must be reassessed daily, it should not be covered with a dressing that is designed to remain in place for a number of days. However, with the possible exception of mechanical debridement using wet-to-dry gauze, there is no evidence to support using products that require daily (or more frequent) removal, and moisture-retentive dressings are recommended for all healable wounds.[2–4,15–18] Therefore, daily wound assessments should be the exception, not the rule. Since the goals of wound care and dressing choices are based on wound characteristics, such as amount of wound exudate, wound depth, and amount of necrotic tissue, these variables should be monitored or formally assessed each time a moisture-retentive dressing is changed.[16,19] Wound monitoring should occur based on patient and wound factors, independent of dress-

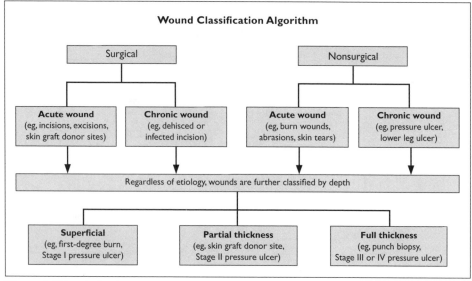

Figure 2. Wound classification algorithm.

ing change needs. Depending on the patient care setting and risk factors for complications, the *condition of the dressing, wound pain,* and *temperature and condition of the surrounding skin* can be monitored as frequently as needed without removing the dressing.[6,20] When a chronic wound is progressing well, in most patient care settings, daily monitoring (without changing the dressing) and regular assessment (at least weekly) are generally recommended.[11–13,20]

Assessing the Wound

General wound classification. The first step in the patient and wound assessment process is to *diagnose and classify the wound*. For this purpose, most wounds can be classified as belonging in one of two general categories. The first category is related to the *cause* (surgical or nonsurgical) and whether the wound is chronic or acute (Figure 2). Despite evolving definitions of the term *chronic wound,* the following continues to be widely used: *a wound that has failed to proceed through an orderly and timely process to produce anatomic and functional integrity or a wound that has proceeded through the repair process without establishing a sustained anatomic and functional result.*[21] Other definitions include a 3-month timeframe for restoration of anatomic and func-

tional integrity.[22] Clinicians should always consider the possibility that a nonsurgical wound is not caused by pressure or by venous or arterial insufficiency. These so-called *atypical ulcers,* for example, wounds caused by inflammatory or metabolic disease, vasculopathy, malignancy, deep infections, or drug reactions, do not meet the general definition of chronic wounds. Similarly, the etiology of some wounds cannot be determined until further testing is done. Regardless, *acute wounds* generally heal more expediently than chronic — or atypical — wounds. Hence, the goals of care are different. Similarly, because superficial and partial-thickness wounds can be expected to take less time to heal and are less likely to develop complications than full-thickness wounds, the second general category is based on *initial wound depth.*[23]

With the exception of the *Clinical, Etiology, Anatomy, Pathophysiology (CEAP) classification system for venous disease,* where all open wounds are classified as class 6 active ulcers,[24,25] most wound classification/staging systems are based on wound depth.[4,26,27] Information about the validity and reliability of these systems is limited. However, their use (eg, pressure ulcer staging) is standard practice in many patient care settings, and the presence of a deeper (more severe) wound is usually associated with worse outcomes and longer healing times than less severe wounds.[13,28] In addition, *diabetic foot ulcer classification systems*, such as the *Wagner Classification* or *University of Texas Wound Classification System*, include other wound-associated variables, such as *the presence of infection, ischemia, and a combination of infection and ischemia*. Therefore, use of these systems may help clinicians perform a more complete wound assessment, particularly at baseline.[25,29]

Choosing a wound assessment method. Clinical wound assessment is not an exact science. It is primarily rooted in clinical observation and hampered by ongoing confusion about commonly used wound-related terms and definitions.[5,19,30] Regardless of the method chosen, the *assessment process*, defined as *collecting, verifying, and organizing data*, will always require the talents of a skilled professional. Since communication, including communicating wound assessment data, is such an integral part of being able to track progress toward achieving the goal of care, standardization of the terminology and techniques used is crucial.

Reliability and validity. Reliability and validity are important clinical concerns. When 2 or more people make the same assessment (*reliability*), it is important that the assessments are similar. For example, with respect to wound measurements, specifying which position the patient should be in when the wound is measured and which type of tape measure or tracing device should be used will greatly increase reliability. The *validity* of an assessment, its ability to assess what it is supposed to, can be increased by choosing the appropriate method. For example, assessing wound depth by looking at a photograph is not as valid as measuring actual depth.

Qualitative, descriptive, and quantitative methods. A wound assessment method can be descriptive, qualitative, or quantitative. The use of descriptive and qualitative methods alone (eg, the wound has improved and is smaller than last week) is not acceptable for determining a plan of care or evaluating outcomes. For some wound variables, clinicians have no choice but to describe the observation (eg, wound odor), but if a valid and reliable quantitative method exists, it should be used in order to facilitate communication and continuity of care.

Prepare to assess. A wound assessment cannot be performed if loose debris, particulate matter, or dressing residue is present. Therefore, *wound cleansing* is an important early step in the wound assessment process. For assessment purposes, rinsing the wound with saline will usually suffice. However, when particulate matter is adherent to the wound bed, other forms of debridement may be necessary, including irrigation at safe pressures (between 4 and 15 pounds per square inch).[2-4]

Assessing and measuring wound depth. Wound depth assessment and measurement are important because they affect the goal and wound care plan of care (treatment modality) and help monitor treatment effectiveness. Deep wounds take longer to heal than partial-thickness wounds.[13] It is important to differentiate *staging* (which is a description of depth) from *measuring* the actual depth of the wound. When a wound has sufficient depth (eg, a stage III pressure ulcer), recording ulcer stage during the first assessment does not replace the need for measuring actual depth. If a wound is covered with eschar, wound depth cannot be assessed. In these instances, document "unable to stage" or "unable to assess wound depth" and explain why.[4] Also, the exact depth of wounds with sinus tracts or tunnels may be difficult to assess because the bottom of the tunnel cannot be seen. These wounds can be classified as full-thickness (Table 1), and the amount of wound care product needed to fill the tract or tunnel can be used as a gauge for determining the extent of tissues involved.

Many wounds do not fit into simple depth categories and contain areas of partial-thickness and full-thickness dermal involvement. When using a pressure ulcer or foot ulcer staging system, the stage corresponding with the deepest area of the wound should be documented. Similarly, a wound containing areas of partial- and full-thickness dermal involvement is classified as a full-thickness wound.

Burn wounds are classified based on *depth* and *area*. For example, partial-thickness wounds are classified as superficial or deep second-degree burns, and wound area is defined as total body surface area involved. As mentioned, classification systems for diabetic foot ulcers also include a description of wound depth. Pressure ulcer staging

Table I. Staging and describing the extent of tissue damage	
Structures Involved	**Examples of Wounds, Commonly Used Wound Descriptions, Classification, or Staging Systems**
• Epidermis (stratum corneum, granulosum, spinosum, and germinativum)	Superficial wound Category/stage I pressure ulcer* Grade 0 (or 0) diabetic foot ulcer** First-degree burn
• Epidermis • Dermis (hair follicles, apocrine and sebaceous glands, blood and lymph vessels, nerve endings)	Partial-thickness wound Shave biopsy abrasion Skin graft donor site Category/stage II pressure ulcer* Grade 1 (or I) diabetic foot ulcer** Category Ib, IIa, IIb, and III skin tear*** Second-degree burn
• Epidermis • Dermis • Subcutaneous tissue/superficial fascia (fat, fibrous and elastic tissue, deeper blood vessels)	Full-thickness wound Punch biopsy Penetrating wound Category/stage III pressure ulcer* Grade 2 (or I) diabetic foot ulcer** Category Ia skin tear*** Third-degree burn
• Epidermis • Dermis • Subcutaneous tissue • Deep fascia/underlying structures (muscle, tendon, bone)	Full-thickness wound Dehisced surgical wound Category/stage IV pressure ulcer* Grade 3 (or II/III) diabetic foot ulcer** Third-degree (sometimes called fourth-degree) burn

*European Pressure Ulcer Advisory Panel and National Pressure Ulcer Advisory Panel. Prevention and treatment of pressure ulcers: quick reference guide. Washington, DC: National Pressure Ulcer Advisory Panel; 2009. **Wagner FW Jr. The dysvascular foot: a system for diagnosis and treatment. *Foot Ankle.* 1981;2(2):64–122 or (text in parentheses) Lavery LA, Armstrong DG, Harkless LB. Classification of diabetic foot wounds. *Ostomy Wound Manage.* 1997;43(2):44–53. ***Payne RL, Martin ML. Defining and classifying skin tears: need for a common language. *Ostomy Wound Manage.* 1993;39(5):16–20.

systems, on the other hand, are solely based on the depth of tissue injury. Assessing the extent of dermal involvement can be particularly difficult because dermal thickness varies with age (thin at birth and after the fifth decade of life), sex (thicker in men than in women), and anatomical location (ranging from less than 1 mm on the eyelids to greater than 4 mm on the back).[31]

Another limitation is that few wound classification systems have been tested for validity and reliability, which causes problems with accuracy when used in clinical practice.[32,33] Finally, stag-

ing systems were not designed to capture changes that occur during the healing process, and they should be used to facilitate admission diagnostic procedures only. Just as we do not change the admission assessment of a deep second-degree burn to a superficial second-degree burn when it is healing, pressure ulcers should not be downstaged or backstaged as they heal.

If there is sufficient depth, all wounds, including pressure ulcers, should be measured at the initial and follow-up assessments.

How To

Assessing and measuring wound depth, undermining, and tunneling. When trying to assess and describe the extent of tissue damage, it may be helpful to find *markers of wound depth*. For example, islands of epithelium in the wound bed may be indicative of a superficial or partial-thickness wound (Table 1). When underlying structures, such as fascia or tendon, are visible, the wound extends down through the dermis and can be classified as full-thickness. The presence of fibrin slough on the wound bed is usually indicative of a full-thickness injury. It helps to remember that dermal thickness ranges from approximately 1 mm to 4 mm; thus, most wounds that are deeper than 4 mm involve subcutaneous tissue and can be classified as full-thickness wounds.[31] Finally, document if the wound bed is irregular, for example: "Lateral aspect of wound extends through subcutaneous tissue. Proximal aspect of the wound contains dermis." The depth of full-thickness wounds is most commonly measured and quantified by gently inserting a sterile swab into the wound at a 90° angle or perpendicular to the surrounding skin. Find the deepest point and put a gloved forefinger on the swab at skin level. Remove the swab and place it next to a measuring guide, calibrated in centimeters.[34] The presence or absence of *undermining*, a space between the surrounding skin and wound bed, and tunneling also can be determined in this manner. The depth of a *tunnel* or *pocket* of undermining can be measured using the same technique as described for wound depth. The validity and reliability of this method depends on clinician skills and documentation.

First, determine if you need assistance to help the patient remain in the position required to perform the assessment and make sure that you have all the equipment (eg, ruler, pen, paper) at hand. Second, the value of the measurement for evaluating change (reliability) also depends on documenting how (patient position) and where (eg, most lateral area) in the wound it was obtained. If tunneling or undermining is present, estimate and record the percentage of the wound margin involved and the location. If it is difficult to describe where the measurement was obtained, draw a picture of the wound and mark the area or use a "clock" system. For example, for all assessment findings, the area of the wound closest to the patient's head is 12 o'clock. There are no limitations on how many depth measurements can be made, and it may be helpful to take 2 or 3 measurements in different areas to get a clear picture of the wound dimensions. Taking multiple measurements close together and recording the average may improve accuracy. Insertion of any object into the wound may cause trauma, and if cotton swabs are used, particles can remain in the wound bed. A variety of disposable wound probes with or without attached foam tips and ruled measurement sticks are commercially available and, unlike cotton swabs, will not deposit particulates in the wound bed. Technological advances also have led to the development and increased availability of handheld devices designed to scan and measure wound size and depth and to calculate volume.[35–37] If valid and reliable, these devices may help standardize assessment and documentation practices. In clinical practice, at this time, wound volume is rarely included as an important wound assessment variable. Measuring wound volume is complicated, and calculating it based on area and depth is generally unreliable.[37] Most importantly, it does not help clinicians decide which treatment to use and it has not been shown to predict treatment outcome.

Regardless of how depth is measured, once a method has been chosen for a particular wound, *standardizing the procedure is crucial to evaluate whether the wound is moving in the direction of the goal of care*.

Assessing wound area/size. Measuring and recording wound size upon admission are crucial to helping clinicians develop the goal of care and patient care plan. First, initial wound size affects healing time. Large wounds take more time to heal than small wounds.[14,38] Second, ongoing wound measurements quantify change in wound area/size to help answer the question, "Is the wound healing?" In fact, percentage reduction in wound size during the first 2 to 4 weeks of care has consistently been found to be an independent predictor of whether a chronic wound is going to heal. These observations have been made for diabetic foot ulcers,[39] venous leg ulcers,[40,41] and full-thickness pressure ulcers.[14,38] Given the consistency and strength of this evidence, it is recommended that clinicians reevaluate the plan of

Table 2. Commonly used methods to measure wounds in the clinic

Method	Description	Advantages	Disadvantages	Comments
Tape measure or ruler	• Length (longest area of tissue breakdown) and width (longest measurement perpendicular to the length) are measured using a disposable measuring guide/ruler calibrated in centimeters • Record length, width, method of measurement, patient position at time of assessment	• Easy • Inexpensive • Fast • Good inter-rater and intra-rater reliability • Provides a clinically reliable record of changes in wound size over time	• May be difficult to determine wound edge • Length x width usually does not provide actual wound size • Reliability decreases with increasing wound size • Method may not be suitable for research purposes	• Good correlation between ruler measurements, tracings, and perimeter measurements has been found
Tracing	• Disposable acetate sheet, measuring guide, or plastic bag is held over the wound while tracing the edges with a permanent, fine-tip marker; add location markers (eg, head, toes), date, patient number • Clean the sheet or remove contaminated side of plastic bag/measuring guide • Attach tracing to chart and/or calculate area using 1.0-cm or 0.5-cm grid paper* • Record area, method of obtaining and calculating measurement, patient position at time of measurement	• Easy • Expense is determined by materials used • Fast • Excellent interrater and intrarater reliability	• May be difficult to see wound margins • If transparency does not contain grid, tracing has to be copied to grid paper to calculate area • Manual counting of squares on grid paper may cause over- or underestimation of actual area	• Tracings can be a valuable part of patient records and changes in wound area can easily be compared

* Some measuring guides incorporate a 1.0-cm or 0.5-cm grid. See Figure 3.

care if a chronic wound does not exhibit a size reduction of 20% to 50% after 2 to 4 weeks of care.[2–4,16,17]

How To

The most commonly used techniques for measuring wound area/size in the clinical setting include *tape measurements* and *tracings* (Table 2, Figure 3). Both measurement methods have advantages and disadvantages (Table 2), and their accuracy depends to a large extent on defining and recognizing the wound edge — a well documented challenge.[30] Before developing and implementing a wound measurement protocol, the following limitations should be considered. *All 2-dimensional measurement techniques only*

provide an index of wound area. Even though length x width calculations provide valuable information about the progress of a wound, the actual number obtained when multiplying length and width measurements is accurate only if the wound has a regular geometric shape. Ruler-based measurements are less accurate for irregular or large wounds.[42] In addition, research shows that measuring the longest measurement of the wound (length) followed by the longest measurement perpendicular to the length (width) yields more reliable results than using the "clock" method (head-to-toe = length and side-to-side = width).[43] As with other assessments, *patient position at the time of measurement, recording how the measurements were obtained* (see measuring wound depth), and *method consistency* are important. For example, if patient positioning limitations necessitate moving the surrounding skin in order to visualize and measure the wound (as may be the case with wounds in the gluteal cleft area), this should be documented. In these instances, wound measurements can vary considerably and short-term (eg, weekly) comparisons are unlikely to be valid. Fortunately, research also has shown that when using paper tape or a grid transparency, wound measurements take approximately 1 minute to complete.[44]

Some devices that measure wound depth also measure wound area,[35–37] and in addition to tape measures and acetate tracings (Figure 3), devices that use electronic or computerized planimetry and digital photography using computerized planimetry are also available. These methods of measurement show improved accuracy and high interrater and intrarater reliability,[45,46] although measurements are more accurate for large than for small wounds.[47]

Color photographs, most commonly used for documentation, also can be used to measure wound area/size, as long as the wound is not on a curved surface.[48] Photographs can be taken using a regular 35-mm or digital camera with a linear

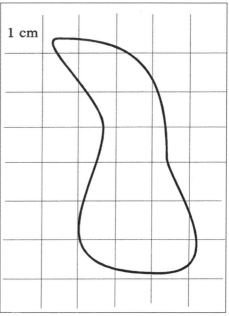

Figure 3. Using a 1.0-cm grid to determine wound size, count the crosspoints that fall completely within the ulcer. This ulcer measures 13 cm². When using a 0.5-cm grid, count the crosspoints and divide the number by 4.

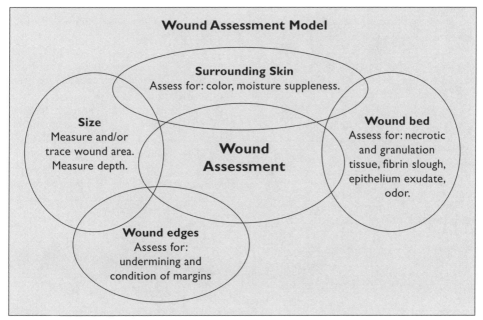

Figure 4. Wound assessment model. ©1994 Krasner and van Rijswijk.

measurement scale next to the wound and/or at a standard distance. Similar to regular wound measurement methods, the accuracy of the measurement depends to a large extent on the definition and identification of the wound edge.[49] In addition, **standard photographs** or **digital images** can be a useful addition to the patient chart (see documentation) and digital images can be used for telemedicine. Although specialty cameras with grid film or photography using ruler measurement have reasonable degrees of accuracy, **stereophotogrammetry**, using a video camera and special computer software, has been found to be precise.[50] Despite limitations, photographs may help wound care experts assess wounds, including estimating wound size, when a bedside assessment cannot be performed.[45] The equipment needed to utilize these measuring techniques may not be readily available or prove too costly in the clinical setting. For the most part, manual measurements are most practical and economical. Better still, after measuring the wound, a simple calculation ([(baseline area − current area) / baseline area] x 100%) will provide the clinician with an estimate of percent reduction in wound area since the start of treatment, which will help answer the question, "Is the wound healing?"[2,4,14,38–41]

Assessing the wound bed. After cleansing and measuring the dimensions of the wound, the appearance of the wound bed needs to be assessed and documented (Figure 4) because wound bed appearance affects both the goal and the wound care plan of care (treatment modality) and helps monitor treatment effectiveness.[2–5,16–18] Research using a tool that includes rating the predominant tissue type in a wound (eg, granulation tissue, slough, necrotic tissue) has shown this tool to be sensitive to change in tissue type and correlates well with overall improvement.[51] In another pressure ulcer healing instrument study, change in tissue type was predictive of outcome (healing) but not as important as the presence of pockets (undermining) or change in wound area.[52] At this time, many wound assessment recommendations are based on limited levels of evidence. However, more evidence is likely to become available with increasing research of wound healing instruments and wound care algorithms that typically include several wound assessment variables.

In order to develop a wound care plan of care

and monitor its effect in clinical practice, simply noting the presence or absence of granulation tissue, necrotic tissue, and fibrin slough is insufficient because this method will not capture changes in the wound bed until the process is complete (eg, completely free of necrotic tissue). Also, as previously mentioned, confusion about wound terminology and qualitative descriptors remains an important concern and potential impediment to optimal wound assessment.[5,19,30,49] Hence, clear descriptions and, if possible, quantification are important because many wounds contain a combination of granulation and necrotic tissue or fibrin slough (Figure 5).

Estimating tissue percentage range (eg, less than 25% necrotic tissue or 25%–50% necrotic tissue) was first studied as part of the **Pressure Sore Status Tool**, later revised as the **Bates-Jensen Wound Assessment Tool (BWAT)**.[53] Subsequent research has shown that, in clinical practice, percentage description of necrotic tissue/fibrin slough is a valid concept for determining which type of dressing to use and whether debridement is needed and has prospective validity when used in wound assessment tools.[5,13,15]

How To

After cleansing the wound, carefully inspect all aspects of the wound bed and estimate what percentage of the wound bed is covered with necrotic tissue, granulation tissue, and newly formed epithelium. The latter can be visible on the wound edges and in the wound bed of partial-thickness or superficial wounds. Necrotic tissue can be described as dry or moist and may vary in color from black to yellow, gray, tan, or brown. Soft, yellow necrotic tissue is often described as fibrin slough. The amount and aspect of granulation tissue should be estimated and described (Figure 5). Healthy granulation tissue has a pebbled texture and is shiny red or pink. Depending on anatomical location, it is not uncommon for muscle tissue, tendon, ligaments, or bone to be visible in deep wounds. This, too, should be noted. In persons with diabetic foot ulcers, for example, the ability to probe to bone is considered predictive of osteomyelitis and, although not very specific, further diagnostic tests should be considered.[54]

Assessing the wound edges and surrounding skin. In addition to assessing the extent

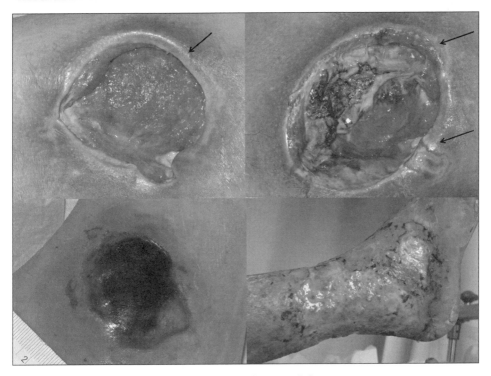

Figure 5. Wound bed presentations. Clockwise from top left:
a) Full-thickness wound contains 95% healthy granulation tissue. Note rolled wound edge and area of undermining (arrow).
b) Full-thickness wound containing 50% necrotic tissue (including slough). Note rolled wound edges and areas of breakdown suggesting undermining.
c) Wound depth cannot be assessed; > 80% of wound bed covered with dry necrotic tissue. Note erythema of surrounding skin and evidence of recent bleeding suggesting trauma/inflammation.
d) Wounds containing 100% necrotic tissue (fibrin slough). Unable to assess depth.

and depth of undermining, the condition of the *wound edges* should be noted. Both assessments influence the patient course and wound care plan of care. For example, when wound edges are undermined, the application of a primary wound filler dressing to reduce wound dead space is usually required,[2,15] and pressure ulcers with undermining and pockets may take longer to heal than ulcers without undermining.[52] Similarly, in one venous ulcer study, the absence of a healing wound edge with evidence of re-epithelization was a predictor of increased time to healing.[55]

The condition of the *surrounding skin* also may provide important information about the status of the wound and the effects of treatment.

Surrounding skin assessment includes evaluating *color, induration, edema*, and *suppleness* (Figure 4). If the surrounding skin is white/pale, it may be macerated, suggesting that wound exudate has overwhelmed the dressing or that moisture from the outside (eg, urine) was able to penetrate the dressing. Redness of the surrounding skin may be suggestive of unrelieved pressure or prolonged inflammation.[2] Inflammation/vasodilation will cause an increase in skin temperature. A temperature difference between the skin immediately surrounding and a short distance from the wound can be assessed using the back of the hand or finger. Also, *redness, tenderness, warmth, and swelling of the surrounding skin are the classic clini-*

cal signs of infection.[56] Results of one study in patients with venous ulcers showed a significant correlation between a 2°F increase in surrounding skin temperature and clinical signs of wound infection.[57] Digital infrared thermometers, such as the one used in this study, could help provide early warning signs of wound infection. However, clinicians should be aware of the many environmental and patient-related factors that can influence the accuracy of these thermometers.[57] As with wound bed assessments, it is important to remember that most wound edge and surrounding skin assessment information is based on expert opinion and consensus.

How To

After cleansing the wound, examine the *distinctness, degree of attachment to the wound base, color, and thickness of the wound edge*. If it is difficult to see where the wound ends and the surrounding skin starts, re-epithelization may be taking place, and this observation should be charted. Thick ("rolled") and unattached wound margins, commonly described as *epibole* or "*closed wound edges*," are believed to hinder the normal migration of epithelial cells across the wound bed. When observed, this is usually an indication that the wound has been present for some time and that the newly formed epithelial cells have migrated down and around the wound edge because they did not find moist, healthy, granulation tissue to resurface in the wound bed. Callus formation around the wound in a person with a diabetic foot ulcer may be an important indicator of unrelieved pressure.

Irritation of the surrounding skin, which also may impair wound healing, can result from contact with feces or urine, from a reaction to the dressing or tape used, or from a reaction to frequent or inappropriate dressing/tape removal. In patients with darkly pigmented skin, skin color changes (eg, a difference between the patient's usual skin color and the color of the skin surrounding the wound) should be noted.[4] *Signs of maceration include pale, white, or grey periwound skin*, and in patients with leg ulcers, the surrounding skin may exhibit signs of *capillary leakage* (hemosiderin pigmentation, lipodermatosclerosis) or *ischemia* (absence of hair growth; cool, clammy skin).[3,25] Assessing and documenting *suppleness* of the sur-

rounding skin is important because overly moist as well as overly dry skin (commonly seen in patients with impaired peripheral perfusion) is more prone to injury. *Induration* (an abnormal firmness of the tissues) and *edema* are assessed by gently pressing the skin within approximately 4 cm of the wound edge. Document the location and the extent (in centimeters) of induration and edema as well as pitting or nonpitting characteristics. In one study that evaluated a pressure ulcer assessment instrument, the presence of induration was associated with delayed healing.[58]

Assessing exudate and odor. The type and amount of wound exudate should be assessed because these characteristics provide important information about wound status and the most appropriate treatment.[59] Change in the amount of exudate also may be a sign of healing.[58] However, at this time, no reliable and valid wound exudate assessment tool exists. Some suggestions include rating/describing the amount of moisture in the wound bed and the condition of the surrounding skin.[16,53] Other suggestions include using the type of dressing needed to control exudate as a "yardstick," eg, wounds with scant exudate are those that can be covered with a nonabsorptive dressing for up to 7 days.[55] Clinically, rating the amount of wound exudate will be useful only if a description of each rating is provided. The content and construct validity of the following descriptors, but not their prospective validity or reliability, has been established.[5,15,53] When the wound is dry, there is no exudate. A moist wound contains scant or small amounts of exudate — enough to keep the wound moist but not wet. A moderately exuding wound is wet/saturated and a highly exuding wound is bathing in fluid. In addition to amount, the type of exudate should be described. Most commonly, exudate type is recorded as *serous* (clear fluid without blood, pus, or debris); *serosanguineous* (thin, watery, pale red to pink fluid); *sanguineous or bloody* (bloody, bright red); and *seropurulent or purulent* (thick, cloudy, yellow, or tan).[53] Regardless of which assessment is chosen, consistent and clear descriptions will help achieve the goal of wound assessment to monitor progress.

Traditionally, the presence of *wound odor* (and pus) was used to diagnose infection. Hence, when moisture-retentive dressings were first used, the odor that inevitably accompanied their removal was sometimes mistaken for infection. All wounds, particularly after they have been occluded, will emit an odor, and as with all wound assessment variables, cleansing is important prior to assessing odor. Necrotic wounds tend to have an offensive odor, and wounds infected with anaerobic bacteria tend to produce a distinct acrid or putrid smell.[60] Pseudomonas infection often produces a characteristic fruity or sweet odor. Odor is a subjective assessment and cannot be quantified. However, a descriptive odor assessment can provide important information, because a change in the type or amount of odor may be indicative of a change in wound status. As with all assessment parameters, standardizing what to assess, how to assess, and how to document it will increase their usefulness. Odor assessments can include a *description of the odor* (eg, sweet, like fresh blood, putrid) as well as a *description of the amount of odor* (eg, filled the room, could only smell it immediately following dressing removal, disappeared when dressing was discarded).

How To

Using the information provided, adopt an existing or develop a *wound exudate and odor assessment instrument* that meets the requirements of the clinical practice site. Combined with other wound assessments, consistent use will help guide topical wound care decisions and monitor outcomes.

Clinical wound assessment for signs of infection. All wounds are contaminated with a variety of organisms. Determining when these organisms have invaded the tissues and multiplied to cause cellular injury (infection) can be very challenging in patients with chronic wounds. The classic clinical signs of infection — redness, tenderness, warmth, swelling of the surrounding skin, the presence of pus, and skin anesthesia or sloughing[56] — are usually easy to identify in acute wounds. In chronic wounds, however, unrelieved pressure, chronic inflammation, and allergic reactions to dressings also can cause redness, tenderness, warmth, and swelling of the surrounding skin. At the same time, signs of infection in chronic wounds are often blunted. In one study, 7 of 20 persons with diabetic foot ulcers and no clinical symptoms of infection had biopsy-confirmed osteomyelitis.[54] Thus, infections in

chronic wounds can easily be overdiagnosed or underdiagnosed. For example, when wound care specialists were asked to diagnose infection by looking at the photographs of 120 nonhealing wounds, the percentage of correctly diagnosed infections ranged from 37% to 90%, indicating great variability and low reliability.[61]

For chronic wounds, the following variables for assessing wound infection have been proposed: *increasing pain; the presence of erythema, edema, warmth, purulent exudate, sanguinous exudate, serous exudate, and delayed healing; discoloration of granulation tissue; friable granulation tissue; pocketing at the base of the wound; foul odor; and wound breakdown*.[60,62] Not surprisingly, given the complexity of chronic wound healing, in a study of persons with diabetic foot ulcers, none of these individual wound variables predicted actual microbial load, but a composite of these variables did have some diagnostic validity.[62] In another study, an examination of basically the same wound variables in patients with leg or foot ulcers showed that wounds with debris, increased exudate, and friable tissue were 5 times more likely to have scant or light bacterial growth, whereas wounds with elevated temperature were 8 times more likely to have moderate or heavy bacterial growth.[63] While direct evidence remains sparse, the literature is consistent in that a combination of the aforementioned wound observations should raise concerns about the possibility that a chronic wound is infected. Specifically, most evidence-based guidelines of care include recommendations to assess the patient and review the patient's history for risk of infection and at least 4 signs of clinical infection, for example:

- Inflammation, increased pain, increased exudate, or pyrexia[64]
- Increase in amount or change in characteristics of exudate, decolorization and friability of granulation tissue, undermining, abnormal odor, epithelial bridging (a bridge of epithelial tissue across a wound bed) at the base of the wound, or sudden pain[65]
- Elevated temperature, purulent exudate, foul purulent wound exudate, increasing wound pain, cellulitis, increasing wound size, undermining of the wound, or peripheral wound induration[15,16]
- Erythema, edema, odor, purulent or foul-

smelling exudate, increase in ulcer pain and exudate, fever, or friable or irregular granulation tissue.[2]

In addition to some of these variables, the EPUAP/NPUAP guideline includes an increase in the amount of necrotic tissue as a possible sign of infection.[4] If the wound is not healing and the aforementioned wound changes are observed, most guidelines recommend a *quantitative tissue, swab, or bone culture* be obtained, providing this approach is consistent with the patient goal of care.[2,4] At all times, it is crucial to remember that a patient's overall health condition affects his or her risk of infection, confirming the observation of Louis Pasteur (1822–1895) that "the germ is nothing — the milieu [the environment within] is everything."

How To

Following the patient and wound assessment, recommendations described together with careful documentation and evaluation of findings will result in prompt recognition of wound changes or a lack of progress that could signal the presence of infection. If baseline patient and wound assessment findings or a change in the patient's overall health condition suggests an increased risk of infection, consider increasing the frequency with which the wound is assessed. If an infection is suspected, additional diagnostic tests — including quantitative tissue, swab, or bone biopsy for culture — should be ordered.

Documentation evaluation and wound healing instruments. All wound and patient assessment variables must be carefully documented and evaluated. The assessments provide the (documented) foundation for the plan of care (treatment modality), but in order to evaluate the effectiveness of the wound care plan of care, assessments must be reviewed over time. For example, measuring the wound on a regular basis is useless unless wound area and percent change are calculated weekly or once every 2 weeks. Many facilities utilize separate wound assessment forms that facilitate evaluation of the observations. As long as wound assessment protocols are clearly defined and changes in all observations are consistently reviewed, the overall goal of clinical wound assessments can be met.

For documentation purposes, regular or digital wound photographs can be taken to serve as a permanent record. Prior to developing a wound photograph guideline, it is important to carefully review the guideline rationale and all procedures. Compliance with the Health Insurance Portability and Accountability Act in the United States and other regulatory and legal standards is essential. Healthcare institutions and systems often have photography guidelines that must be followed by individual practitioners. A wound photograph guideline should include descriptions on what to include in the photograph (labels), how to maximize clinical information in the photograph itself, and whether or not the photograph should be accompanied by a written report.[66,67]

Meeting the second objective of wound assessment — to monitor treatment effectiveness — may be facilitated by using a wound healing instrument. Most are not designed to guide care and cannot replace the need to assess the wound variables discussed. However, their use will not involve additional patient care procedures as long as the wound assessment definitions used in the setting's wound care protocol are similar to those used in the wound assessment instrument. For example, almost all instruments used to measure healing contain wound size, wound bed aspects, and exudate as variables for assessment. Hence, these observations can all be simply transferred to a wound healing instrument. A careful review of 10 different wound healing instruments concluded that the use of wound healing instruments cannot be generally endorsed but that the *BWAT (previously Pressure Sore Status Tool)* and *PUSH (Pressure Ulcer Scale for Healing)* have been validated to the greatest extent for use with different types of chronic wounds.[68] In addition, content and prospective validity of BWAT variables also has been established,[5,13,15] and additional research using the PUSH tool for use in a variety of chronic wounds[51] and the *DESIGN-R instrument* for pressure ulcer monitoring has been conducted.[52] In light of increased emphasis on standardized documentation and outcomes evaluations, it can be anticipated that research using these instruments will continue providing clinicians with the data they need to develop and implement evidence-based guidelines for wound assessment and documentation.

Conclusion

Wound assessments are the foundation for establishing patient goals and wound care plans of care and are the only means of determining the effectiveness of interventions. Regular reassessments also may motivate patients and caregivers and will help clinicians develop their own treatment outcome database. Knowledge about the appropriateness, validity, and reliability of commonly used assessment terms and methods to describe wounds, develop wound care plans of care, and ascertain outcomes has increased substantially in recent years. While much remains unknown, application of existing knowledge will help clinicians provide evidence-based care and optimize outcomes in all patient care settings.

Practice Pearls

- A thorough wound assessment includes a complete patient evaluation.
- Treatment is predicated on the results of the wound assessment.
- In clinical practice, consistency of assessment methods used is key.

Self-Assessment Questions

1. Commonly assessed wound characteristics include:
   A. Wound depth, wound size, tissue type, etiology, and tissue perfusion
   B. Wound depth, tissue perfusion, surrounding skin condition, and wound odor
   C. Tissue type, amount of exudate, wound depth, surrounding skin condition, wound etiology, and contamination
   D. Tissue type, amount of exudate, wound depth and size, odor, surrounding skin condition, and wound edges

2. Wound size is an important characteristic to assess on a regular basis because:
   A. It helps clinicians select the right dressing
   B. Documentation of wound size affects reimbursement rates
   C. Change in wound size is a predictor of healing
   D. A change in wound size correlates with a change in patient status

3. The process of wound assessment can best be defined as:
   A. Collecting, verifying, and organizing information about the wound for the purpose of evaluating the effectiveness of the plan of care
   B. Watching and tracking changes in the wound for the purpose of documenting its status
   C. Keeping track of information about the wound so as to facilitate communication
   D. Collecting wound status information for the purpose of selecting the most appropriate treatment modalities

Answers: 1–D, 2–C, 3–A

References

1. van Rijswijk L, Gray M. Evidence, research, and clinical practice: a patient-centered framework for progress in wound care. *Ostomy Wound Manage.* 2011;57(9):26–38.
2. Association for the Advancement of Wound Care (AAWC). Association for the Advancement of Wound Care guideline of pressure ulcer guidelines. Malvern, PA: Association for the Advancement of Wound Care (AAWC); 2010.
3. Registered Nurses Association of Ontario (RNAO). Assessment and management of venous leg ulcers: guideline supplement. Toronto, ON: Registered Nurses Association of Ontario (RNAO); 2007.
4. National Pressure Ulcer Advisory Panel, European Pressure Ulcer Advisory Panel. Pressure ulcer treatment recommendations. In: Prevention and treatment of pressure ulcers: clinical practice guideline. Washington, DC: National Pressure Ulcer Advisory Panel; 2009:51–120.
5. Beitz JM, van Rijswijk L. A cross-sectional study to validate wound care algorithms for use by registered nurses. *Ostomy Wound Manage.* 2010;56(4):46–59.
6. van Rijswijk L. Frequency of reassessment of pressure ulcers. *Adv Wound Care.* 1995;8(4):suppl 19–24.
7. *Merriam-Webster's Collegiate Dictionary.* 11th ed. Springfield, MA: Merriam-Webster, Inc; 2010.
8. van Rijswijk L. The language of wounds. In: Krasner DL, Rodeheaver GT, Sibbald RG, eds. *Chronic Wound Care: A Clinical Source Book for Healthcare Professionals.* 4th ed. Malvern, PA: HMP Communications; 2007:25–28.
9. Spilsbury K, Nelson A, Cullum N, Iglesias C, Nixon J, Mason S. Pressure ulcers and their treatment and effects on quality of life: hospital inpatient perspectives. *J Adv Nurs.* 2007;57(5):494–504.
10. Schultz GS, Wysocki A. Interactions between extracellular matrix and growth factors in wound healing. *Wound Repair Regen.* 2009;17(2):153–162.
11. Karim RB, Brito BL, Dutrieux RP, Lassance FP, Hage JJ. MMP-2 assessment as an indicator of wound healing: a feasibility study. *Adv Skin Wound Care.* 2006;19(6):324–327.

12. Ennis WJ, Meneses P. Wound healing at the local level: the stunned wound. *Ostomy Wound Manage.* 2000;46(1A Suppl):39S–48S.

13. Bolton L, McNees P, van Rijswijk L, et al; Wound Outcomes Study Group. Wound-healing outcomes using standardized assessment and care in clinical practice. *J Wound Ostomy Continence Nurs.* 2004;31(2):65–71.

14. Polansky M, van Rijswijk L. Utilizing survival analysis techniques in chronic wound healing studies. *WOUNDS.* 1994;6(5):150–158.

15. Beitz JM, van Rijswijk L. Using wound care algorithms: a content validation study. *J Wound Ostomy Continence Nurs.* 1999;26(5):238–249.

16. ConvaTec. SOLUTIONS wound care algorithm. Princeton, NJ: ConvaTec; 2008. Available at: www.guideline. gov.

17. Steed DL, Attinger C, Colaizzi T, et al. Guidelines for the treatment of diabetic ulcers. *Wound Repair Regen.* 2006;14(6):680–692.

18. Centers for Medicare & Medicaid Services. OASIS-C Process-Based Quality Improvement Manual. Baltimore, MD: Centers for Medicare & Medicaid Services; 2010.

19. Beitz JM, van Rijswijk L. Developing evidence-based algorithms for negative pressure wound therapy in adults with acute and chronic wounds: literature and expert-based face validation results. *Ostomy Wound Manage.* 2012;58(4):50–69.

20. van Rijswijk L, Lyder CH. Pressure ulcer prevention and care: implementing the revised guidance to surveyors for long-term care facilities. *Ostomy Wound Manage.* 2005 Apr;Suppl:7–19.

21. Lazarus GS, Cooper DM, Knighton DR, et al. Definitions and guidelines for assessment of wounds and evaluation of healing. *Arch Dermatol.* 1994;130(4):489–493.

22. Mustoe TA, O'Shaughnessy K, Kloeters O. Chronic wound pathogenesis and current treatment strategies: a unifying hypothesis. *Plast Reconstr Surg.* 2006;117(7 Suppl):35S–41S.

23. Clark RA. Cutaneous tissue repair: basic biological considerations. I. *J Am Acad Dermatol.* 1985;13(5 Pt 1):705–725.

24. Eklöf B, Rutherford RB, Bergan JJ, et al; American Venous Forum International Ad Hoc Committee for Revision of the CEAP Classification. Revision of the CEAP classification for chronic venous disorders: consensus statement. *J Vasc Surg.* 2004;40(6):1248–1252.

25. Bolton L, Corbett L, Bernato L, et al; Government and Regulatory Task Force, Association for the Advancement of Wound Care. Development of a content-validated venous ulcer algorithm. *Ostomy Wound Manage.* 2006;52(11):32–48.

26. Doupis J, Veves A. Classification, diagnosis, and treatment of diabetic foot ulcers. *WOUNDS.* 2008;20(5):117–126.

27. Lavery LA, Armstrong DG, Harkless LB. Classification of diabetic foot wounds. *Ostomy Wound Manage.* 1997;43(2):44–53.

28. Oyibo SO, Jude EB, Tarawneh I, Nguyen HC, Harkless LB, Boulton AJ. A comparison of two diabetic foot ulcer classification systems: the Wagner and the University of Texas wound classification systems. *Diabetes Care.* 2001;24(1):84–88.

29. Frykberg RG, Zgonis T, Armstrong DG, et al; American College of Foot and Ankle Surgeons. Diabetic foot disorders. A clinical practice guideline (2006 revision). *J Foot Ankle Surg.* 2006;45(5 Suppl):S2–S66.

30. Van Poucke S, Nelissen R, Jorens P, Vander Haeghen Y. Comparative analysis of two methods for wound bed area measurement. *Int Wound J.* 2010;7(5):366–377.

31. Odland GF, Short JM. Structure of the skin. In: Thomas B, Arndt KA, Fitzpatrick WH, eds. *Dermatology in General Medicine.* New York, NY: McGraw-Hill Book Co; 1971.

32. Defloor T, Schoonhoven L, Katrien V, Weststrate J, Myny D. Reliability of the European Pressure Ulcer Advisory Panel classification system. *J Adv Nurs.* 2006;54(2):189–198.

33. Buntinx F, Beckers H, De Keyser G, et al. Inter-observer variation in the assessment of skin ulceration. *J Wound Care.* 1996;5(4):166–170.

34. Krasner D. Wound measurements: some tools of the trade. *Am J Nurs.* 1992;92(5):89–90.

35. Hammond CE, Nixon MA. The reliability of a hand-held wound measurement and documentation device in clinical practice. *J Wound Ostomy Continence Nurs.* 2011;38(3):260–264.

36. Romanelli M, Magliaro A. Objective assessment in wound healing. In: Kirsner RS, Falabella AF, eds. *Wound Healing.* Boca Raton, FL: Taylor & Francis Group; 2005:671–679.

37. Little C, McDonald J, Jenkins MG, McCarron P. An overview of techniques used to measure wound area and volume. *J Wound Care.* 2009;18(6):250–253.

38. Edsberg LE, Wyffels JT, Ha DS. Longitudinal study of Stage III and Stage IV pressure ulcer area and perimeter as healing parameters to predict wound closure. *Ostomy Wound Manage.* 2011;57(10):50–62.

39. Sheehan P, Jones P, Caselli A, Giurini JM, Veves A. Percent change in wound area of diabetic foot ulcers over a 4-week period is a robust predictor of complete healing in a 12-week prospective trial. *Diabetes Care.* 2003;26(6):1879–1882.

40. Kantor J, Margolis DJ. A multicentre study of percentage change in venous leg ulcer area as a prognostic index of healing at 24 weeks. *Br J Dermatol.* 2000;142(5):960–964.

41. van Rijswijk L. Full-thickness leg ulcers: patient demographics and predictors of healing. Multi-Center Leg Ulcer Study Group. *J Fam Pract.* 1993;36(6):625–632.

42. Keast DH, Bowering CK, Evans AW, Mackean GL, Burrows C, D'Souza L. MEASURE: a proposed assessment framework for developing best practice recommendations for wound assessment. *Wound Repair Regen.* 2004;12(3 Suppl):S1–S17.

43. Bryant JL, Brooks TL, Schmidt B, Mostow EN. Reliability of wound measuring techniques in an outpatient wound center. *Ostomy Wound Manage.* 2001;47(4):44–51.

44. Liskay AM, Mion LC, Davis BR. Comparison of two devices for wound measurement. *Dermatol Nurs.* 1993;5(6):437–441,434.

45. Houghton PE, Kincaid CB, Campbell KE, Woodbury MG, Keast DH. Photographic assessment of the appearance of chronic pressure and leg ulcers. *Ostomy Wound Manage.* 2000;46(4):20–30.

46. Sugama J, Matsui Y, Sanada H, Konya C, Okuwa M,

Kitagawa A. A study of the efficiency and convenience of an advanced portable Wound Measurement System (VISITRAK). *J Clin Nurs.* 2007;16(7):1265–1269.

47. Shaw J, Hughes CM, Lagan KM, Bell PM, Stevenson MR. An evaluation of three wound measurement techniques in diabetic foot wounds. *Diabetes Care.* 2007;30(10):2641–2642.

48. Plassman P, Melhuish JM, Harding KG. Methods of measuring wound size: a comparative study. *WOUNDS.* 1994;6(2):54–61.

49. Terris DD, Woo C, Jarczok MN, Ho CH. Comparison of in-person and digital photograph assessment of stage III and IV pressure ulcers among veterans with spinal cord injuries. *J Rehabil Res Dev.* 2011;48(3):215–224.

50. Langemo DK, Melland H, Hanson D, Olson B, Hunter S, Henly SJ. Two-dimensional wound measurement: comparison of 4 techniques. *Adv Wound Care.* 1998;11(7):337–343.

51. Hon J, Lagden K, McLaren AM, O'Sullivan D, Orr L, Houghton PE, Woodbury MG. A prospective, multicenter study to validate use of the PUSH in patients with diabetic, venous, and pressure ulcers. *Ostomy Wound Manage.* 2010;56(2):26–36.

52. Matsui Y, Furue M, Sanada H, et al. Development of the DESIGN-R with an observational study: an absolute evaluation tool for monitoring pressure ulcer wound healing. *Wound Repair Regen.* 2011;19(3):309–315.

53. Bates-Jensen BM, Vredevoe DL, Brecht ML. Validity and reliability of the Pressure Sore Status Tool. *Decubitus.* 1992;5(6):20–28.

54. Schwegler B, Stumpe KD, Weishaupt D, et al. Unsuspected osteomyelitis is frequent in persistent diabetic foot ulcer and better diagnosed by MRI than by 18F-FDG PET or 99mTc-MOAB. *J Intern Med.* 2008;263(1):99–106.

55. Falanga V, Saap LJ, Ozonoff A. Wound bed score and its correlation with healing of chronic wounds. *Dermatol Ther.* 2006;19(6):383–390.

56. Stevens DL, Bisno AL, Chambers HF, et al; Infectious Diseases Society of America. Practice guidelines for the diagnosis and management of skin and soft-tissue infections. *Clin Infect Dis.* 2005;41(10):1373–1406.

57. Fierheller M, Sibbald RG. A clinical investigation into the relationship between increased periwound skin temperature and local wound infection in patients with chronic leg ulcers. *Adv Skin Wound Care.* 2010;23(8):369–379.

58. Bates-Jensen BM. The Pressure Sore Status Tool a few thousand assessments later. *Adv Wound Care.* 1997;10(5):65–73.

59. Baranoski S. Wound assessment and dressing selection. *Ostomy Wound Manage.* 1995;41(7A Suppl):7S–12S.

60. Cutting KF, Harding KG. Criteria for identifying wound infection. *J Wound Care.* 1994;3(4):198–201.

61. Lorentzen HF, Gottrup F. Clinical assessment of infection in nonhealing ulcers analyzed by latent class analysis. *Wound Repair Regen.* 2006;14(3):350–353.

62. Gardner SE, Hillis SL, Frantz RA. Clinical signs of infection in diabetic foot ulcers with high microbial load. *Biol Res Nurs.* 2009;11(2):119–128.

63. Woo KY, Sibbald RG. A cross-sectional validation study of using NERDS and STONEES to assess bacterial burden. *Ostomy Wound Manage.* 2009;55(8):40–48.

64. Australian Wound Management Association Inc., New Zealand Wound Care Society Inc. Australian and New Zealand Clinical Practice Guideline for Prevention and Management of Venous Leg Ulcers. Port Melbourne, VIC, Australia: Cambridge Publishing; 2011.

65. Institute for Clinical Systems Improvement (ICSI). Pressure ulcer prevention and treatment. Health care protocol. Bloomington, MN: Institute for Clinical Systems Improvement (ICSI); 2010.

66. Phillips K. Incorporating digital photography into your wound care practice. *Wound Care Canada.* 2006;4(2):16–18.

67. Knowlton SP, Brown G. Legal aspects of wound care. In: Baranoski S, Ayello EA, eds. *Wound Care Essentials: Practice Principles.* 3rd ed. Ambler, PA: Lippincott Williams & Wilkins; 2012.

68. Pillen H, Miller M, Thomas J, Puckridge P, Sandison S, Spark JI. Assessment of wound healing: validity, reliability and sensitivity of available instruments. *Wound Practice and Research.* 2009;17(4):208–217.

Nutritional Strategies for Pressure Ulcer Management

Mary E. Posthauer, RD, CD, LD;
Jos M.G.A. Schols, MD, PhD

Objectives

The reader will be challenged to:
- Define the direct and indirect roles of nutrients in the wound healing process
- Analyze the role of nutrition in pressure ulcer prevention and healing
- Establish an interprofessional approach to wound care, including nutrition.

Introduction

No one will argue the importance of adequate nutrition for preserving skin and tissue viability and promoting tissue repair processes like wound healing. Good nutritional status generally reflects a healthy condition and adequate body power. However, despite this assumption, little scientific evidence about the relationship between nutrition or nutrition intervention and wound healing is available. Most studies that have been performed are related to the problem of pressure ulcers. Hence, this chapter focuses on nutritional strategies for pressure ulcer management.

Prevalence of Pressure Ulcers

Pressure ulcers are common across all healthcare sectors throughout the world and have been described as one of the most costly and physically debilitating care problems. A survey by the European Pressure Ulcer Advisory Panel (EPUAP) found an overall prevalence of 18.1% in 5 different European countries, and a study of the National Pressure Ulcer Advisory Panel (NPUAP) found a similar prevalence of 15% together with an incidence of 7% in American hospitals.[1,2] The Agency for Healthcare Research and Quality (AHRQ) in the United States noted that pressure ulcer-related hospitalizations increased by 80% from 1993 to 2006. Specifically, the prevalence figures are highest among vulnerable populations, such as frail and disabled residents in long-term care facilities, individuals receiving palliative care, and medically complex patients in intensive care units.[3]

Posthauer ME, Schols J. Nutritional strategies for pressure ulcer management. In: Krasner DL, Rodeheaver GT, Sibbald RG, Woo KY, eds. *Chronic Wound Care: A Clinical Source Book for Healthcare Professionals.* Vol 1. 5th ed. Malvern, PA: HMP Communications; 2012:117–130.

The impact of pressure ulcers is significant to individuals and the healthcare system.[4] Individuals with pressure ulcers have increased awareness about their pain, reduced quality of life, and limited abilities to participate in activities and rehabilitation. The amount of healthcare resources to manage the care of individuals with pressure ulcers in addition to frequent hospital stays is staggering.[5] The *pressure ulcer cost-of-illness* has been calculated to be at least 1% of the total Dutch healthcare budget and 4% of the United Kingdom healthcare budget.[6,7] In the United States, the Centers for Medicare & Medicaid Services (CMS) reported that the cost of treating a pressure ulcer in acute care, as a secondary diagnosis, in 2008 was $43,180.00 per hospital stay.[8–10] In the United States, the cost of litigation adds to the burden of healthcare costs, especially in long-term care, where 87% of settlements against facilities are awarded to the plaintiffs.[11] Therefore, addressing the overall management of pressure ulcers is now a prominent national healthcare issue in many western countries. Despite advances in healthcare, pressure ulcers remain a major cause of morbidity and mortality.

Both *poor nutritional intake* and *poor nutritional status* have been identified as the key risk factors for pressure ulcer development and protracted wound healing. Notwithstanding methodological shortcomings, cross-sectional and prospective studies suggest a fairly strong correlation between malnutrition and pressure ulcer development.[12–15] Malnutrition is a status of nutrition in which a deficiency, excess, or imbalance of energy, protein, and other nutrients causes measurable adverse effects on tissue, body structure, body function, and clinical outcome. The studies related to pressure ulcers have mostly focused on the relationship between pressure ulcers and undernutrition. Multivariate analysis of epidemiological data indicates that poor nutritional status and related factors, such as low body weight and poor oral food intake, are independent risk factors for pressure ulcer development.[16–18] Moreover, it appears that many acute and chronically ill as well as elderly individuals at risk for pressure ulcer development or with established pressure ulcers suffer from undesired weight loss.[17–20] A recent study from Shahin et al on the relationship between malnutrition parameters and pressure ulcers

in German hospitals and nursing homes clearly established a significant relationship between the presence of pressure ulcers and undesired weight loss (5%–10%). Inadequate and poor nutritional intake was strongly related to the presence of pressure ulcers in both healthcare settings as well.[21]

These findings confirm the importance of adequate nutritional care in individuals prone to pressure ulcer development, especially since malnutrition is a reversible risk factor for wounds (including pressure ulcers), unless the individual has a terminal illness.

Pathophysiology

In the NPUAP and EPUAP clinical practice guideline on pressure ulcer prevention and treatment, a pressure ulcer is defined as a localized injury to the skin and/or underlying tissue, usually over a bony prominence, as a result of pressure or pressure in combination with shear.[22] The external mechanical loading of the skin can be a force perpendicular to the skin surface (direct pressure), a force parallel to the skin surface (shear), or a combination of both. Depending on the magnitude, time duration, and type of the mechanical load, the mechanical and geometrical properties of the tissues, as well as the susceptibility of the individual, ischemia as a result of the deformation of the tissues will lead to hypoxia. In addition, blocking of the nutrient supply and blocking of waste product removal combined with a subsequent change in pH will eventually lead to tissue damage. Finally, reperfusion after a period of ischemia may increase the ultimate cell death damage. The resultant tissue necrosis may cause local injured tissue alterations and even further exacerbate the damage.[22]

The development of pressure ulcers depends on extrinsic and intrinsic risk factors. The most important extrinsic risk factors are pressure, shear, and friction, which lead to mechanical loading and secondary damage to the skin and soft tissue. Intrinsic factors have an effect on tissue viability and consequently influence the pathophysiological response to mechanical loading. Studies have found significant associations with age, sex, limited activity, care dependency, incontinence (bowel and bladder), acute disease (eg, infection), and nutritional status. The relative influence of each of these intrinsic risk factors is still unclear.[22]

Pressure Ulcer Risk Assessment, Prevention, and Treatment

Pressure ulcer risk assessment. Based on targeted parameters, risk assessment aimed at identifying susceptible individuals is of utmost importance in daily clinical practice. Next to the overall clinical assessment of general health status and, related to this, the possible diseases affecting tissue perfusion and sensory perception (eg, cardiovascular diseases, diabetes, and neurological diseases), pressure ulcer risk assessment should be performed in a structured, interprofessional way and should include activity, mobility, the skin's viability and moisture, and nutritional status.

Pressure ulcer risk assessment scales can be used to support risk assessment. Several widely used risk assessment scales include the Waterlow pressure sore risk scale and the Braden scale, which consists of 6 items referring to sensory perception, skin moisture, activity, mobility, nutritional status, and the extent of friction and shear forces.[23,24] In scientific research, risk assessment scales in general appear to have a poor predictive value, yet the advice is to incorporate them in the daily care process because they can be regarded as a means of alerting healthcare professionals to the possibility of pressure ulcers. Their use indeed may lead to structural systematic assessment and a stimulus for treatment of pressure ulcer risk within the healthcare organization.

Pressure ulcer prevention.[22] After establishing pressure ulcer risk or pressure ulcer diagnosis, preventive measures should be initiated. Relevant preventive measures include:

- Regular inspection of the skin for signs of redness in individuals identified as being at risk of pressure ulceration together with the use of skin emollients to hydrate dry skin
- Reduction of the duration and magnitude of pressure on vulnerable areas of the body by repositioning at-risk individuals in combination with using pressure redistribution surfaces, such as mattresses, beds, seats, and cushions
- Optimization of the individual's general health condition, including improvement of mobility and nutritional status.

Pressure ulcer treatment.[22] In the case of a confirmed pressure ulcer, therapeutic measures must be taken directly and in agreement with an additional comprehensive assessment of the individual involved. During the course of the treatment, the aforementioned preventive measures remain in force.

Curative intervention consists primarily of appropriate wound care to encourage tissue repair as much as possible. This process includes cleaning the wound (removal of any necrosis, disinfection, and cleansing of the wound) and application of appropriate wound dressings. Sometimes surgical interventions may be indicated.

In addition, attention must be paid to the individual's general health status, the management of secondary infection, pain, and psychosocial suffering, and, last but not least, adequate nutritional care.

Basic Aspects of Wound Healing

Healing of pressure ulcers is a complex process directly influenced by the status of the local wound environment and also by the overall physical condition of the individual. The wound healing process involves the overlapping sequential stages of blood coagulation, inflammation, migration and proliferation of defense and repair cells (eg, neutrophils, macrophages, lymphocytes, endothelial cells, fibroblasts, and keratinocytes), remodelling of tissue structure, scar formation, and maturation. To promote wound healing, several endogenous factors are crucial. One such factor is the body's ability to generate an adequate inflammatory and defense response to manage the bacterial burden of the wound and to create the required enzymatic environment needed for the various wound repair tasks. These tasks include prevention of ischemia-reperfusion damage and counteracting of oxidative damage; removal of devitalized tissue; prevention of cell migration; epidermal-mesenchymal interactions during keratinocyte migration; angiogenesis; remodelling of newly synthesized connective tissue during maturation; and regulation of growth factor activities. In the total process of wound repair, nutrients also play an important role.

Role of Nutrients in Wound Healing

Carbohydrates, fats, and proteins supply the energy source (kilocalories) for the body. Consumption of adequate kilocalories supports collagen and nitrogen synthesis for healing. External consumption also promotes anabolism by sparing the body's endogenous protein from being used as an energy source.[25] When the energy from carbohydrates and fats fails to meet the body's requirements, glucose is synthesized by the liver and kidney from non-carbohydrate sources, such as protein or amino acids. Gluconeogenesis occurs when the nitrogen is removed from the amino acid that is part of the protein structure leaving the carbon skeleton that can be used as an energy source by the body. When visceral protein stores in the muscle are converted to glucose, the caloric requirement needed to promote anabolism and reverse catabolism (a breakdown of protein and other body energy sources) is increased. The decline in lean body mass can lead to muscle wasting, loss of subcutaneous tissue, and poor wound healing.

Fat. Fat, the most concentrated source of kilocalories, transports the fat-soluble vitamins (A, D, E, and K) and provides insulation under the skin and padding to bony prominences. Meats, eggs, dairy products, and vegetable oils contain fat.

Protein and amino acids. Protein is the only nutrient containing nitrogen and is composed of amino acids that form the building blocks of protein. Protein is important for tissue perfusion, preservation of immune function, repair and synthesis of enzymes involved in wound healing, cell multiplication, and collagen and connective tissue synthesis. Protein is required to compensate for the nitrogen lost through pressure ulcer skin breakdown and exudate.[26]

Foods that provide all 9 essential amino acids, such as meat, poultry, fish, eggs, milk products, and soybeans, are considered complete proteins. Essential or indispensable amino acids must be obtained from the diet. The body requires an adequate supply of the essential amino acids plus enough nitrogen and energy to synthesize the 11 other amino acids. Legumes, grains, and vegetables contain incomplete proteins, meaning they are lacking or low in one or more of the essential amino acids.

During periods of stress or trauma, such as injury, wound healing, or sepsis, certain amino acids, such as arginine and glutamine, become conditionally essential. *L-arginine*, which is 32% nitrogen, has been shown in some studies to increase concentrations of hydroxyproline, which is an amino acid that is a constituent of collagen and an indicator of collagen deposition and protein in the wound site.[27,28] Desneves et al conducted a randomized controlled trial to measure pressure ulcer healing for 3 groups of subjects using the Pressure Ulcer Scale for Healing (PUSH) scores. One group received a standard hospital diet. A second group received the standard hospital diet plus 2 high-calorie supplements totalling 500 Kcalories, 18 g of protein, 72 mg of vitamin C, and 7.5 mg of zinc. The third group received the standard diet plus 2 high-calorie supplements totalling 500 Kcalories, 21 g of protein, 9 g of added arginine, 500 mg of vitamin C, and 50 mg of zinc. The third group noted a reduction in the PUSH score (indicating clinical improvement) when they consumed the oral nutritional supplement containing arginine.[29] This was a small study of 16 people. In a randomized controlled trial, van Anholt et al discovered significantly reduced PUSH scores and significantly faster wound healing in non-malnourished individuals aged 18 to 90 years with normal body mass indices (BMIs), no undesired weight loss, and stage III or stage IV pressure ulcers who received an oral nutritional supplement with arginine, protein, zinc, ascorbic acid, and vitamin E.[30] Additional research is needed to determine the impact of using arginine alone or combined with other nutrients.[31]

While it has been shown that inflammatory cells within the wound use *glutamine* for proliferation and as a source of energy, studies on the effectiveness of consuming supplements containing glutamine are inconclusive.[32]

Water. Water is distributed throughout the body in our intracellular, interstitial, and intravascular compartments and serves as the transport medium for moving nutrients to the cells and removing waste products. Fluids are the solvent for minerals, vitamins, amino acids, glucose, and other small molecules, thus enabling them to diffuse into and out of cells.

Individuals with draining wounds, emesis, diarrhea, increased insensible loss due to elevated temperature, or increased perspiration require additional fluids to replace lost fluid.[33] Water constitutes 60% of an adult's body. The elderly individual generally has increased body fat and decreased lean body mass, resulting in a decreased percentage of water stored. The decrease in water stored coupled with a declined sense of thirst places the elderly at risk for dehydration. Schols et al noted that illness and warm weather are contributing factors to dehydration in the elderly.[34] Hydration needs are met with liquids plus the water content of food, which accounts for 19% to 27% of the total fluid intake of healthy adults.[35] Adequate intake of fluids for healthy adults is 2.7 L/day for women and 3.7 L/day for men. This includes all beverages as well as the moisture content of food.

Vitamins and minerals. The role of micronutrients that are assumed to promote wound healing is debatable. Ascorbic acid (vitamin C), a water-soluble vitamin, is a cofactor with iron during the oxidation of proline and lysine in the production of collagen. Hence, a deficiency of vitamin C prolongs the healing time and contributes to reduced resistance to infection.[36] The Dietary Reference Intake (DRI) of 70–90 mg/day of vitamin C is achieved with the consumption of fruits and vegetables, such as citrus fruits, tomatoes, potatoes, and broccoli. Most oral nutritional supplements provide ascorbic acid along with calories, protein, and other vitamins and minerals. Mega doses of ascorbic acid have not resulted in accelerated pressure ulcer healing.[37]

Vitamin A and vitamin E are fat-soluble vitamins, and the dietary intake of these vitamins comes from a variety of foods. Vitamin A acts as a stimulant during the wound healing process to increase collagen formation and promote epithelization. Mega doses of vitamin A above 3,000 ug of the DRI's Tolerable Upper Limit (UL), the maximum level of daily nutrient intake that is likely not to pose concern, should not be recommended without consultation with the physician. Vitamin E acts as an antioxidant, and the DRI can easily be met with food and/or a multivitamin, unless a deficiency is confirmed.

Zinc, a cofactor for collagen formation, also metabolizes protein, liberates vitamin A from storage in the liver, and assists in immune function. Individuals who have large draining wounds, poor dietary intake over an extended time, or excessive gastrointestinal losses may trigger a zinc deficiency. Unless a deficiency is confirmed, elemental zinc supplementation, above the UL of 40 mg/day, is not recommended for individuals with pressure ulcers.[38,39] *Copper* is an essential mineral for collagen cross-linking. Zinc and copper com-

pete for the same binding site on the albumin molecule, thus high serum zinc levels interfere with copper metabolism, inducing a copper deficiency.[40,41] If deficiencies are suspected, a multivitamin with minerals may be appropriate. Check the nutrient analysis of oral nutritional supplements or enteral formulas recommended to individuals with pressure ulcers, since they usually contain additional micronutrients.

Nutritional Screening and Assessment

Screening and assessment of nutritional status should be part of the prevention and treatment plan for individuals at risk for pressure ulcer development and those with pressure ulcers.

Nutritional screening. Unless the individual has a terminal illness, under-nutrition is a reversible risk factor for pressure ulcer development, making early identification and management critical. Individuals at risk for pressure ulcer development may also be in danger of under-nutrition, so nutritional screening should be completed.[17–20,26,42] Healthcare organizations should have a policy on nutritional screening and its frequency. Screening should be completed upon admission to a healthcare setting and with each condition change. Since individuals frequently move from one healthcare setting to another, the screening results must be documented and communicated from one care setting to another.[26,43] Screening tools should be quick and easy to use, validated, and reliable for the patient population served.[44] Any qualified healthcare professional may complete a screening. Validated screening tools are more widely used in Europe than in the United States. In a cross-sectional study, Langkamp-Henken et al noted an advantage to using the *Mini-Nutritional Assessment (MNA)* and the *MNA short form (MNA-SF)* over using visceral protein when screening and assessing nutritional status.[45,46] The MNA-SF was revised to 6 questions and revalidated for adults age 65 and older and has an 80% sensitivity and specificity and a 97% positive predictive value according to clinical status.[47] The *Malnutrition Universal Screening Tool (MUST)* was validated in acute care, long-term care, and the community and identifies those individuals who are underweight or at risk for under-nutrition.[48] The MUST tool uses

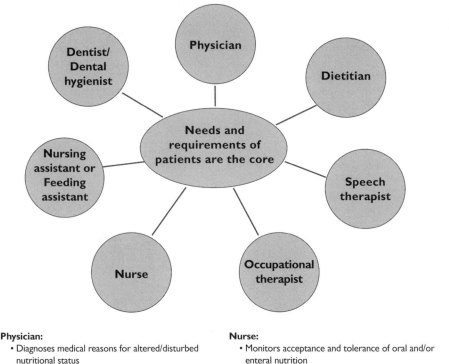

Physician:
- Diagnoses medical reasons for altered/disturbed nutritional status
- Responsible for ordering all medications and treatments

Dietitian:
- Completes nutrition assessment and estimates nutrition/hydration requirements
- Provides dietary recommendations and monitors nutritional status

Speech Therapist:
- Screens and evaluates chewing and swallowing ability
- Determines training compensation and recommends food/fluid consistency

Occupational Therapist:
- Assesses feeding skills and/or recommends techniques to improve motor skills
- Recommends appropriate position for eating and/or self-help feeding devices, ie, special utensils

Nurse:
- Monitors acceptance and tolerance of oral and/or enteral nutrition
- Alerts physician, dietitian, and patient of changes in nutritional status, such as meal refusal, and changes in weight or hydration status

Nursing Assistant or Feeding Assistant:
- Delivers food (trays) and provides feeding assistance, if needed
- Alerts nurse and/or other team members of refusal of or decline in oral intake

Dentist/Dental Hygienist:
- Assesses oral/dental status (eg, inflamed gums, oral lesions, denture problems)
- Offers oral healthcare

Figure 1. Nutrition for pressure ulcer prevention and treatment is interprofessional care.

5 steps to establish nutritional risk and determine a plan of care. First, the height and weight are recorded to determine BMI. In step 2, percentage of unplanned weight loss is recorded. In step 3, established acute disease effect is scored. In step 4, the previous 3 scores are added to obtain the overall risk of malnutrition, and step 5 uses either the management guide or local policy to develop a plan of care.

When the screening tool triggers a nutrition assessment, timely referral to the appropriate professionals is critical. Conditions requiring immediate assessment and intervention include unplanned weight loss, dysphagia, poor appetite or the inability to consume adequate food or fluid, and pressure ulcers or other wounds. The registered dietitian (RD) completes the nutrition assessment and collaborates and communicates with the other healthcare team members. In addition to the RD, the members of the nutritional team include the speech therapist who is responsible for screening, evaluating, and treating swallowing problems; the occupational therapist who works to strengthen the individual's ability to feed him or herself; and the nursing staff whose responsibilities include monitoring factors, such as mood, pain, and dentition, which can affect oral intake. The physician is responsible for the overall care of the individual and ordering any treatments recommended by the team (Figure 1).

Nutrition assessment. Nutrition assessment is a methodical process of obtaining, verifying, and interpreting data in order to make decisions about the basis of nutrition-related problems. The American Dietetic Association (ADA) Nutrition Care Process includes 4 steps:

- Nutrition assessment
- Nutrition diagnosis
- Nutrition intervention
- Nutrition monitoring and evaluation.[49]

The assessment includes obtaining anthropometric measurements; evaluating visual signs of poor nutrition, oral status, chewing/swallowing ability, and/or diminished ability to eat independently; and interpreting and analyzing medical, nutritional, and biochemical data along with food-medication interactions.

Anthropometrics. Anthropometric measurements include height, weight, and BMI. Obtaining accurate height and weight is important, since these values are the basis for calculating BMI and caloric requirements. Individuals should be weighed on a calibrated scale at the same time of the day and wearing the same amount of clothing. Specialty beds often are equipped with a device to weigh an immobile individual. The RD evaluates the severity of the weight loss, considering the effect of recent surgery, diuretic therapy, and other traumatic events. Significant weight loss places an individual at increased nutritional risk and has a negative effect on wound healing. Several studies support the theory that *unintentional weight loss of 5% in 30 days or 10% in 180 days is a predictor of mortality in the elderly.*[50–53] During the interview with the individual or care-

giver, the RD/clinician asks what the usual body weight has been over the past few months. Usual body weight is used to calculate the percentage of weight lost or gained over time thus determining the significance of any weight change.

BMI, an index of an individual's weight in relationship to his or her height, is calculated as weight (kg)/height (m^2), or weight (lb)/height (in^2) x 705. BMI is highly correlated with body fat, but increased lean body mass or a large body frame can also increase the BMI. It is generally agreed that a normally hydrated individual with a BMI $\geq$ 30 is obese and an individual with a BMI less than 20 is considered underweight. The National Pressure Ulcer Long Term Care Study (NPULS) of residents in nursing homes who were at risk for developing a pressure ulcer reported that more than 50% of the residents had a 5% weight loss during a 12-week study, and 45.6% were considered underweight (defined by a BMI of 22 or less). Residents with the highest percentage of weight loss more often had a recent pressure ulcer.[54] Under-nutrition has been defined in the literature as protein and energy deficiency often associated with coexisting deficiencies of micronutrients, which is reversed solely by nutrients.[55] Unintentional weight loss, poor food intake, and the inability to eat independently impact the healing process.[56]

The obese individual is also at risk for pressure ulcer development, and healing may be delayed when the diet consumed is inadequate in nutrients, including protein. When pressure ulcer healing is the goal, the interprofessional team should evaluate the risks versus the benefits of recommending a low-calorie diet.

Nutrition-focused clinical examination. The interprofessional team, including the RD, should examine the individual for physical signs of under-nutrition and protein depletion as evident by changes in the hair, skin, or nails, such as thin, dry hair; brittle nails; or cracked lips. Individuals with missing or decayed teeth or ill-fitting dentures often reduce their intake of difficult-to-chew protein foods, thus restricting their caloric intake and increasing the chance for weight loss. If untreated, individuals with swallowing problems or dysphagia may become dehydrated, lose weight, and develop pressure ulcers. Loss of dexterity and/or the ability to self-feed is a risk factor

Table 1. Recommendations of the NPUAP/EPUAP Guideline[22]

Adapted with permission of the European Pressure Ulcer Advisory Panel and the National Pressure Ulcer Advisory Panel. Prevention and treatment of pressure ulcers: quick reference guide. Washington, DC: National Pressure Ulcer Advisory Panel; 2009.

Nutrition for Pressure Ulcer Prevention

General Recommendations

1. Screen and assess the nutritional status of every individual at risk for pressure ulcer development in each healthcare setting.
    1.1. Use a valid, reliable, and practical tool for nutritional screening that is quick and easy to use and acceptable to both the individual and the healthcare worker.
    1.2. Establish and implement a nutritional screening policy in all healthcare settings, along with recommended frequency of screening.
2. Refer each individual with nutritional risk and pressure ulcer risk to a registered dietitian and also, if needed, to a multidisciplinary nutritional team that includes a registered dietitian, a nurse specializing in nutrition, a physician, a speech and language therapist, an occupational therapist, and, when necessary, a dentist.
    2.1. Provide nutritional support to each individual with nutritional risk and pressure ulcer risk, following the nutrition cycle. This support should include:
    • Nutritional assessment
    • Estimation of nutritional requirements
    • Comparison of nutrient intake with estimated requirements
    • Provision of appropriate nutritional intervention, based on appropriate feeding route
    • Monitoring and evaluation of nutritional outcome, with reassessment of nutritional status at frequent intervals while the individual is at risk.
    2.2. Follow relevant and evidence-based guidelines on enteral nutrition and hydration for individuals at risk for pressure ulcer development who show nutritional risk or nutritional problems.
    2.3. Offer each individual with nutritional risk and pressure ulcer risk a minimum of 30–35 kcal/kg/day, with 1.25–1.5 g/kg/day protein and 1 mL of liquid intake per kcal per day

Specific Recommendations: Nutrition Prevention

1. Offer high-protein mixed oral nutritional supplements and/or tube feeding, in addition to the usual diet, to individuals with nutritional risk and pressure ulcer risk because of acute or chronic diseases or following surgical intervention (strength of evidence = A).
    1.1. Administer oral nutritional supplements and/or tube feeding in between the regular meals to avoid reduction of normal food and fluid intake during regular mealtimes (strength of evidence = C).

often resulting in poor oral intake. All of these conditions are roadblocks to wound healing.

Biochemical data. Analysis of current laboratory values is one component of the nutrition assessment. Biochemical assessment data must be used with caution because values can be altered by hydration, medication, and changes in metabolism. There is not one specific laboratory test that can expressly determine an individual's nutritional status. Serum hepatic proteins including albumin, prealbumin (transthyretin), and transferrin may not correlate with the clinical observation of nutritional status.[57] Serum albumin has a long half-life (12–21 days), and multiple factors, such as infection, acute stress, hydration, and excess cortisone, decrease the albumin level, making it a poor indicator of visceral protein status. Edema depresses albumin levels and dehydration falsely elevates both prealbumin and albumin levels. Low albumin levels may manifest the presence of inflammatory cytokine production or other comorbidities rather than poor nutritional status (eg, from the local wound bed or a systemic inflammatory process).[58] Prealbumin also decreases

Table 1. Recommendations of the NPUAP/EPUAP Guideline[22] *continued*

Adapted with permission of the European Pressure Ulcer Advisory Panel and the National Pressure Ulcer Advisory Panel. Prevention and treatment of pressure ulcers: quick reference guide. Washington, DC: National Pressure Ulcer Advisory Panel; 2009.

Nutrition for Pressure Ulcer Healing

Role of Nutrition in Pressure Ulcer Healing

1. Screen and assess nutritional status for each individual with a pressure ulcer at admission and with each condition change and/or when progress toward pressure ulcer closure is not observed (strength of evidence = C).

    1.1. Refer all individuals with pressure ulcers to the dietitian for early assessment and intervention for nutritional problems (strength of evidence = C).

    1.2. Assess weight status for each individual to determine weight history and significant weight loss from usual body weight (≥ 5% change in 30 days or ≥ 10% in 180 days) (strength of evidence = C).

    1.3. Assess the individual's ability to eat independently (strength of evidence = C).

    1.4. Assess the adequacy of total nutrient intake (food, fluid, oral supplements, enteral/parenteral feedings) (strength of evidence = C).

2. Provide sufficient calories (strength of evidence = B).

    2.1. Provide 30–35 kcal/kg for individuals with a pressure ulcer under stress. Adjust formula based on weight loss, weight gain, or level of obesity. Individuals who are underweight or who have had significant unintentional weight loss may need additional kilocalories to cease weight loss and/or regain lost weight (strength of evidence = C).

    2.2. Revise and modify (liberalize) dietary restrictions when limitations result in decreased food and fluid intake. These adjustments are to be managed by a dietitian or medical professional (strength of evidence = C).

    2.3. Provide enhanced foods and/or oral supplements between meals if needed (strength of evidence = B).

    2.4. Consider nutritional support (enteral or parenteral nutrition) when oral intake is inadequate. This must be consistent with the individual's goals (strength of evidence = C).

3. Provide adequate protein for positive nitrogen balance for an individual with a pressure ulcer (strength of evidence = B).

    3.1. Offer 1.25–1.5 g/kg/day protein for an individual with a pressure ulcer when compatible with the goals of care and reassess as condition changes (strength of evidence = C).

    3.2. Assess renal function to ensure that high levels of protein are appropriate for the individual (strength of evidence = C).

4. Provide and encourage adequate daily fluid intake for hydration (level of evidence = C).

    4.1. Monitor individuals for signs and symptoms of dehydration: changes in weight, skin turgor, urine output, elevated serum sodium, or calculated serum osmolality (strength of evidence = C).

    4.2. Provide additional fluid for individuals with dehydration, elevated temperature, vomiting, profuse sweating, diarrhea, or heavily draining wounds (strength of evidence = C).

5. Provide adequate vitamins and minerals (strength of evidence = B).

    5.1. Encourage consumption of a balanced diet that includes good sources of vitamins and minerals (strength of evidence = B).

    5.2. Offer vitamin and mineral supplements when dietary intake is poor or deficiencies are confirmed or suspected (strength of evidence = B).

with metabolic stress, inflammation, infection, and surgical trauma. Studies indicate that hepatic proteins may correlate with the severity of illness rather than with nutritional status.[58-65]

Since the blood carries oxygen to the wound bed, anemia may have an adverse effect on wound healing. Blood loss, poor dietary intake, malabsorption, and increased iron needs are causes of anemia. Biochemical data used to diagnose iron-deficiency anemia include low hemoglobin and hematocrit, low mean corpuscular volume (MCV), low serum iron, low ferritin, and elevated total iron-binding capacity (TIBC). Treatment for iron-deficiency anemia is oral iron therapy.

Older adults often have pernicious anemia or *vitamin B12 deficiency* that is caused by inadequate intrinsic factor. The prevalence of anemia[66] increases with each decade of life after age 70. Without adequate intrinsic factor, vitamin B12 cannot be properly absorbed. Laboratory results include low hemoglobin, hematocrit, and serum B12; normal or elevated MCV; and elevated serum iron, ferritin, folate, and homocysteine. There are several ways to supply vitamin B12, but the monthly injection is most effective. Some individuals with low B12 levels respond to daily intake of oral B12 with the suggested dose of 1000 IU or to the use of nasal sprays or patches.

Diet history. The *diet history* includes consultation with the individual and/or caregivers to determine the type, quantity, and frequency of food usually consumed by the individual. Questions about any vitamin, mineral, or herbal supplements taken by the individual should also be noted. The healthcare team should consider any factors that may influence the individual's decision about nutrition, such as culture, tradition, religion, and belief systems of ethnic and minority groups. Often, culture or religion strongly influence food intake and may affect nutritional status. Since the individual is the center of the wound care model, recommendations for nutritional interventions should incorporate the values and beliefs of the individual.

Nutrition Intervention

Ultimately, the nutrition assessment will lead to a nutrition diagnosis and nutritional support.

The cycle for both prevention and treatment should include:
• Nutrition assessment
• Estimation of nutritional requirements
• Comparisons of intake with estimated requirements
• Provision of appropriate nutrition intervention, based on appropriate feeding route
• Monitoring and evaluation of nutritional outcome, with reassessment of nutritional status at frequent intervals.

Early nutrition intervention and subsequent monitoring of the nutritional plan can reverse poor outcomes associated with under-nutrition and promote healing. Caloric, protein, and fluid requirements should be individualized and increased or decreased, depending on the assessed requirement of the individual. Hypermetabolic conditions, such as infection, stress, and trauma, require calories above the baseline requirements. *Renal function should be assessed routinely to ensure that high levels of protein are appropriate.*[67] The interprofessional team should frequently review the type and amount of food and fluid consumed by the individual to determine when fortified foods and/or oral nutritional supplements should be incorporated into the treatment plan. Fortified foods include commercial products, such as cereal, soup, cookies, or dairy products enriched with additional calories and protein, or enriched menu items prepared by the staff of a care facility.

Research supports the theory of providing oral nutritional supplements to reverse under-nutrition, prevent pressure ulcer occurrence, and promote pressure ulcer healing.[68-70] As previously noted, *oral nutritional supplements* provided in addition to the diet for non-malnourished individuals also decreased the healing time.[30] One study noted that individuals who consume oral nutritional supplements between meals, in addition to the usual diet, experience better absorption of nutrients.[71]

Therapeutic or restricted diets often result in unappealing meals that are refused, thus delaying wound healing. The American Dietetic Association's 2010 position statement noted that "the quality of life and nutritional status of older adults residing in healthcare communities can be enhanced by individualization to the least restrictive diet appropriate."[72]

When normal oral intake is inadequate to promote healing, **enteral or parenteral nutrition** is considered if it is consistent with the individual's goal of overall treatment. The interprofessional team should discuss the risks and benefits with the individual or his or her caregiver. When the gut is functioning, enteral feeding via oral nutritional supplements in addition to the diet or total tube feeding is the preferred route. Provision of an adequate nutrient supply can lower the incidence of metabolic abnormalities, reduce septic morbidity, and improve survival rates. However, research fails to show the benefit of initiating enteral tube feeding to improve pressure ulcer healing rates.[73,74]

The **NPUAP/EPUAP guideline** on prevention and treatment of pressure ulcers is the most recently published international guideline on pressure ulcer care.[22] The guideline was developed following a systematic, comprehensive review of peer-reviewed, published research on pressure ulcers from January 1998 to January 2008 and will be updated routinely as new research becomes available. This guideline also gives the most relevant recommendations regarding nutritional care for individuals prone to pressure ulcer development (Table 1).

Conclusion

Nutrition is a key element in pressure ulcer prevention and the treatment of individuals with pressure ulcers. The early identification of under-nutrition and the correction of nutritional deficits prevent pressure ulcer occurrence, promote pressure ulcer healing, and improve the individual's quality of life. Nutritional care has to be incorporated into integrated and multidisciplinary pressure ulcer care, performed by a dedicated interprofessional team. In order to achieve optimal nutrition for each individual prone to pressure ulcer development, goals should be evaluated frequently and revised with each condition change or when progress toward healing is not occurring. The amount and type of nutritional support should be consistent with medical goals and the individual's wishes. While each member of the interprofessional team has a distinct role in the care and treatment of the individual prone to pressure ulcer development, collaboration, communication, complementariness, and continuity are fundamental to benefit the individuals involved.

Practice Pearls
- Screen and assess the nutritional status of individuals at risk for or with pressure ulcers and determine appropriate interventions.
- Encourage consumption of a balanced diet, which includes good sources of calories, protein, vitamins, and minerals.
- Provide enriched food and/or oral nutritional supplements between meals, if appropriate and consistent with the person's overall plan of care.

Self-Assessment Questions

1. The appropriate daily kilocalories for an individual with a category/stage IV pressure ulcer weighing 120 pounds (54.5 kg) is:
   A. 1,100 kilocalories
   B. 1,650 kilocalories
   C. 1,909 kilocalories
   D. 1,275 kilocalories

2. The non-malnourished individual with a category/stage III pressure ulcer may benefit from:
   A. An oral nutritional supplement with calories, protein, vitamin A, and copper
   B. A balanced 2,200 kilocalorie diet plus a vitamin supplement
   C. A 1,200 kilocalorie diet plus 1,000 mg of ascorbic acid and 220 mg of zinc sulfate
   D. An oral nutritional supplement with added protein, arginine, zinc, vitamin C, and vitamin E

3. Mr. B has a wound infection, a draining pressure ulcer, and a fever. Wound healing can be facilitated by increasing:
   A. Fluid
   B. Vitamin C
   C. Iron
   D. Protein

Answers: 1-C, 2-D, 3-A

References

1. Vanderwee K, Clark M, Dealey C, Gunningberg L, Defloor T. Pressure ulcer prevalence in Europe: a pilot study. *J Eval Clin Pract.* 2007;13(2):227–235.
2. National Pressure Ulcer Advisory Panel. Cuddigan J, Ayello EA, Sussman C, eds. *Pressure Ulcers in America:*

Prevalence, Incidence, and Implications for the Future. Reston, VA: NPUAP; 2001.

3. Russo CA, Steiner C, Spector W. Hospitalizations related to pressure ulcers among adults 18 years and older, 2006. Available at: http://www.hcup-us.ahrq.gov/reports/statbriefs/sb64.jsp. Accessed December 22, 2008.

4. Hopkins A, Dealey C, Bale S, Defloor T, Worboys F. Patient stories of living with a pressure ulcer. *J Adv Nurs.* 2006;56(4):345–353.

5. Allman RM, Goode PS, Burst N, Bartolucci AA, Thomas DR. Pressure ulcers, hospital complications, and disease severity: impact on hospital costs and length of stay. *Adv Wound Care.* 1999;12(1):22–30.

6. Severens JL, Habraken JM, Duivenvoorden S, Frederiks CM. The cost of illness of pressure ulcers in The Netherlands. *Adv Skin Wound Care.* 2005;15(2):72–77.

7. Bennet G, Dealey C, Posnett J. The cost of pressure ulcers in the UK. *Age Ageing.* 2004;33(3):230–235.

8. Centers for Medicare & Medicaid Services. Proposed fiscal year 2009 payment, policy changes for inpatient stays in general acute care hospitals. Available at: http://www.cms.hhs.gov/apps/media/press/factsheet.asp?Counter=3045&intNumPerPage=10&checkDate=&checkKey=&srchType=1&numDays=3500&srchOpt=0&srchData=&keywordType=All&chkNewsType=6&intPage=&showAll=&pYear=&year=&desc=&cboOrder=date. Accessed December 3, 2008.

9. Centers for Medicare & Medicaid Services. Medicare program; proposed changes to the hospital inpatient prospective payment systems and fiscal year 2009 rates; proposed changes to disclosure of physician ownership in hospitals and physician self-referral rules; proposed collection of information regarding financial relationships between hospitals and physicians; proposed rule. Federal Register. 2008;73(84):23550. Available at: http://edocket.access.gpo.gov/2008/pdf/08-1135.pdf. Accessed December 3, 2008.

10. Dorner B, Posthauer ME, Thomas D; National Pressure Ulcer Advisory Panel. The role of nutrition in pressure ulcer prevention and treatment: National Pressure Ulcer Advisory Panel white paper. *Adv Skin Wound Care.* 2009;22(5):212–221.

11. Voss AC, Bender SA, Ferguson ML, Sauer AC, Bennett RG, Hahn PW. Long-term care liability for pressure ulcers. *J Am Geriatr Soc.* 2005;53(9):1587–1592.

12. Pinchcofsky-Devin GD, Kaminski MV Jr. Correlation of pressure sores and nutritional status. *J Am Geriatr Soc.* 1986;34(6):435–440.

13. Thomas DR. The role of nutrition in prevention and healing of pressure ulcers. *Clin Geriatr Med.* 1997;13(3):497–511.

14. Berlowitz DR, Wilking SV. Risk factors for pressure sores. A comparison of cross-sectional and cohort-derived data. *J Am Geriatr Soc.* 1989;37(11):1043–1050.

15. Green SM, Winterberg H, Franks PJ, Moffatt CJ, Eberhardie C, McLaren S. Nutritional intake in community patients with pressure ulcers. *J Wound Care.* 1999;8(7):325–330.

16. Guenter P, Malyszek R, Bliss DZ, et al. Survey of nutritional status in newly hospitalized patients with stage III or stage IV pressure ulcers. *Adv Skin Wound Care.*

2000;13(4 Pt 1):164–168.

17. Thomas DR, Verdery RB, Gardner L, Kant A, Lindsay J. A prospective study of outcome from protein-energy malnutrition in nursing home residents. *JPEN J Parenter Enteral Nutr.* 1991;15(4):400–404.

18. Mathus-Vliegen EMH. Clinical observations: nutritional status, nutrition, and pressure ulcers. *Nutr Clin Pract.* 2001;16:286–291.

19. Ek AC, Unosson M, Larsson J, Von Schenck H, Bjurulf P. The development and healing of pressure sores related to the nutritional state. *Clin Nutr.* 1991;10(5):245–250.

20. Kerstetter JE, Holthausen BA, Fitz PA. Malnutrition in the institutionalized older adult. *J Am Diet Assoc.* 1992;92(9):1109–1116.

21. Shahin ES, Meijers JM, Schols JM, Tannen A, Halfens RJ, Dassen T. The relationship between malnutrition parameters and pressure ulcers in hospitals and nursing homes. *Nutrition.* 2010;26(9):886–889.

22. National Pressure Ulcer Advisory Panel and European Pressure Ulcer Advisory Panel. Prevention and treatment of pressure ulcers: clinical practice guideline. Washington, DC: NPUAP; 2009.

23. Bergstrom N, Braden BJ, Laguzza A, Holman V. The Braden Scale for Predicting Pressure Sore Risk. *Nurs Res.* 1987;36(4):205–210.

24. Jalali R, Rezaie M. Predicting pressure ulcer risk: comparing the predictive validity of 4 scales. *Adv Skin Wound Care.* 2005;18(2):92–97.

25. Clark M, Schols JM, Benati G, et al; European Pressure Ulcer Advisory Panel. Pressure ulcers and nutrition: a new European guideline. *J Wound Care.* 2004;13(7):267–272.

26. Stratton RJ, Green CJ, Elia M. *Disease-Related Malnutrition: An Evidence-Based Approach to Treatment.* Oxon, UK: CABI Publishing; 2003.

27. Kirk SJ, Hurson M, Regan MC, Holt DR, Wasserkrug HL, Barbul A. Arginine stimulates wound healing and immune function in elderly human beings. *Surgery.* 1993;114(2):155–160.

28. Barbul A, Lazarou SA, Efron DT, Wasserkrug HL, Efron G. Arginine enhances wound healing and lymphocyte immune responses in humans. *Surgery.* 1990;108(2):331–337.

29. Desneves KJ, Todorovic BE, Cassar A, Crowe TC. Treatment with supplementary arginine, vitamin C and zinc in patients with pressure ulcers: a randomised controlled trial. *Clin Nutr.* 2005;24(6):979–987.

30. van Anholt RD, Sobotka L, Meijer EP, et al. Specific nutritional support accelerates pressure ulcer healing and reduces wound care intensity in non-malnourished patients. *Nutrition.* 2010;26(9):867–872.

31. Langer G, Schloemer G, Knerr A, Kuss O, Behrens J. Nutritional interventions for preventing and treating pressure ulcers. *Cochrane Database Syst Rev.* 2003;(4):CD003216.

32. Ziegler TR, Benfell K, Smith RJ, et al. Safety and metabolic effects of L-glutamine administration in humans. *JPEN J Parenter Enteral Nutr.* 1990;14(4 Suppl):137S–146S.

33. Thomas DR, Cote TR, Lawhorne L, et al; Dehydra-

tion Council. Understanding clinical dehydration and its treatment. *J Am Med Dir Assoc.* 2008;9(5):292–301.

34. Schols JM, De Groot CP, van der Cammen TJ, Olde Rikkert MG. Preventing and treating dehydration in the elderly during periods of illness and warm weather. *J Nutr Health Aging.* 2009;13(2):150–157.

35. Institute of Medicine of the National Academies. Dietary Reference Intakes: Water, Potassium, Sodium, Chloride, and Sulfate. Available at: http://iom.edu/Reports/2004/Dietary-Reference-Intakes-Water-Potassium-Sodium-Chloride-and-Sulfate.aspx. Accessed June 5, 2010.

36. Ronchetti IP, Quaglino D Jr, Bergamini G. Ascorbic acid and connective tissue. In: Harris JR, ed. *Subcellular Biochemistry Volume 25 Ascorbic Acid: Biochemistry and Biomedical Cell Biology.* New York: Plenum Press; 1996:249–264.

37. Ter Riet G, Kessels AG, Knipschild PG. Randomized clinical trial of ascorbic acid in the treatment of pressure ulcers. *J Clin Epidemiol.* 1195;48(12):1453–1460.

38. Institute of Medicine of the National Academies. *Dietary Reference Intakes: The Essential Guide to Nutrient Requirements.* Washington, DC: The National Academies; 2006.

39. Cataldo CB, DeBruyne LK, Whitney EN. *Nutrition and Diet Therapy, Principles and Practice.* Belmonth, CA: Wadsworth; 2003.

40. Reed BR, Clark RA. Cutaneous tissue repair: practical implications of current knowledge. II. *J Am Acad Dermatol.* 1985;13(6):919–941.

41. Goode HF, Burns E, Walker BE. Vitamin C depletion and pressure sores in elderly patients with femoral neck fracture. *BMJ.* 1992;305(6859):925–927.

42. Elia M, Zellipour L, Stratton RJ. To screen or not to screen for adult malnutrition? *Clin Nutr.* 2005;24(6):867–884.

43. Kondrup J, Allison SP, Elia M, Vellas B, Plauth M; Educational and Clinical Practice Committee, European Society of Parenteral and Enteral Nutrition (ESPEN). ESPEN guidelines for nutrition screening 2002. *Clin Nutr.* 2003;22(4):415–421.

44. Ferguson M, Capra S, Bauer J, Banks M. Development of a valid and reliable malnutrition screening tool for adult acute hospital patients. *Nutrition.* 1999;15(6):458–464.

45. Langkamp-Henken B, Hudgens J, Stechmiller JK, Herrlinger-Garcia KA. Mini nutritional assessment and screening scores are associated with nutritional indicators in elderly people with pressure ulcers. *J Am Diet Assoc.* 2005;105(10):1590–1596.

46. Hudgens J, Langkamp-Henken B, Stechmiller JK, Herrlinger-Garcia KA, Nieves C. Immune function is impaired with a mini nutritional assessment score indicative of malnutrition in nursing home elders with pressure ulcers. *JPEN J Parenter Enteral Nutr.* 2004;28(6):416–422.

47. Kaiser MJ, Bauer JM, Ramsch C, et al; MNA-International Group. Validation of the Mini Nutritional Assessment short-form (MNA-SF): a practical tool for identification of nutritional status. *J Nutr Health Aging.* 2009;13(9):782–788.

48. BAPEN (British Association of Parenteral and Enteral Nutrition) Malnutrition Advisory Group, The MUST Report, Nutritional screening of adults: a multidisciplinary responsibility. Available at: http://www.bapen.org.uk/must_tool.html. Accessed June 3, 2011.

49. American Dietetic Association. *International Dietetics & Nutrition Terminology (IDNT) Reference Manual: Standardized Language for the Nutrition Care Process.* 3rd ed. Chicago, IL: The American Dietetic Association; 2011.

50. Landi F, Onder G, Gambassi G, Pedone C, Carbonin P, Bernabei R. Body mass index and mortality among hospitalized patients. *Arch Intern Med.* 2000;160(17):2641–2644.

51. Ryan C, Bryant E, Eleazer P, Rhodes A, Guest K. Unintentional weight loss in long-term care: predictor of mortality in the elderly. *South Med J.* 1995;88(7):721–724.

52. Sullivan DH, Johnson LE, Bopp MM, Roberson PK. Prognostic significance of monthly weight fluctuations among older nursing home residents. *J Gerontol A Biol Sci Med Sci.* 2004;59(6):M633–M639.

53. Murden RA, Ainslie NK. Recent weight loss is related to short-term mortality in nursing homes. *J Gen Intern Med.* 1994;9(11):648–650.

54. Horn SD, Bender SA, Bergstrom N, et al. Description of the National Pressure Ulcer Long-Term Care Study. *J Am Geriatr Soc.* 2002;50(11):1816–1825.

55. ASPEN Board of Directors and the Clinical Guidelines Task Force. Guidelines for the use of parenteral and enteral nutrition in adult and pediatric patients. *JPEN J Parenter Enteral Nutr.* 2002;26(1 Suppl):1SA–138SA.

56. Gilmore SA, Robinson G, Posthauer ME, Raymond J. Clinical indicators associated with unintentional weight loss and pressure ulcers in elderly residents of nursing facilities. *J Am Diet Assoc.* 1995;95(9):984–992.

57. Myron Johnson A, Merlini G, Sheldon J, Ichihara K; Scientific Division Committee on Plasma Proteins (C-PP), International Federation of Clinical Chemistry and Laboratory Medicine (IFCC). Clinical indications for plasma protein assays: transthyretin (prealbumin) in inflammation and malnutrition. *Clin Chem Lab Med.* 2007;45(3):419–426.

58. Mahan LK, Escott-Stump S, eds. *Krause's Food, Nutrition, & Diet Therapy.* St Louis, MO: WB Saunders (Elsevier); 2008.

59. Shenkin A. Serum prealbumin: Is it a marker of nutritional status or of risk of malnutrition? *Clin Chem.* 2006;52(12):2177–2179.

60. Lim SH, Lee JS, Chae SH, Ahn BS, Chang DJ, Shin CS. Prealbumin is not a sensitive indicator of nutrition and prognosis in critical ill patients. *Yonsei Med J.* 2005;46(1):21–26.

61. Robinson MK, Trujillo EB, Mogensen KM, Rounds J, McManus K, Jacobs DO. Improving nutritional screening of hospitalized patients: the role of prealbumin. *JPEN J Parenter Enteral Nutr.* 2003;27(6):389–395.

62. Bachrach-Lindstrom M, Unosson M, Ek AC, Arnqvist HJ. Assessment of nutritional status using biochemical and anthropometric variables in a nutritional intervention study of women with hip fracture. *Clin Nutr.* 2001;20(3):217–223.

63. Fuhrman MP, Charney P, Mueller CM. Hepatic proteins and nutrition assessment. *J Am Diet Assoc.* 2004;104(8):1258–1264.

64. Steinman TI. Serum albumin: its significance in patients with ESRD. *Semin Dial.* 2000;13(6):404–408.

65. Dutton J, Campbell H, Tanner J, Richards N. Pre-dialysis serum albumin is a poor indicator of nutritional status in stable chronic hemodialysis patients. *EDTNA ERCA J.* 1999;25(1):36–37.

66. American Medical Directors Association (AMDA). *Anemia in the Long-Term Care Setting.* Columbia, MD: American Medical Directors Association; 2007.

67. Clinical practice guidelines for nutrition in chronic renal failure. K/DOQI, National Kidney Foundation. *Am J Kidney Dis.* 2000;35(6 Suppl 2):S1–S140.

68. Horn SD, Bender SA, Ferguson ML, et al. The National Pressure Ulcer Long-Term Care Study: pressure ulcer development in long-term care residents. *J Am Geriatr Soc.* 2004;52(3):359–367.

69. Bergstrom N, Horn SD, Smout RJ, et al. The National Pressure Ulcer Long-Term Care Study: outcomes of pressure ulcer treatments in long-term care. *J Am Geri-*

atr Soc. 2005;53(10):1721–1729.

70. Bourdel-Marchasson I, Barateau M, Rondeau V, et al. A multi-center trial of the effects of oral nutritional supplementation in critically ill older inpatients. *Nutrition.* 2000;16(1):1–5.

71. Wilson MM, Purushothaman R, Morley JE. Effect of liquid dietary supplements on energy intake in the elderly. *Am J Clin Nutr.* 2002;75(5):944–947.

72. Dorner B, Friedrich EK, Posthauer ME; American Dietetic Association. Position of the American Dietetic Association: individualized nutrition approaches for older adults in health care communities. *J Am Diet Assoc.* 2010;110(10):1549–1553.

73. Henderson CT, Trumbore LS, Mobarhan S, Benya R, Miles TP. Prolonged tube feeding in long-term care: nutritional status and clinical outcomes. *J Am Coll Nutr.* 1992;11(3):309–325.

74. Mitchell SL, Kiely DK, Lipsitz LA. The risk factors and impact on survival of feeding tube placement in nursing home residents with severe cognitive impairment. *Arch Intern Med.* 1997;157(3):327–332.

How to Read, Understand, and Interpret Quantitative Research

M. Gail Woodbury, PhD, BScPT, MAPWCA;

Jack Meintjes, MBChB, DOM, FCPHM(SA) Occ Med, MMed(Occ Med);

Christina Lindholm, PhD, RN

Objectives

The reader will be challenged to:

- Analyze how the research question determines the research study design and how the design affects interpretation of the results
- Consider how even with the best study design the project may be poorly conducted and how this affects the study's interpretation and usefulness for guiding practice
- Reflect on how situations with less than the best study designs have been used, how such studies may provide at least preliminary information about a topic, and how one would interpret these studies for practice, eg, case study or case series rather than randomized controlled trials (RCT) to provide information about the intervention
- Analyze the use of appropriate outcome measures or endpoints in studies and the effect of their use on interpretation of studies
- Gain comprehension of a few biostatistical basics.

Introduction

Evidence-based practice (EBP) is the goal of health-care practitioners across all professions who are working in wound care around the world. Evidence-based medicine (EBM), a term that can be used interchangeably with EBP, originally was defined as the "conscientious, explicit, and judicious use of current best evidence in making decisions about the care of individual patients." It involves "integrating individual clinical expertise with the best available external clinical evidence from systematic research" and patient choice.[1] Patient choice involves the patient's values — preferences, concerns, and expectations — as well as circumstances, ie, clinical state and clinical setting.[2]

How does one achieve EBP? It requires practitioners to read, understand, and interpret research literature and then to use it to inform practice. Greenhalgh said that EBP requires practitioners to read the *right papers* at the *right time*, to alter their behavior, and then to influence the behavior of other people — which is often more difficult — in the light of what they found.[3]

The objectives of this chapter are to provide some basic information about research evidence, to discuss how research quality affects interpretation of findings (acceptance, rejection, or caution), and to excite interest in gaining these important skills. Using the topic of *therapy*, we will indicate the best study designs and explain how the studies should be interpreted when conducted well and how the studies should be interpreted when conducted poorly or if

Woodbury MG, Meintjes J, Lindholm C. How to read, understand, and interpret quantitative research. In: Krasner DL, Rodeheaver GT, Sibbald RG, Woo KY, eds. *Chronic Wound Care: A Clinical Source Book for Healthcare Professionals.* Vol 1. 5th ed. Malvern, PA: HMP Communications; 2012:131–140.

Table 1. Sample size determination based on considerations	
Consideration	**Explanation**
Type I error	Risk of finding significance by chance alone: Usually the significance or alpha (α) level is set at 0.05, which means that 5 times out of 100 or 1 out of 20, significance will be found by chance rather than because of a true difference. Sometimes the α level is set higher, at $P = .10$, when the researcher is looking for associations between variables.
Type II error	Risk of not finding significance when there is a true difference: The beta (β) level is usually set at 0.20, which gives 80% statistical power. This means that 20% of the time, a true difference will not be detected statistically. When the impact of missing finding a difference is vital, the statistical power might be set as high as 90%, but the disadvantage is the need for a much larger sample.
Clinically important difference	Amount of difference that is relevant, set by the investigator: A big difference is hard to detect. A small difference may not be real or relevant.
Feasibility	The number of subjects that can be recruited realistically.

other than the best study designs are used. We will also discuss endpoints or outcomes that are most appropriate and the effect on study interpretation when less than the best outcomes are used. Finally, we will present some biostatistical issues and their interpretations as they apply to therapy.

Study Designs: What They Are and Why They Matter

Each research study is designed to answer a specific research question. The research question should include information about the *Population* (patients/subjects), *Intervention* that is applied, *Comparison* (or control) group, *Outcomes* (outcome measures), and *Time* (if applicable), ie, *PICO(T)*.[3] Different types of research questions are best answered by specific research designs.[4]

Clinicians need to assess various research designs when they read and critically evaluate individual studies or integrated studies (studies in which the information from individual studies has been synthesized). Levels of evidence have been proposed based on the appropriateness of the research study design to answer the research question within each category of research (eg, therapy, diagnosis, prognosis). The Oxford Centre for Evidence-Based Medicine produced

one of the best known classification systems for evidence and in 2011 released a newly revised version.[5] The study designs, their potential flaws, and their strengths for answering various research questions will be discussed within the therapy research category.

Therapy and Study Design

Healthcare clinicians are particularly interested in the therapies or interventions that are reputed to "work," ie, to be efficacious. The best individual study research design for evaluating therapy is the *randomized controlled trial (RCT)* because it has the least potential of introducing bias. The RCT is a prospective, experimental study design in which as many aspects of the study as possible are controlled, eg, subject selection, random allocation, implementation of the study intervention and control intervention (or placebo), follow-up of subjects, blinding, and measurement of outcome. Sample subjects from a target population are allocated randomly to receive an intervention of interest or comparison intervention, which might be a placebo or sham. Sometimes there are more than 2 groups with group outcomes measured and compared. An appropriate sample size to aid interpretation of

	Table 2. The Oxford 2011 Levels of Evidence for Therapy[5]
1	Systematic review of randomized trials or n-of-1 trials
2	Randomized trial or observational study with dramatic effect
3	Non-randomized controlled cohort/follow-up study
4	Case-series, case-control studies, or historically controlled studies
5	Mechanism-based reasoning

the results of a statistical hypothesis test is determined in advance. When a statistical test is done, if too big a sample has been used, a difference could be detected even if there is not one. If too small a sample is used, it will not be possible to detect a difference even if there is one. (Table 1 lists considerations for the determination of sample size. *Power analysis* is defined in the glossary.) Random allocation is required in an effort to achieve equivalence of the groups, ie, to reduce the differences in demographic and clinical variables between the groups that might affect outcome and thus mask or exaggerate the effect of the intervention.

Systematic error or bias is the difference between the true treatment effect and the observed effect that is measured in a study. Although we can never really know the true effect, researchers make every effort to minimize bias in all its forms through careful research study design. The potential for systematic error exists in all research studies and designs and will be discussed for each design.

The individual study at the top of the *evidence hierarchy* for therapy is the RCT. This design is regarded as providing the most robust individual study evidence for superiority or inferiority of, for example, devices for wound management. Table 2 lists the Oxford 2011 Levels of Evidence for therapy.[5] Sometimes several individual studies are combined and the topic synthesized to provide clinicians with a pre-appraised topic. For example, a *systematic review of RCTs* provides a higher level of evidence as illustrated in Table 2. The sample size is larger, and therefore, the ability to detect a treatment effect, if one exists, is greater.

For therapy, a systematic review of homogeneous RCTs is considered the highest level of evidence. Clinicians who use the findings of a systematic review accept that the critical appraisal done by others, eg, the Cochrane group or other individuals, was done appropriately.

After the RCT, for individual studies, the next levels of evidence are *observational studies*, ie, cohort studies and case-control studies, in which the interventions and comparisons are naturally occurring. The investigator does not conduct the interventions but rather finds situations in which they occur naturally and documents what is being done (the treatment and control situations) and the outcomes that result.

A *cohort study* is usually prospective (looking forward in time). When used to evaluate therapy, a cohort study involves following a sample of subjects who are treated perhaps in different settings with different interventions, eg, an intervention of interest in one facility and a comparison intervention or no intervention in another facility. Outcomes of both situations are compared. These studies lack the kinds of controls that are possible in a RCT. For example, the groups are not likely to be equivalent, and this on its own could affect outcome. The interventions are unlikely to be conducted uniformly, and the comparisons also will not be uniform. This means that in order to see an effect, these studies usually must be very large. The greatest concern is the possibility that other variables, called *confounding variables*, will interfere in the study and the confounding variables — rather than the interventions — will produce the observed results. Therefore, a key component of these studies must be statistical handling and

Table 3. Examples of outcomes or endpoints[6]
Biomarkers
Change in wound condition
Circulation
Costs and resources used
Dressing performance
Infection signs (reduction of infection signs)
Bioburden
Quality of life
Pain reduction
Symptoms, signs
Reduction rate (eg, wound size, edema)
Wound closure
Healing time

discussion of potentially confounding variables.

Case-control studies are usually retrospective (looking backward in time). There are 2 groups: the case group includes subjects who have a particular outcome and the control group includes subjects who do not have the outcome. Working backward from the outcomes, the groups are studied to determine the extent to which they have been treated or not treated using the intervention of interest, another intervention, or none for comparison. Often these studies are done by chart review to determine the relationship of the outcome, which could be healing versus non-healing, to the subject characteristics and interventions that were done in the past. A major limitation of case-control studies is the inadequacy of patient charts and the inability to direct the information that is available. Similar to cohort studies, a major consideration in

case-control studies is the potential influence of confounding variables, so these must be recognized, handled appropriately using statistics, and discussed realistically.

A therapy or intervention can be evaluated using *observational study designs*, such as cohort studies and case-control studies. However, the risk of bias is greater with observational study designs than with RCTs. Circumstances that might necessitate the use of observational study designs include situations where randomization is unethical or when the cost of conducting an RCT is prohibitive. Sometimes a very good cohort or case-control study provides more accurate information than a poorly conducted RCT. *All of these studies — RCTs, cohort studies, and case-control studies — have comparison or control groups. This is essential for attributing causation — that the intervention was the cause of the outcome.* Without the comparison group, eg, case study or case series, this point cannot be made.

To interpret the results of cohort studies and case-control studies used to evaluate an intervention, several factors must be considered. If sources of bias are minimized, confounding variables are accounted for, and there is a large effect, the results can be accepted with considerable confidence. In the Oxford 2011 levels of evidence document from the Oxford Centre for Evidence-Based Medicine, such a study would be considered as highly as a good RCT.[5] However, if sources of bias are not controlled and confounding variables are not accounted for, whether there was a large effect or not, the results would have to be interpreted with great caution.

All of the aforementioned studies are examples of *quantitative research* that is done to determine if a therapy or intervention works or at least helps, and quantitative researchers want to obtain the most unbiased answer. *Qualitative research* cannot answer this question in relation to therapy, but it is done to add meaning. It is particularly suited for certain wound-related research questions that are subjective, eg, pain.

There are different types of qualitative studies. For example, *phenomenology* investigates an experience as it is lived. *Grounded theory* investigates social problems. *Ethnography* investigates cultures. Historical studies provide a narrative description of past events.

Endpoints or Outcomes in Wound Research Evaluating Therapy

Gottrup et al[6] thoroughly discussed the question of endpoints and outcomes. Table 3 lists some wound research outcomes or endpoints.

Appropriate Study Endpoints or Outcome Measures

Examples of primary outcomes of interest to clinicians include wound healing, reduction of exudate or malodor, and pain reduction. Wound healing might be the primary outcome, but there may be other outcomes, including **surrogate endpoints** (see the glossary). The research question determines the correct endpoints or outcomes. For example, for evaluating silver dressings, the primary outcome should not necessarily be wound healing but rather reduction of wound surface critical colonization. For evaluating treatment of malignant wounds, reduction of odor or bleeding may be an important primary endpoint rather than healing. The primary outcome as well as secondary and surrogate outcomes should be clearly stated in the study purpose and methodology sections. Rapid wound closure might not always be the prime outcome.

Appropriate Comparison

At different stages in our understanding of the effect of an intervention, different control or comparison groups are needed. In early stages, research questions of **efficacy and safety** might be needed for regulatory purposes (The Medical Devices Directive MDD 93/42/ECC), and the comparison would probably be a placebo or sham control group. In situations testing a variation of an intervention that is known to be effective, it would not be appropriate to use a sham control. From an ethical perspective, the new variation would have to be tested in relation to the intervention used in standard practice. Another issue is whether the device is **cost effective** in clinical use. An RCT is not always mandatory for regulatory purposes but sometimes is mandatory for reimbursement. Choice of control or comparison group should be based on the best available product, which might vary

from country to country. In many studies, gauze dressings act as a control. This has been questioned, since gauze dressings are no longer the treatment of choice in most cases.

Biostatistics for RCTs

Biostatistics, as a field of study, refers to:

1. Mathematical figures that summarize and describe a group of patients or subjects in a study (eg, proportion with ulcers, mean number of healed ulcers), referred to as **sample statistics**
2. Estimated numbers in the target populations to which the findings of a specific study could be applied or generalized, referred to as **population parameters**.

In addition to bias or systematic error, the other threat to research studies is random error, and this is accounted for using biostatistics. In the analysis of an RCT, a comparison is made between the treatment group and the control group. Depending on the outcome in which the researcher is interested, the analysis can be done in a number of ways:

1. Comparing the incidence rates (or incidence densities) of a specific outcome (eg, healing of a wound) in the treatment group to the control group by dividing the incidence rate (or incidence density) of the intervention group by the incidence rate (or incidence density) of the control group: If the **relative risk**, as this is called, is equal to one, it means that the incidence rates (or incidence densities) in both groups are equal. If the value is larger than one, it means that the incidence rate (or incidence density) in the intervention group is larger than what was found in the control group.
2. Comparing the incidence rates (or incidence densities) of a specific outcome (eg, wound healing) in the treatment group to the control group by subtracting the incidence rate (or incidence density) found in the control group from what was found in the intervention group: If the **risk difference**, as this is called, is equal to zero, it means that the incidence rates (or incidence densities) in both groups are equal. If the value is larger than one, it means that the incidence rate (or incidence density) in the intervention group is larger.

3. If numerical data are used in the analysis, another summary measure could be used in the comparison, eg, a *comparison of the means*. In a study of electrical stimulation (ES) compared with sham ES applied to chronic leg ulcers, Houghton et al[7] reported the outcome in terms of mean decrease from initial wound surface area over the 4-week treatment period. The ES group showed a mean decrease of 44.3%, which was more than 2 times greater than that observed in wounds treated with sham units (mean decrease 16.0%).[7]

Interpreting Results

For each study you read, ask yourself the following questions:

- **What is the research question?** Do I know everything I need to know, ie, PICO(T)?
- **Has the appropriate study design been used to answer the question?**
  o If so, has the study been done well?
  o If not utilizing the best study design, is the study conducted in such a way that it will answer the research question?
  o For both instances, does the research include the following: adequate sample size (justified), reasonable comparison, appropriate outcome measures, correct statistical handling, and sensible interpretation by paper authors in relation to study limitations?

Examples of Studies and Interpretation

Consider the following questions: Is compression therapy beneficial for healing in patients with leg ulcers? What is the best method of compression? Franks et al[8] provided an example of a good "real life" or effectiveness study in which subjects were not chosen for their ability to show a good outcome. A total of 166 subjects with leg ulcers were randomly allocated to one of two class II below-knee types of marketed compression stockings. The 18-month recurrence rate was 24% of 92 subjects in one group and 32% of 74 subjects in the other group. The rate is the number of people who experienced

recurrence divided by the total number of people times 100 to express the rate as a percentage, ie, 22/92 x 100 = 24% and 24/74 x 100 = 32%. The statistical difference between these rates has a P value, $P = .353$. Because the P value is greater than .05, the difference in recurrence rate between the 2 groups is not statistically significant. There is no difference. (See Appendix for information about rates and P values.)

Another finding in the study was an *overall relative risk (RR) of recurrence* of 1.16 with 95% confidence interval (CI) of 0.65 to 2.04.[8] Relative risk equalling 1.0 would indicate that using compression stockings made no difference to the recurrence rate. The observed value of 1.16 really is not different from 1.0, and the 95% CI from 0.65 to 2.04 includes 1.0 and confirms this. Based on the information observed in this sample, we would say that we are 95% confident that the population value, the true value, lies between 0.65 and 2.04 and this interval contains 1.

However, in a systematic review that involved the combined results of 39 RCTs, O'Meara et al[9] found that ulcers healed more rapidly with the use of multi-component compression than with single-component compression but that even single-component compression was more effective than not using compression. This systematic review is much more informative, because by combining the findings of several studies, it indicates the types of compression that are effective.

In another RCT example, negative pressure wound therapy (NPWT) was compared with advanced moist wound therapy (AMWT).[10] It was reported that NPWT is more effective in achieving diabetic wound closure and preventing secondary amputations: 10.2% of patients in the AMWT comparison group versus 4.1% in the NPWT group ($P = .035$). The interpretation of this P value for the sample is that the NPWT group had significantly fewer secondary amputations than the comparison group that was receiving standard care.

Vermeulen et al conducted a systematic review to determine whether silver-containing agents should be advocated for the treatment of infected or contaminated wounds. No significant difference in complete wound healing was found for subjects treated with silver-containing agents compared with standard foam dressings.[11] This review, therefore, did not provide conclusive evidence to support the use of silver-containing agents. Does this mean that silver dressings do not work? Does it mean that possibly there are better outcome measures that might have been used or that the studies in the review were too small or heterogeneous? The review highlights the need for additional well designed studies on this topic.

Conclusion

Evidence-based wound care should be based on best available scientific evidence, clinical experience, and patients' values.[1] Keeping up with the deluge of research literature is a challenge, but understanding it is a greater challenge that requires ongoing learning. Recognizing and differentiating study designs is a first step. Research study designs and their potential sources of bias are well described in research textbooks and many references.[6,12–14]

It is important to understand that not all research is equal — some studies are well conducted and others are less well conducted. All researchers try to do the best they can, but the reality of research is that it is hard to get a large enough sample, that subjects are really just patients with all their complexities, that staff conducting projects have competing responsibilities and skill levels, that the best outcome measures vary according to the audience for the study and country, and that statistics cannot fix everything. However, we need the best evidence in wound care that we can create.

The study of wounds is relatively new, and evidence to justify the use of various therapies is limited. In addition, the quality of existing studies is affected by small sample sizes, inadequate follow-up periods, non-random allocation to groups, lack of blinding, lack of control or comparison groups, or poor description or interventions.[6] More wound research is needed, and everyone in the wound community needs to help. Clinicians can help by telling researchers their clinical questions, and researchers can help clinicians by providing reasonable interpretations of research results and bringing them to the bedside. We all need to gain a better understanding of research so that we can interpret what we read intelligently.

Practice Pearls

- The research question dictates the best research study design. To evaluate if a therapy works, the RCT is considered the best individual study design because bias is minimized.
- Non-randomized and observational research designs, considered lower levels of evidence, can be appropriate if their potential limitations are expertly handled in the conduct, statistical analysis, and discussion of the study.
- Biostatistics explain the magnitude of research study results.

Glossary

Power refers to the statistical probability that the null hypothesis will be rejected (finding significance) if it is false (when there is no difference).

Power analysis is conducted to determine the statistical power of a study in which a statistical effect or difference has not been detected. A calculation is done using the considerations for sample size (Table 1) with power $(1 - \beta)$ being the determination of interest. The power would be expressed as 80% or 67%. Researchers usually try to achieve at least 80% power.

Surrogate endpoints are easily measurable outcomes, such as physical signs or lab findings that are not primary endpoints but reflect important endpoints. The classical example in medical clinical studies is the use of the immediate and simple outcome reduction in blood pressure instead of reduction in stroke or heart attacks.

Type I error refers to the error of rejecting a true null hypothesis, ie, finding significance when there is not a true difference.

Type II error refers to the error of failing to reject a false null hypothesis, ie, not finding significance when there is a true difference.

Appendix

What is a rate?

A rate is a quotient of 2 numbers. The numerator and denominator are usually assessed in the same time.

A rate is used to describe the rapidity of

events and can be used for quantities of the same or of different natures. It describes the speed of events over time, for example:
- 30 runs in 5 cricket overs indicates a run rate of 6 runs per over
- 6 failed students for every 100 enrolled students indicates an expected failure rate of 6% per year
- 76 heart beats in 60 seconds indicates a heart rate of 76 beats per minute
- 22 of 92 = 24% and 24 of 74 = 32% in the Franks et al article.[8]

Notice that the **same time** applies to the numerator and denominator. The runs and the overs in the cricket example occurred in the same time; the students who are enrolled and the students who fail do so in the same year, etc.

What does the *P* value mean?

A *P* value is used to indicate something about the population (ie, persons who will see the researcher in the future and not the persons who were in the study). A *P* value is the result of a statistical hypothesis test, of which there are many (eg, Chi-squared, McNemar, Student's t-test). The actual calculation of the *P* value is beyond the scope of this text, but the basics of statistical hypothesis testing follow.

After a researcher has performed a study in which 2 groups of participants (A and B) were compared, the researcher would have calculated one of the measures of association to compare the values found in the 2 groups of participants. If the researcher found that (for instance) the incidence rate in group A differs from the incidence rate in group B, he would like to know whether this difference is also true for the population (ie, patients who were not part of the study but who will be seen in the future). The statistician can perform a hypothesis test to indicate what is likely to be seen in the population.

The statistician will consider 2 hypotheses, called the **null-hypothesis (H_0)** and the **alternative hypothesis (H_A)**. After performing the appropriate hypothesis test and finding the *P* value, the researcher can then make certain statements about H_0. Irrespective of the specific findings in the study participants, H_0 will always assume that there is no difference between the 2 measures that are compared *in the population*. For our hypothetical example, the 2 hypotheses will be the following:

	Hypotheses	Meaning/Interpretation
H_0	A = B	The incidence rate of the population represented by group A in the study is exactly the same as the incidence rate of the population represented by group B in the study.
H_A	A ≠ B	There is a difference between the incidence rates of the population as represented by group A and group B in the study (the one incidence rate is larger or smaller than the other one).

Using the *P* value:

After stating the 2 hypotheses and performing the statistical hypothesis test, the researcher can now make a decision about the null-hypothesis, based on the *P* value.

If the *P* value is small (by convention, "small" means $P < .05$), the null-hypothesis is *rejected*. If the *P* value is large (by convention, "large" means $P > .05$), the null-hypothesis is *not rejected*.

The following facts should be noted:
- The hypothesis test uses the study data to say something about patients who will be seen in the future. The *P* value thus refers to future patients and not to the findings of the study (for which the real data exist).
- If a study is not performed correctly, the statistician can still calculate a *P* value, but this may not represent the "truth" in future patients. The *P* value should thus be interpreted with caution and always within the context of the study that was done.
- Neither H_0 nor H_A is ever "accepted." It is thus not possible to say with 100% certainty that the findings are correct (unless the whole population was studied). The *P*

value thus gives the researcher an indication of where to put his faith (in H_0 or H_A) based on the information provided by the study participants.

- If the null-hypothesis is rejected, we would then normally assume that the 2 values in the population are likely to be different. If the null-hypothesis is not rejected, we assume that the values in the population are likely to be the same.
- If the P value is small ($P < .05$), it does not indicate whether the difference between the 2 populations is large or small. It merely indicates whether there is a difference or not. This means that a P value of .00001 does not indicate a bigger difference than a P value of .02.

Examples

The following findings were published in a medical journal.

Example A: *Wound complications on the first visit were 44.4% in group A and 30.4% in group B ($P = .816$).*

Interpretation: In the study that was performed, group A had 14% more wound complications on the first visit than what was found in group B. However, when comparing the people in the population that is represented by group A and group B, there is likely no difference in the wound complications on the (future) first visit.

Example B: *The average pain intensity score was reduced from 6.3 at baseline to 2.8 at week 4 ($P < .001$).*

Interpretation: In the study that was performed, the average pain score for the study participants at baseline was 3.5 scores higher than the average pain score at week 4. For patients who will be seen in the future, the pain score at baseline is likely to be different from the pain score at week 4.

Example C: *Patients from the intervention group had in total 97% pressure ulcer-free days versus 94% in the control group ($P < .001$).*

Interpretation: In the study that was performed, it was found that participants who received the intervention had 3% more pressure ulcer-free days than those participants who did not have the intervention. For patients who will

receive the intervention in the future, there is likely to be a difference in the percentage of pressure ulcer-free days when they are compared to patients who will not receive the intervention in the future.

Self-Assessment Questions

1. Which of the following statements about research design for evaluating the effectiveness of therapy is correct?
   - A. The only appropriate individual study design is the RCT.
   - B. Observational study designs should never be used to evaluate therapy.
   - C. The RCT is the best individual study design for evaluating therapy because bias is minimized.
   - D. Case studies can be used to evaluate effectiveness of therapy.

2. How does one know if the research design for a study is correct?
   - A. The correct research design is the one that most appropriately answers the research question with the least bias.
   - B. The correct research design is the one that the researcher can afford.
   - C. The correct research design is the one that requires thousands of subjects.
   - D. The correct research design is the one that takes the least time.

Answers: 1–C, 2–A

References

1. Sackett DL, Rosenberg WM, Gray JA, Haynes RB, Richarson WS. Evidence based medicine: what it is and what it isn't. *BMJ*. 1996;312(7023):71–72.
2. Straus SE, Richardson WS, Glasziou P, Haynes RB. *Evidence-Based Medicine. How to Practice and Teach EBM*. 3rd ed. Toronto: Elsevier Churchill Livingstone; 2005.
3. Greenhalgh T. *How to Read a Paper. The Basics of Evidence-based Medicine*. 4th ed. West Sussex, UK: Wiley-Blackwell/BMJ Books; 2010.
4. Woodbury MG, Ayello EA, Harding K, Orsted HL, Queen D, Woo KY, Sibbald RG. Assessing and Measuring Evidence – Rethinking Gold Standards. Presented at the Symposium on Advanced Wound Care and Wound Healing Society Meeting in San Diego, CA, April 24–27, 2008.
5. Centre for Evidence-Based Medicine. CEBM (Centre for Evidence-Based Medicine) Levels of Evidence. Available at: http://www.cebm.net/mod_product/

design/files/CEBM-Levels-of-Evidence-2.1.pdf. Accessed November 7, 2011.

6. Gottrup F, Apelqvist J, Price P; European Wound Management Association Patient Outcome Group. Outcomes in controlled and comparative studies on non-healing wounds: recommendations to improve the quality of evidence in wound management. *J Wound Care*. 2010;19(6):237–268.

7. Houghton PE, Kincaid CB, Lovell M, et al. Effect of electrical stimulation on chronic leg ulcer size and appearance. *Phys Ther*. 2003;83(1):17–28.

8. Franks PJ, Oldroyd MI, Dickson D, Sharp EJ, Moffatt CJ. Risk factors for leg ulcer recurrence: a randomized trial of two types of compression stocking. *Age Aging*. 1995;24(6):490–494.

9. O'Meara S, Cullum NA, Nelson EA. Compression for venous leg ulcers. *Cochrane Database Syst Rev*. 2009;(1):CD000265.

10. Blume PA, Walters J, Payne W, Ayala J, Lantis J. Comparison of negative pressure wound therapy using vacuum-assisted closure to advanced moist wound therapy in the treatment of diabetic foot ulcers: a multicenter randomized controlled trial. *Diabetes Care*. 2008;31(4):631–636.

11. Vermeulen H, van Hattem JM, Storm-Versloot MN, Ubbink DT. Topical silver for treating infected wounds. *Cochrane Database Syst Rev*. 2007;(1): CD005486.

12. Margolis DJ. Wound care epidemiology. In: Krasner DL, Rodeheaver GT, Sibbald RG, eds. *Chronic Wound Care: A Clinical Source Book for Healthcare Professionals*. 4th ed. Malvern, PA: HMP Communications; 2007.

13. Bolton L, Dotson P, Kerstein MD. Controlled clinical trials versus case studies: why wound care professionals need to know the difference. In: Krasner DL, Rodeheaver GT, Sibbald RG, eds. *Chronic Wound Care: A Clinical Source Book for Healthcare Professionals*. 4th ed. Malvern, PA: HMP Communications; 2007.

14. Woodbury MG. Research 101: developing critical evaluation skills. *Wound Care Canada*. 2004;2(2):32–38.

The Outpatient Wound Clinic

Laurel A. Wiersema-Bryant, APRN, BC, CWS;
Linda A. Stamm, APRN, BC, CWS;
Jennifer A. Berry, FNP-BC;
John P. Kirby, MD, FCCWS, FACS

Objectives

The reader will be challenged to:

- Appraise the need for a dedicated outpatient facility for the coordination and care of patients with wounds
- Assess a wound clinic's ability to coordinate care across medical specialties and to concentrate the use of available resources, both personnel and supplies, to optimally heal wounds
- Fulfill the increased patient demand for wound care excellence as the field develops as an interprofessional specialty.

Introduction

This chapter presents the development of an outpatient wound clinic for the care and management of nonhealing and chronic wounds. The coordinated management of patients with wounds is the focus of an outpatient wound clinic. The concept of an interprofessional team approach to the care of patients with wounds is not new. Utilization of the team approach in the care and management of wounds has been encouraged in acute care and long-term care for some time. Data exist to support the influence of the team approach in achieving cost-effective outcomes.[1] Patients with wounds increasingly are being cared for in the outpatient arena. Reimbursement by third-party payers is largely for wound care given in the outpatient setting. A quick look at the practices in which these patients are being managed traditionally reveals home care, general practitioner offices, general surgery offices, dermatology, rheumatology, hematology/oncology, internal medicine, plastic surgery, orthopedic surgery, cardiology, and vascular surgery. Management of these patients is as varied as the practice settings, so coordination of care can be difficult.

In response to the increasing number of patients with nonhealing and chronic wounds, more wound clinics are being developed. A recent Internet search with the key word "wound clinic" was answered with 4,800,000 results in 0.17 seconds. The key word "wound center" was answered with 25,000,000 results in 0.13 seconds. While there were certainly duplicates in the responses, clearly the concept of moving the challenging wound care patient to a focused

Wiersema-Bryant LA, Stamm LA, Berry JA, Kirby JP. The outpatient wound clinic. In: Krasner DL, Rodeheaver GT, Sibbald RG, Woo KY, eds. *Chronic Wound Care: A Clinical Source Book for Healthcare Professionals.* Vol 1. 5th ed. Malvern, PA: HMP Communications; 2012:141–150.

Table 1. Client attributes for consideration

Attribute	Facility/Room Design	Equipment Needs
Ambulatory	• Routine • Easy access to parking helpful	• Standard
Wheelchair dependent	• ADA compatible • May need lift assist or ceiling-mounted lift • Evaluate width of doorways and ability to turn into rooms/hallways • Restrooms accessible	• Valet parking helpful • Wheelchairs near entrance • Lift equipment or lift orderlies/techs; check facility for lift policy • Consider ceiling lift in new construction
Stretcher/ambulance	• Easy access for ambulance to deliver • May require more time or additional space for wait for return trip	• Stretcher or bed
Weight challenged	• Exam rooms to accommodate bariatric furniture • Waiting room furniture to accommodate bariatric patients • Doorway/hallway access accommodates bariatric wheelchair/bed/stretcher • Bariatric restroom	• Bed or standing scale that weighs to 1,000 lb • Assorted sizes of blood pressure cuffs • Patient gowns in size 5X to 8X
Cultural diversity	• Exam room furniture to accommodate language interpreter, privacy curtain, etc.	• Mobile video phone if interpreter cannot be physically present

care center is widely accepted. A well planned, well coordinated wound care clinic provides comprehensive assessment, medical and surgical management, state-of-the-art treatment, and follow-up care. The clinic should not be conceived as a place of last resort for treatment failures but as a central place for the management of wounds and patient/caregiver education. This chapter will discuss the process of establishing a wound clinic, ongoing management of the clinic, and areas for further support for the practice of wound care and caring.

Establish the Need

The hospital and/or individuals planning for a wound healing center have several options when developing a model for the practice.[2] A hospital planning for a wound healing center may have the staff and financial support to develop the practice with little or no outside or commercial support. It is estimated that *opening a new practice may cost approximately $350,000 US to $500,000 US* in equipment, space construction/remodeling, and furnishings. The hospital planning committee will also need to develop procedure man-

uals, documentation tools, training costs for staff, recruitment and hiring of staff to supplement current employees, and a plan for ongoing salary needs. The hospital planning group will also want to plan for monitoring of outcomes and collection of data to monitor cost data and to identify persons skilled in maximizing reimbursement and insurance authorization.

Alternatively, *the planning group may elect to work with a commercial company to develop and manage the wound healing center*. The commercial entity then provides the staff, training, and practice policies and assumes the burden of the start-up costs and, in many cases, the salary expenses. This option transfers the cost of start-up and equipment needs to the industry sponsor. In return, the wound care company enters into a fee sharing or monthly management fee to operate the center.

A hybrid of the aforementioned options exists when a planning group retains a consultant to set up the wound healing center. This option allows the facility to maintain ownership of the practice while utilizing procedure manuals, quality assurance programs, documentation systems, and access to established treatment algorithms. The hospital retains ownership of the facility, equipment, billing, and staff hiring and salaries.

The business plan should incorporate the data obtained during the market research phase of the project. Key elements of the business plan include the introduction, vision and mission of the clinic, description of the business, market and competition analysis, product development, marketing and distribution plan, organizational plan, development schedule, financial plan, and executive summary. In determining the direction and focus of the wound clinic, it is important to write a mission statement. The **mission statement** should be global in scope and provide a shared sense of purpose, direction, and achievement both in terms of focusing the clinic and for team building among the clinic staff. Once written, the mission statement will help to define and focus the remainder of the plan. The plan should include both short-term (1 year) and long-term (3 to 5 years) goals. The **goals** should include, but not be limited to, patient visit volume projections, growth in the type of services provided, continued professional development of the clinic staff, research opportunities, monitors for success of the clinic, and cost savings to the institution (if hospital-based). Assuming the market research phase has supported the need for the wound clinic, there are a few additional operational issues that need to be assessed. These issues include the size and type of space needed by the expected population to be served, any special equipment that will be needed, and staffing needs.

A careful and critical look at the business side of the wound healing center is necessary early in the planning process. The selection of a strategy for the formation of the practice and business aspects of the center (or clinic) may prevent struggles in the future.

Needs Assessment

The initial step in the development of a wound clinic is the identification of the need for such a service. Market research must provide clear, concise information about the need for the clinic. *Utilize a marketing department, if available, to assist in the needs assessment process.* In gathering demographic information, a variety of sources may be used:

- Hospital/facility/health authority demographics of patient types
    - o Determine the geographic area of the population to be targeted for care
    - o Drill down to understand clinical needs of the population to be served (Table 1)
    - o Where are patients currently receiving care?
    - o Is there sufficient physician/provider commitment for appropriate patient referrals to maintain a stable patient volume?
- Demographic studies by the Centers for Disease Control and Prevention (CDC)/ consensus data
- Prevalence data on people with diabetes that may be included in the American Diabetes Association (ADA) database
- State and county health department databases
- American Association of Retired Persons (AARP) database

In essence, the marketing research refines the clinical needs of the patients the center will serve, how many patients the center will serve, and how they will reach the center.

The formation of a center for wound management and healing is a must for most hospitals, as the challenge of chronic wounds is complex and involves multifactorial problems and interprofessional solutions.

Services Offered

The identified needs of the population to be served must be carefully evaluated. The characteristics of the population to whom services will be offered will help to define the professional staff, support/clerical staff, physical design, and location of the wound healing center.

The wound healing center should have available the equipment and staff needed to perform the majority of diagnostic evaluations and treatment modalities within or in close proximity to the clinic. *Universal precautions should be employed for the entire patient population as indicated by the individual facility's policy and procedures.* Diagnostics needed may include radiologic evaluation, vascular laboratory testing, laboratory testing including analysis of blood chemistry and hematology, wound culture (quantitative), and

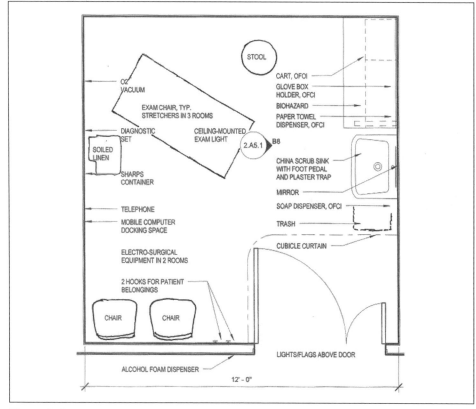

Figure 1. Basic room design.

pathology. Treatment modalities may include surgical intervention and debridement, hyperbaric oxygen, ultrasound therapy, offloading of the neuropathic foot/limb, application of tissue substitutes and grafts, and compression therapy. Planning should include a view to the future with respect to diagnostics and treatment modalities not yet available in clinical practice.

A survey monitoring *the evolving wound care clinic identified 6 basic themes with respect to practice expansion*.[3] The 6 themes are summarized as:

1. Increasing clinic volume
2. Addition of services not currently provided
3. Development of new clinic sites linked to the parent clinic
4. Addition of physician specialists to the clinic staff
5. Increased education
6. A contract with a management company.

Physical Space

The space needed requires a careful, thorough evaluation of the expected patient population. Figure 1 represents a standard exam room that will accommodate a standard exam table, a stretcher, a podiatric chair, or a bariatric exam table/chair. Other configurations exist for multiplace hyperbaric chambers and room configurations from a variety of online resources.

The current obesity epidemic highlights the need for logistical forethought to accommodate patients with special needs or handicaps. This information should be available as a result of the market research data. The following questions must be explored:

• Is existing space available for the clinic?
• Where is the space located?
• If the space is a multifunctional area, is the time needed to efficiently run the clinic available?
• If the clinic is open for patients on a part-

time basis, how will emergency calls/visits be handled?

- How and by whom is the staff to be trained? How will ongoing education be provided?
- How accessible is the location to patients?
- Do you anticipate patients arriving by ambulance, by wheelchair, or ambulatory?
- If the patients are wheelchair- or bed-bound, are stretcher-beds available for them in the facility?
- Is space available to accommodate stretcher- or bed-bound patients?
- If a patient requires lift or transfer assistance, is the clinic able to properly provide this?
- Is public transit available?
- Is accessible parking available?

Portable cautery that can be moved to exam rooms as needed for potential bleeding problems should be made available and staff should be trained on this equipment. Again, universal precautions should be employed for every patient and rooms stocked with protective equipment. Patients of high acuity will most likely need access to parenteral fluids, suction, and oxygen. If every patient exam room does not have these capabilities, patient scheduling is further complicated. If the room space available does not accommodate patients on stretchers, the type of patient seen may need to be restricted to those who are ambulatory or wheelchair-bound. Likewise, *if the appropriate lift equipment is not available, this equipment will need to be added to the start-up costs*. The time to turn a room around will be impacted negatively when patients must be held waiting for lift assistance or ambulance transport.

Staffing and Personnel

Methods of staffing the wound clinic and developing the organizational structure may take on a variety of forms. Generally, staffing requires a medical director and clinic manager, providers representing a variety of specialties, nurses skilled in performing wound care, and a secretary and/or receptionist. Larger clinics may include additional staff (eg, additional physicians specializing in areas not represented by a medical director, physical therapists, a dietitian, an orthoprosthetist, a social worker, home-health nurses, or a combination of these). Providers may be a combination of physicians, nurse practitioners, physician assis-

tants, and others as determined by practice rules as defined by state/country rules. The wound patient population tends to require more nursing time in care and teaching.[4] It may be beneficial to staff the clinic with technical persons who are trained to perform the basics, such as vital signs, dressing removal, and basic wound care. Ancillary staff includes laboratory technicians and financial, legal, supply, and housekeeping personnel. If hyperbaric oxygen therapy is to be offered, trained hyperbaric technicians will need to be added to the treatment team.

The organizational structure establishes the chain of command, and the authority ascribed to the members of the structure can be delineated in the job descriptions. The job descriptions should provide the minimum preparation steps for the position as well as detailed responsibilities for each member of the team. Expectations should be clear and accepted by both the employer and employee. Intervals for performance appraisal should also be identified.

Staffing and Scheduling

The actual daily operations of the wound clinic will depend on a number of factors. If the clinic is set up as a part-time service in a multifunctional area, the time of actual patient visits will be confined to designated hours and day(s) of the week. The opportunity afforded by initially opening as a part-time service takes advantage of existing space and, to some degree, existing staff. This scenario provides low start-up cost relative to hiring staff and renting space for a full-time service. A part-time service also allows for patient volume to build gradually, which is especially important if the volume data gathered during the assessment phase was largely theoretical. One difficulty with a part-time service is providing patients with access to the staff in order to have questions or problems managed after clinic hours. This problem can be easily handled with appropriate telephone triage but needs to be planned prior to the first patient visit (problems or concerns rarely seem to occur during operating clinic hours).

The number of patients scheduled during a given time will depend on the type of visit and the level of acuity. Scheduling is a challenge, as patient visits generally require a disproportionate amount of nursing to physician time. This difficulty can result in lack of efficiency, especially for the physicians/providers. The amount of time needed for direct care, for teaching and support, and for assessment needs to be taken carefully into account. It may be helpful to have a schedule that allows for patient support and teaching after evaluation by the provider(s) and after physician hours in the clinic. Optimally, the reception staff can organize the schedule as it occurs with initial patient evaluations, patients with known time-consuming dressings, or therapies accorded sufficient time. It is helpful to be generous when initially scheduling patients, as well as allowing a greater amount of time for initial visits than for follow-up visits.

The patient visit will be further expedited if additional information is available prior to the visit. If testing is required, it is beneficial to schedule the test to allow time for the results to be obtained by the clinic staff prior to the patient's next appointment. Ideally, noninvasive testing can be performed at the time of the initial visit. Patients referred to the wound clinic may arrive with test results from their referral source, which further facilitates the visit. When testing is required, the patient may require an appointment of several hours in duration; this needs to be considered in the schedule.

Another opportunity for scheduling is managing time for patients participating in clinical trials. In general, the visits for participation in clinical trials are longer and require separate documentation and additional procedures from what may be routine in the clinic. This needs to be communicated to the person scheduling patient visits.

Patients with special needs must have these details communicated to the scheduler. For example, when a patient arrives on a stretcher, requiring a specific exam room, this information should be communicated and the appropriate room reserved. Perhaps a patient is bed-bound and needs to be weighed. With appropriate planning, an appropriate bed scale can be available, as well as the staff to perform the weighing procedure. Patients requiring special assistance may be coded on the schedule to allow for further efficiency in, for example, lift assistance, a specific exam room, testing, and procedures. Other special needs of the patient may also be obtained prior to the visit, including, but not limited to:

• An interpreter for non-English-speaking patients

• An interpreter for the hearing impaired
• Family members if the patient is cognitively impaired
• Coordination with appointments in the facility.

Optimal scheduling requires good communication between the office staff and the clinical staff.

Management of Referrals

The management of patient referrals to the wound clinic depends on timely communication with the referring source. The referral source may be a self-referral, but more likely, it is from a physician or other healthcare provider. *One common complaint about specialty-type clinics is that of inadequate communication with referral sources.* A plan to provide such communication should be in place before the first patient is seen. Another method of minimizing "referral anxiety" is to establish the wound clinic as a "consult" service by stressing that it does not intend to take over primary care of the patient but assists with the management of the patient only with respect to wound care. In fact, in a busy wound clinic, many chronically ill patients can overload the clinic with non-direct wound care activities. Having the primary care physician manage these problems improves wound clinic flow and patient outcome. Rapid communication of the wound care plan and progress to the primary care physician leads to optimal care and future referrals. Unless the wound clinic plans to provide primary care, it is important that all patients seen have a primary care physician.

A wound clinic evaluation plan should be in place from the inception and planning phases. The goal of the evaluation process is to measure progress, monitor outcomes, and evaluate established goals and objectives. Program evaluation may include such issues as infection rate, time to wound closure, recidivism rate, rehospitalization rate, and others. Another aspect of the program to monitor is in the area of demographics. How closely does the actual patient population match the projected statistic? This information is useful for concurrent planning and for the marketing department that may have facilitated the research during the planning phase. Conflicts are minimized if the original mission statement is adhered to and alternative agendas are rejected. Finally, it is helpful to have *periodic team meetings* to discuss the evaluation of findings. Staff meetings provide the opportunity to hear the data, comment on the results, and formulate ideas for future research.

Clinical Management

Assessment. Patient assessment and, specifically, wound assessment can take many forms. As previously described, the first portion of the assessment begins with the receptionist scheduling the patient. *Upon presentation to the clinic, the intake evaluation forms should include an assessment of the history of the wound, any associated pain, and the patient's expectations for the visit.* A wound clinic operating as an outpatient clinic of a hospital will likely have required assessments and forms already in place. A careful medical history and physical exam should be performed. Laboratory studies, including routine hematology, chemistries, nutritional indices, as well as wound culture and possibly tissue for pathology, may be ordered. A nutritional history is also helpful, as is assessment for familial medical history. During the initial interview, it is helpful to obtain social information with respect to smoking, alcohol consumption, exercise regimen, and the availability of support persons. Finally, it is suggested to take an inventory of past and current wound care. When eliciting this information, it is most helpful to identify actual wound care being performed, as this may differ considerably from the current order. The wound profile should be carefully documented. Both quantitative and qualitative information should be gathered.

Quantitative information includes wound size and depth, surface area, a photograph of the wound and surrounding skin, and wound perimeter tracing. If the wound is venous in nature, additional information regarding leg volume with ankle and calf circumference measurements is appropriate. The patient with a diabetic foot ulcer may need neurosensory testing, pressure mapping of the foot, and assessment of the non-involved foot. Tools to assist in quantitative assessment continue to be developed and may be integrated into practice as they become available for bedside use.

Qualitative information includes wound description, description of the peri-wound skin, odor, exudate, edema, anatomic location, pain, type of tissue exposed, and color. (Pain should be quantified with a self-report using a pain scale if possible; we include this assessment as the "5th" vital sign when recording vital signs.)

Depending on the differentiation of wound by type, other testing may be required. Wounds with a potential vascular origin may require vascular testing. Vascular testing generally involves noninvasive testing of pulses, Doppler waveform analysis, ankle brachial Doppler pressure, and transcutaneous oxygen analysis. Invasive vascular testing may involve arteriography. Other vascular testing may be indicated based on clinical assessment. Diagnostic radiography may be indicated to rule out the presence of osteomyelitis. This testing may require plain films, bone scan, or magnetic resonance imaging (MRI). If infection is suspected, a wound bone biopsy may be indicated with operative debridement of the wound.

Many documentation systems exist, including utilization of one of the commercially available computerized tools. A facility may opt to purchase an existing computer-based documentation system or develop a computer database internally. Whichever system is chosen, it should facilitate data management for the tracking of clinical outcomes, cost of care, and other facility needs.

Guidelines. Applicable institutional guidelines may be utilized to the extent to which they fit the needs of the clinic. Applicable general policies may include patient scheduling, staffing, medical authority, documentation, and infection control. The wound clinic team will want to develop guidelines specific to the service. These guidelines may include wound cleansing and debridement, use of sedation, wound culturing, topical wound care, and use of adjuvant management, such as sequential compression therapy, orthotic devices, and pressure relief.

Financial considerations. The responsible provider needs to consider the reimbursement pattern for the expected patient volume. The probable mix of private pay, private insurance, Medicare, Medicaid, and healthcare contracts is important to assess. If an outpatient facility depends heavily on negotiated contracts, it is critical that those in the position of negotiating the contracts be aware of the proposed service. Recommended treatments may not be covered, resulting in potentially suboptimal clinical outcomes and frustrated clients who are unable to obtain supplies and adjuvants for care. Furthermore, these payer mixes and reimbursement contracts are not static and need to be reviewed regularly to align them. Assumptions need to be made from the geographic and demographic information regarding the anticipated volume of patients to be seen during years 1 to 5. The projected volume of service should be described by visit type, procedures, and diagnostic codes so that the capabilities of the clinic can meet (or exceed) the anticipated patient population needs. Another aspect of volume projection is the opportunity for secondary inpatient admissions, surgical procedures, and referrals to other ancillary services as a result of the clinic volume. For example, there should be an anticipated increase in the volume of outpatient vascular studies documenting a wound patient's blood flow. *Cost justification will be apparent to the parent institution through a reduction of inpatient days and hospital re-admission.* Does the proposed patient population require expanded services, such as lymphedema care or hyperbaric oxygen therapy? The field of wound care is an evolving interprofessional specialty and as such needs continued administrative support, physician leadership, and nursing expertise.

When appropriate, individuals may be referred to home care services to provide the wound care needed. Home care then responds by assisting the patient and the family with caring for the wound and assisting with obtaining necessary supplies. If home care is not available, the family and/or significant other is instructed on wound care, and supplies can be ordered through an outside durable medical equipment company.

Additional potential influences on the success of the clinic require one to take a critical look at future trends in healthcare that may impact the clinic. These trends may include but are not limited to political, legal, economical, and social arenas. The economics of a clinic are complex and require the clinician and financial analyst to be clear on financial targets. As clinicians, we advocate that a comprehensive wound clinic is cost effective in managing the patient with a chronic wound. However, from a financial perspective, concentrating this population in one area looks expensive. When the costs of caring for this population are dispersed throughout the healthcare setting, the actual cost of care is offset by those patients whose

care is not as expensive in terms of both dollars and resource utilization. Therefore, this concept, which concentrates the care of the wound patient, now exposes these costs, and the clinician may be faced with developing a strategy to "lose less money" rather than to break even or potentially show a profit.

Billing issues can be a concern for the facility and the practitioner. How the billing will be managed needs to be addressed at this stage of development. Will there be one bill to the patient, which includes professional services as well as facility procedure and dressing charges, or will there be separate professional and facility charges? Standard office reimbursements may not cover the cost of the dressings, which redirects the need for careful discussion with the insurance providers before the clinic opens.

Summary

Running an outpatient wound clinic can be an exciting process. The concept is continuing to evolve. The vitality that can be brought to such a setting will make a difference for the staff, patients, and caregivers. A center focused on the care and management of people with nonhealing and chronic wounds brings together interested professionals who are willing to learn, to teach, and to share with the patient a coordinated approach to an often difficult to manage problem. It is an area where clinical research can be accomplished with a coordinated team effort.

This chapter has focused on the process of formalizing an idea and bringing it to reality with careful research and planning. It is our hope that the concepts presented in this chapter will facilitate the process of opening a wound clinic for those individuals contemplating such a service. Certainly, additional areas could be covered, including the development and use of guidelines for both diagnosis and topical wound care. For additional information on these aspects of operating a wound clinic, we recommend other chapters of this source book and other articles on selecting treatment modalities and wound healing and repair (Table 2).

Conclusion

It should be stressed that there are many methods for achieving organized treatment of nonhealing and chronic wounds. Establishing an outpatient

Table 2. Resources for the clinician

Publications:	Today's Wound Clinic Journal of Wound Care WOUNDS	Advances in Skin and Wound Care Ostomy Wound Management Wound Care Canada
Guidelines:	AHRQ Clinical Practice Guidelines AMDA Clinical Practice Guideline: Pressure Ulcers EPUAP NPUAP Pressure Ulcer Guidelines Medical Algorithms Project International Pressure Ulcer Prevention Guidelines International Pressure Ulcer Treatment Guidelines World Union of Wound Healing Societies Best Practice Consensus Statements Wound Healing Society Guidelines Wound Ostomy Continence Nursing Society Guidelines Association for the Advancement of Wound Care (AAWC) Wound Care Clinic Directory	
Organizations:	Association for the Advancement of Wound Care American Professional Wound Care Association Canadian Association of Wound Care European Pressure Ulcer Advisory Panel National Pressure Ulcer Advisory Panel National Alliance of Wound Care World Union of Wound Healing Societies Wound Healing Society Wound Ostomy Continence Nursing Society	

wound clinic is simply one of these ways. Even with respect to the wound clinic, the structure may take many different forms from the model presented here or from any of a number of variations including a "virtual" clinic. The clinic, if it is to be successful, must meet the needs of the population to be served. Therefore, careful analysis of that population cannot be underestimated. Likewise, a careful, realistic appraisal of potential referral sources and competitors needs to be completed. The best designed, best planned clinic will not survive without patients. However, a properly positioned clinic offering a comprehensive approach for patients and their wounds is an opportunity for clinical excellence with cost savings for the institution, improved outcomes for the patients, and continued professional development for the involved clinicians.

While the primary goal for most wound clinics is achieving wound healing, that goal is not realistic for some of our patients. The team needs to acknowledge that not all patients have wounds that will heal or remain healed. The team should have a plan for those patients who are not following a "healing" trajectory. These patients may require a palliative approach or even referral to other centers. In all instances, qualitative management of wound-related symptoms and wound pain should be recognized as a component of care in the wound clinic.[5]

Self-Assessment Questions

1. What are the key elements in identification of the need for an outpatient wound clinic?
   A. Physician commitment to support and re-

Practice Pearls

• Information gathered from the past and evolved-present allows the team to expand the scope of service and ask the appropriate questions as a new full-time facility is planned.

• The costs to care for the wound population continue to rise as reimbursement continues to fall.

• Concentrating the costs to one area allows the financial experts to identify reimbursement strategies as well as determine long-term survival and viability of the project.

ferral is lacking

B. Market analysis identifies an existing wound center in a nearby facility

C. The demographics of the population to be served match the proposed service plan

D. All of the above

2. What are the necessary components of the mission statement?

A. It is based on one person's ideas

B. The mission statement is global in scope with a shared sense of purpose, direction, and achievement

C. The mission statement contains only short-term goals

D. Team building of staff is not essential in planning for the clinic

3. The business plan should include the following:

A. Concern regarding costs of operation is not considered in the business plan

B. Billing issues are not a concern for the facility or practitioner

C. The marketing plan does not influence the business plan

D. The economics of a wound clinic are complex and require the clinician and financial analyst to be clear on financial targets

Answers: 1–C, 2–B, 3–D

References

1. Seaman S. Outpatient wound care in a capitated environment: quality care for the patient and an ideal practice for the wound specialist. *Today's Wound Clinic.* 2011;July/August:12–15.

2. Pruneda RC. Development of a wound healing center. In: Sheffield PJ, Smith APS, Fife CE, eds. *Wound Care Practice.* Flagstaff, Ariz: Best Publishing Company; 2004:731–746.

3. Fife C. Reader survey: monitoring the changing wound care clinic. *Today's Wound Clinic.* 2011;July/August:16–18.

4. Sheehan DD, Zeigler MH. Developing an outpatient wound care clinic in an acute rehabilitation setting. *Rehabil Nurs.* 2010;35(3):91–98.

5. Woo K, Sibbald G, Fogh K, et al. Assessment and management of persistent (chronic) and total wound pain. *Int Wound J.* 2008;5(2):205–213.

Wound Care in Home Care: The Global Perspective

Ben Peirce, RN, BA, CWOCN;
Hiske Smart, RN, MA, PG Dip(UK), IIWCC(Toronto);
Keryln Carville, RN, STN(Cred), PhD;
Connie Harris, RN, ET, IIWCC, MSc

Objectives
The reader will be challenged to:
- Compare and contrast home care systems in different countries
- Analyze the strengths and weaknesses of each system
- Consider piloting ideas that may improve local wound home care services.

Introduction

Healthcare differs dramatically between countries. This chapter highlights the differences among home healthcare nurses who care for patients with wounds in South Africa, Australia, Canada, and the United States. The authors outline how home care is provided in each of these countries and describe the challenges and successes they have experienced. The authors' insights provide valuable information for community-based providers around the world.

The South African Experience

In South Africa, the healthcare delivery system consists of a large public health sector and a smaller private health sector. The former is free of charge, consumes about 11% of the government's total budget, and provides a service to roughly 80% of the South African population, which is an estimated 50.5 million people.[1] The public sector is divided into primary, secondary, and tertiary layers. The primary service, which has a preventive and basic community focus, is extremely limited in resources.[2] The secondary layer includes access to regional hospitals and serves as the referral point to specialist care in well resourced tertiary hospitals or back to basic community care. The public and private sectors provide no formalized home healthcare services.

Registered nurses are allowed to act as independent practitioners[3] within their scope of nursing practice in South Africa. These private nurse practitioners are most often contracted by patients themselves and will render an individual-

Peirce B, Smart H, Carville K, Harris C. Wound care in home care: the global perspective. In: Krasner DL, Rodeheaver GT, Sibbald RG, Woo KY, eds. *Chronic Wound Care: A Clinical Source Book for Healthcare Professionals.* Vol 1. 5th ed. Malvern, PA: HMP Communications; 2012:151–157.

ized home care service, which may be covered by patients' medical insurance or paid for by the patients themselves.

The lack of healthcare services in the home setting provided the impetus for the Wound Healing Association of Southern Africa[4] to conduct a study in the remote rural area of Whembe in Limpopo Province, South Africa, where an HIV project is instituted. This project provides a non-government, home-based care system to about 5.5 million people.[5,6] The aim of this study[6] was to identify the wound burden that is cared for at home, not in formalized medical care facilities, and also to identify the needs of the care provider working in this setting under the auspices of the provincial administration and USAID.[5]

A qualitative methodology and questionnaire were employed to interview a team of 25 home-based care workers serving as a link between primary health clinics and patients cared for at home. Demographic information included the home-based care workers' gender, age, highest educational level, and comfort in rendering wound care as well as number of current patients receiving care, wound location, treatment, and dressing materials used.

The caseload of patients to care worker was 20:1 (range, 10–24 patients per worker). Of these case loads, at least a third of the patients were seen on a daily basis (range, 4–8), and case workers visited these patients on foot within a range of 25 km a day. At least 50% of the patients under their care had a wound, and 53% of these wounds were on the buttocks/sacrum or lower limb. When asked if they performed the wound care for these wounds, 70% of care workers said that they did. Most wound care was done 3 times a week (50%), 38% of wounds were washed with warm water and soap, and 19% of wounds were cleaned with warm water and salt. The dressing of choice for 49% of respondents was povidone-iodine and dry gauze. When asked if they had received some sort of wound care training, 74% of care workers responded that they had not and that their highest schooling level was Grade 6.

The responsibility of these home care workers to perform wound care compared to their educational levels was the most disconcerting finding in this study. This study identified the need for basic wound care skills training at or below the pri-

mary care level in order to more effectively overcome the challenges of rendering quality wound care with inadequate knowledge and severely limited resources currently faced in home-based care delivery in South Africa.

These findings are troubling in light of the current burden of diseases, such as HIV/AIDS and tuberculosis, found in Africa. The need for wound care training across the basic primary care sector is evident and will empower home-based care workers to do their work more effectively. The patient with a wound will be the person who benefits the most in the long run.

The Australian Experience

Home nursing care in Australia is funded primarily by federal or state governments or fee-for-service arrangements, and significant health problems and complex wounds present no barrier to home healthcare, as governments and insurance funders strive to find less costly alternatives to hospital care.

Variations in services for people with complex wounds or the inability to provide self-care exist across the 8 Australian states and territories. Some home nursing organizations provide wound dressings and devices as a component of care at no additional cost to the patient, while other organizations — especially general practice medical clinics — expect their patients to pay for these consumables. Patients who have to purchase wound dressings obtain them locally, often at inflated costs. The Australian Wound Management Association lobbied the federal government unsuccessfully for the past 3 years for subsidized wound management consumables in order to reduce costs and improve access and equity for all.

For the provision of wound care in homes and clinics, home nursing organizations employ registered nurses with varying levels of knowledge and skills. Nurses employed by Silver Chain in Western Australia currently manage an average of 2,400 wounds daily across the metropolitan Perth area. Half of these are acute post-operative or traumatic wounds, while half are chronic wounds, such as leg ulcers, pressure ulcers, or malignant wounds. Overall, patients with wounds comprise 70% of all clinical cases visited by Silver Chain nurses at home or seen in their wound clinics. To ensure best practice care and optimal outcomes,

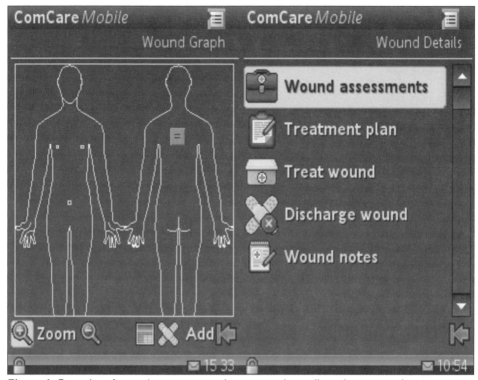

Figure 1. Examples of wound assessment and treatment data collected on smart phones.

participation in competency-based wound educational programs is mandatory for all Silver Chain nurses.

The need to record assessment and treatment outcomes for every wound has led to the development of an innovative electronic data system. ComCare Mobile™ is an application that connects the nurse in the patient's home or in the clinic with Silver Chain's main client record system. ComCare Mobile is designed to run on the current generation of "smart phones" and thus eliminates the need for additional computer technology (Figure 1). Information recorded includes client demographics, comorbidities, and type, etiology, and duration of the wound. Specific wound assessment parameters and treatments used are recorded on a regular basis to support tracking and trending. Individual and collective data can be analyzed and used to determine benchmarks for best practice and cost-effective outcomes across the organization. ComCare Mobile also expedites clinical consultations between the nurse in the home and remote wound specialists, regardless of

their location. This is of paramount importance in a country as vast as Australia.

An adaptation of ComCare Mobile has been used to conduct 4 statewide wound prevalence surveys in all 86 Western Australian public hospitals. Almost 12,000 patient skin and wound inspections and mattress and seating equipment audits were recorded on mobile smart phones by bedside surveyors and transmitted to the central data management system. The WoundsWest surveys revealed that almost 50% of all patients in public hospitals have at least one wound, and many of these patients are discharged into the care of home nursing services for ongoing wound management.

In the community, as in the hospital setting, novice nurses are supported by specialist nurses in wound management, and their titles, including clinical nurse specialist, clinical nurse consultant, and nurse practitioner, are used to differentiate advanced nurse practice roles. The expanded scope of practice for nurse practitioners allows them to prescribe selective medications, order diagnostic tests, perform certain procedures, such as biopsies, and refer patients directly to other health professionals. Wound management specialists in each of these roles have flourished among home nursing organizations in response to advances in evidence, technology, and patient expectations. While clinical governance is officially aligned to the patient's medical practitioner, interprofessional relationships are enhanced by mutual regard for the expertise of all team members.

Attempts to advance wound knowledge and skills among all health providers has led to the development of an interactive, online WoundsWest Education wound program, which is available to all practitioners regardless of location and can be accessed free of cost at www.health.wa.gov.au/woundswest/education. This evidence-based program will ultimately provide access to 16 modules covering various wound types.

In Australia, the number of people with wounds requiring home care is anticipated to increase significantly in line with the aging population. The national challenge is not only to ensure best practice and cost-effective outcomes but also to embrace strategies that promote healthy skin and wound prevention, especially among elderly citizens.

The Southwestern Ontario, Canada, Experience

Canada is divided into 10 provinces and 2 territories. The largest province of Ontario (population 12 million) has 14 regional integrated health networks with associated community care access centers (CCACs) that are the single provider of government-sponsored home care as part of the universality of the Canada Health Act.

The South West Community Care Access Centre (SW-CCAC) provides almost 2 million home visits/hours of service to more than 50,000 individuals annually with more than 50% for wound care. Nursing services represent a significant portion of care delivered by 5 provider agencies contracted to the CCAC with nurses covering 22,000 square kilometers. The wound dressings are initially changed by the nurses, with a "teach the client and reduce nursing visits" mandate, wherever possible. The visits are authorized in a bundle of "X" visits over "X" weeks, based on the types of wounds, giving the flex-

ibility to adjust visits according to the needs of the patient. Daily dressing changes are considered an exceptional situation, and visits are approved only for specific wound criteria. In cases where healing is a realistic goal, identified on the referral by the healthcare practitioner with further input from the nurses, wound status is reported to the CCAC case manager on admission and every 3 weeks. This provides an objective basis for tracking progress and for evaluating the need to modify the plan of care through interprofessional interventions, for example. In addition to home visits by clinicians, advanced wound supplies, cleansing agents, and instruments for sharp debridement are also provided through the CCAC until the time of discharge. When the goal is to teach and discharge to self-care, the client will need to pay for the supplies necessary for continuing care or obtain funding from alternative sources, such as third-party insurance.

Implementing and maintaining wound care educational programs for home care is a challenge. To this end, the SW-CCAC engaged with a wound care industry partner to provide wound care education for 3 years and assisted with the development of the educational content and its delivery.

The SW-CCAC recognized that the provision of educational sessions and resources, such as the Wound Management Program, would not be enough to transfer the new knowledge into practice. "Just in Time" evidence is a strategy used successfully by businesses and involves quick and easy access, with consistent format and focus on implementation in the form of "practice enablers." The development team is combining the creation of practice enablers suited to the SW-CCAC clientele and service providers and a review of the current service delivery model.

Several "Kaizen" events were held in 2010 and 2011. Kaizen is part of the Japanese continuous improvement philosophy and involves improving standardized activities and processes. Groups of CCAC case managers, front-line nurses and managers, clinical educators, and wound care specialists/enterostomal therapy nurses have reviewed the current provision of care for open surgical wounds, pressure ulcers, venous stasis ulcers, diabetic foot ulcers, and ostomies in half-day events for each topic. This has resulted in the development of standardized care plans, patient self-care teaching handouts, and information booklets about the specific etiology and steps that individuals can take to improve their health and ability to manage their own conditions. The patient information booklets are being reviewed to create regional versions that can be used in all settings as part of the South West Regional Wound Care Framework (SWRWCF) project. The Enterostomal Therapy/Wound Care Specialist Nurse Service Delivery model has been reviewed, resulting in a consultative model, also consisting of a block of visits, rather than ongoing visits, to improve access and decrease wait times. Adjunctive therapies, also reviewed using the Kaizen framework, will be available across the whole region for wounds that are not healing according to the expected trajectory, meeting evidence-based criteria.

A larger regional project, the SWRWCF, is intended to standardize evidence-based wound care through education and clinical practice resources across the region within the SW-CCAC, 32 hospital sites, 74 long-term care facilities, and primary care. The SWRWCF is being developed concurrently and synchronously with the SW-CCAC wound initiative. Physicians with interest/expertise in wound care also provided feedback on the content during development.

The SW-CCAC Wound Management Program and the SWRWCF Toolkit are online documents that continue to grow as requests for more tools and more best practice "quick references" are received from physicians and nurses. Both are available at http://www.woundcare.thehealthline.ca.

There is an old African proverb that says that "if you want to go somewhere fast, go alone, but if you need to go a long distance, go with others." The SWRWCF Clinical/Evaluation, Knowledge Translation, and Product Selection/Procurement subcommittees representing acute care and rehabilitation, long-term care, and community sectors have "gone the distance" in envisioning and developing the regional project. Next steps include:

- Education and implementation of the resource toolkit
- Selection and implementation of a wound care database that will be used for documentation at the point of care and for reporting
- Analysis of utilization and trends in all sectors

- The creation of a regional wound care product formulary, which will allow seamless transfer of care and an improved client-centered experience, while improving efficiencies and decreasing costs.

The United States Experience

In the United States, the role of home health in wound care is largely shaped by the Centers for Medicare & Medicaid Services (CMS) Conditions of Participation. Palliative care is covered under a separate benefit and, as a result, is provided by separate agencies. Because CMS is the largest payer in the United States, these guidelines shape who receives home healthcare, what services are provided in the United States, and how care is organized.[7] Additionally, regulations in each state impact home healthcare and can vary significantly.

Services provided by Medicare-certified home healthcare agencies to those who qualify can broadly be described as assessment, treatments, education, and evaluation. Most care provided to patients with wounds falls into the area of treatment and education, as home healthcare clinicians primarily change wound dressings and teach patients and caregivers how to change them as well. Sixty-five percent of home healthcare in the United States is funded by Medicare/Medicaid, 15% by state and local government, 10% by self-payment, 8% by private insurance, and 2% by other sources.[1] Home healthcare clinicians also monitor these wounds to ensure progress is being made and recommend changes to the physician providing oversight. Home healthcare clinicians support patients managing chronic conditions through teaching, problem solving, offering encouragement, and coordinating care. When the patient can be transported and services are available locally, the patient's care team also may include an ambulatory care center or wound clinic that provides diagnostic testing, surgical procedures, and physician oversight.

One of the requirements to be a Medicare-certified home healthcare agency is the ability to collect and transmit basic datasets, called the Outcome and Assessment Information Set (OASIS), for each patient admitted to home healthcare. The CMS uses these datasets to create reports on patient characteristics and on outcomes of the care provided by home healthcare agencies.[8] Results are made available to each home healthcare agency and to the public to support quality transparency. From these OASIS outcome reports, we know that half of all home healthcare patients admitted for care have a wound, though this wound may not be the reason for home healthcare. The most common types of wounds include postoperative surgical incisions or open surgical wounds (49%), pressure ulcers (11%), venous stasis leg ulcers (4%), and the category of "other" (36%), which includes diabetic foot ulcers and lower-extremity arterial disease ulcers.

Initially, the home care nurse focuses on organizing the supplies and providing the treatments, ie, changing the dressings. As soon as possible, the focus of nursing visits changes to teaching the patient or caregiver to change the dressings and then to monitoring progress and, with physician approval, making adjustments to the treatment plan as needed to maintain progress toward goals. This conserves resources while fostering patient independence. Most wound care supplies are covered by CMS and are provided by the home healthcare agency.

Barriers faced by home healthcare agencies include the patient's distance from the provider, limited home healthcare nursing skill in wound care, and ineffective disease self-management among many patients.

Nurse travel time can make coordination of care more difficult and can decrease options available for home healthcare if complications arise. Rising fuel costs have compounded this challenge. Home healthcare agencies endeavor to overcome these barriers via technology, including smart phone access to the medical record, GPS devices, and remote monitoring between visits. Many US home healthcare agencies also ship medical supplies directly to the patient because it reduces nurse travel time.

Limited nursing skill in wound care is also a common barrier. Home healthcare agencies overcome this by providing just-in-time online continuing education and remote support enhanced through shared digital images and by fostering knowledge transfer through professional association memberships.

Finally, ineffective disease self-management is a common and costly barrier to positive wound outcomes. Many complex wounds are associated with chronic illness that must be managed to optimize healing and to avoid wound recurrence. Successful home healthcare agencies overcome this barrier by adopting flexible patient education that can be individualized to the patient's literacy, cultural background, and support system. Continuing education for clinicians in self-management support also has been effective.[9] Self-management may be ineffective due to knowledge deficits, inadequate skills, insufficient motivation, or an ineffective support system.

Despite the challenges faced by home healthcare clinicians caring for patients with wounds, many experts see an important and growing future for home healthcare due to the United States' rapidly aging population and the opportunity for early intervention through home care to avoid wound complications that increase patient pain and suffering and increase the cost of care.

Conclusion

These 4 perspectives from around the world highlight the different approaches taken to care for patients with wounds in the home. Common themes do emerge; however, patients with wounds are common in home care around the world, knowledge and skill in wound care is limited in most home care practitioners, and home care clinicians in each of these countries have taken steps to correct or compensate for this limited knowledge.

> **Practice Pearls**
> - Wounds are a common chronic condition, affecting patients in communities everywhere.
> - Many home care clinicians around the world have limited knowledge and skill in evidence-based practice for patients with wounds.
> - The availability of skilled wound care in the home varies significantly between countries.

Self-Assessment Questions

1. Home care in South Africa is funded through:
   A. The public health sector
   B. The private health sector
   C. Private insurance and patient payment
   D. None of the above

2. The Wound Healing Association of South Africa conducted a survey of the burden of wound care in a rural community because:
   A. Wound care is primarily covered by public health insurance
   B. Home care nurses cannot function independently
   C. There is a general lack of home care services in these communities
   D. None of the above

3. Home care nursing in Western Australia is funded primarily by:
   A. The federal government
   B. State governments
   C. Fee-for-service arrangements
   D. All of the above

4. Individuals caring for patients with complex wounds in the home do not face significant barriers in Australia because:
   A. They are rare in home care
   B. Everyone is seen in outpatient clinics
   C. Payers are eager to find less expensive alternatives to hospitalization for wound management
   D. None of the above

5. Overall, Silver Chain home care patients with wounds represent:
   A. 20% of those served
   B. 40% of those served
   C. 70% of those served
   D. 90% of those served

6. Silver Chain home care in Western Australia developed an EMR to:
   A. Provide patient education
   B. Increase efficiency
   C. Record assessments and outcomes
   D. Improve patient satisfaction

Answers: 1-C, 2-C, 3-D, 4-C, 5-C, 6-C

References

1. Office of the Actuary. Centers for Medicare & Medicaid Services. National Health Care Expenditures. March 2011. Available at: www.cms.gov.
2. Republic of South Africa. National Health Act, 2004 (Act No. 61, 2003). *Government Gazette*. 2004;469(26595).
3. South African Nursing Council. R.2598 of 30 November 1984. Regulations relating to the scope of practice of persons who are registered or enrolled under the Nursing Act, 1978. Available at: http://www.sanc.co.za/regulat/index.html. Accessed May 24, 2011.
4. Wound Healing Association of Southern Africa. Available at: http://www.whasa.org/A_Committee.html. Accessed May 25, 2011.
5. USAID Sub-Saharan Africa. 2005. Youth contribute to home-based HIV/AIDS care. Available at: http://africastories.usaid.gov/search_details.cfm?storyID=396&countryID=29&sectorID=9&yearID=5. Accessed May 24, 2011.
6. Smart H. Uncovering the hidden wound. Presented at the Ubuntu International Wound Care Conference: A Global Wound Healing Initiative in Cape Town, South Africa, September 5–8, 2010.
7. Centers for Medicare & Medicaid Services. Conditions for coverage (CfCs) & conditions of participations (CoPs). Available at: https://www.cms.gov/CFCsAndCoPs/01_Overview.asp#TopOfPage. Accessed June 1, 2011.
8. Centers for Medicare & Medicaid Services. Home health quality initiatives. Available at: http://www.cms.gov/HomeHealthQualityInits/. Accessed June 1, 2011.
9. Bodenheimer T, Lorig K, Holman H, Grumbach K. Patient self-management of chronic disease in primary care. *JAMA*. 2002;288(19):2469–2475.

Best Practice Guidelines, Algorithms, and Standards: Tools to Make the Right Thing Easier to Do

Heather Orsted, RN, BN, ET, MSc; **David Keast**, BSc(Hon), MSc, Dip Ed, MD, CCFP, FCFP; **Heather McConnell**, RN, BScN, MA(Ed); **Catherine Ratliff**, PhD, APRN-BC, CWOCN, CFCN

Objectives
The reader will be challenged to:
- Differentiate between the terms best practice guideline, algorithm, and standard
- Describe the relationship between best practice guidelines, algorithms, and standards
- Identify the stages in the development of best practice guidelines
- Summarize a process to evaluate the quality of existing best practice guidelines
- Analyze barriers to the implementation of best practice guidelines and describe methods to overcome them
- Propose effective interventions aimed at adoption and translation of best practice guidelines into practice.

Introduction

As evidence accumulates regarding healthcare practices, doing things "the way we have always done them" is no longer acceptable. In the past, part of the art and necessity of the practice in healthcare was making decisions on the basis of tradition and, in many cases, inadequate evidence. This often led to variations in practice, inappropriate care, and uncontrolled costs.[1,2] Rapid advances in healthcare make it almost impossible to keep up to date on what is "known." Inadequate care is now a result of inadequate production, evaluation, dissemination, and use of information. The provision of care based on evidence is required to support the creation of best practice cultures that require standards of quality, performance measures, and review criteria.

Comparative effectiveness research helps determine healthcare decisions by providing evidence on the effectiveness, benefits, and harms of different treatment options. Comparative effectiveness research requires the use of a variety of data sources and methods to conduct research and disseminate the results in a form that is quickly usable by clinicians, patients, policymakers, and health plans and other payers.[3]

In the United States, the Effective Health Care Program funds researchers to work together with the *Agency for Healthcare Research and Quality (AHRQ)* to produce effectiveness and comparative effectiveness research for clinicians, consumers, and policymakers. The AHRQ is the federal agency in the United States charged with improving the quality, safety, efficiency, and effectiveness of healthcare for all Americans. The Effective Health Care Program:

Orsted H, Keast D, McConnell H, Ratliff C. Best practice guidelines, algorithms, and standards: tools to make the right thing easier to do. In: Krasner DL, Rodeheaver GT, Sibbald RG, Woo KY, eds. *Chronic Wound Care: A Clinical Source Book for Healthcare Professionals.* Vol 1. 5th ed. Malvern, PA: HMP Communications; 2012:159–170.

- Reviews and synthesizes published and unpublished scientific evidence
- Facilitates the generation of new scientific evidence and analytic tools
- Compiles research findings that are synthesized and/or generated and translates them into useful formats for various audiences.

The AHRQ summary guides are reviews of research findings pertaining to the benefits and harms of different treatment options, and various versions are tailored to clinicians, consumers, or policy makers. Consumer guides provide useful background information on health conditions.

The *National Guideline Clearinghouse™ (NGC)* is a publicly available database of evidence-based clinical practice guidelines available at http://www.guideline.gov. It provides Internet users with weekly updates highlighting new content. The NGC is produced by the AHRQ in partnership with the American Medical Association (AMA) and the American Association of Health Plans (AAHP) Foundation. Key components of the NGC include:

- Structured, standardized abstracts (summaries) about each guideline
- Side-by-side comparisons of two or more guidelines
- Syntheses of guidelines covering similar topics, highlighting similarities and differences in the guidelines
- Links to full-text guidelines, where available, and/or ordering information for print copies
- Annotated bibliographies on guideline development methodology, structure, implementation, and evaluation.

In Canada, the Canadian Medical Association (CMA) maintains a database of clinical practice guidelines along with resources for development, evaluation, and implementation. To be included in the *CMA Infobase*, each guideline must:

1. Include information to help patients and physicians make decisions about appropriate healthcare for specific clinical circumstances. Ethics guidelines are included only if they help in decision-making concerning appropriate care. Guidelines on facilities, management, training, or professional qualifications are not included unless they also contain guidelines on clinical practice.
2. Be produced in Canada by a medical or health organization, professional society, government agency, or expert panel at the national, provincial/territorial, or regional level (clinical practice guidelines produced by individuals are excluded) or be produced outside Canada by one of the foregoing types of groups and officially endorsed by an authoritative Canadian organization.
3. Have been developed or reviewed in the last 5 years (rolling date).
4. Have evidence that a literature search was performed during guideline development.

The CMA Infobase is available at http://www.cma.ca/cpgs.

The *Centre for Evidence-based Medicine (CEBM)* in Oxford, England, promotes evidence-based healthcare and provides resources for clinicians interested in learning more about evidence-based practice. Their goal is to develop, teach, and promote evidence-based healthcare and provide support and resources to doctors and healthcare professionals to help maintain the highest standards of medicine. The CEBM is available at http://www.cebm.net/index.aspx.

Best Practice Approach to Care

Evidence alone is not enough to ensure best practice. In 2000, Sackett et al[4] defined evidence-based medicine (EBM) as follows: "Evidence-based medicine is the integration of best research evidence with clinical expertise and patient values." Kitson, Harvey, and McCormack[5] suggest that a synergy of actions is required to enable successful implementation of the evidence to support best practice. The evidence is required to be scientifically robust, the environment or context has to be ready for change, and the change process has to be appropriately facilitated. Evidence-based medicine is not restricted to randomized trials and meta-analyses but involves finding the best evidence with which to answer clinical questions.[6] See Chapter 3.11.

Best practice needs to be more than a theory. In clinical practice settings, multiple modalities are required to provide and transform the evidence into usable frameworks that enable appropriate facilitation and adoption of best practice by healthcare providers and the agencies in which they work.

Best practice guidelines (BPGs), also sometimes called clinical practice guidelines (CPGs), are systematically developed statements to assist practitioner decisions about appropriate healthcare for specific clinical circumstances.[7] They combine research evidence, experience, and expert opinion to improve patient care through reducing inappropriate variations in practice and promoting the delivery of high-quality, evidence-based healthcare.[8] Guidelines form the framework for practice in supporting policy and procedure recommendations. *Algorithms* or *pathways*, by contrast, are graphic maps that visualize the major cognitive components required to resolve a problem. They can act as clinical decision-making frameworks to guide the implementation of BPGs.[9-11] *Standards* differ in that they are rules or models of care established by professional organizations or regulatory bodies. Standards often set the minimal acceptable level of performance. Some standards may be specific to each discipline and may be enshrined in legislation in certain jurisdictions. Other standards may be flexible and responsive. For example, a common legal standard of care is to compare the care provided to that of a reasonable clinician in similar circumstances.

In practice, BPGs help healthcare clinicians define effective and appropriate practices based on current and extensive scientific research and available evidence; algorithms represent tools or enablers that aid in the implementation of BPGs; and standards set minimal levels of performance. The three, though different, are intimately related.[12]

The BPG, Assessment and Management of Foot Ulcers for People with Diabetes, from the *Registered Nurses' Association of Ontario (RNAO)* illustrates this relationship in many sections. For example, the BPG rationale is presented under the heading "Background Context" and then accompanied by an algorithm (Pathway to Diabetic Foot Ulcers) to enable further understanding of the concepts discussed. The same document contains a discussion relating to sharp debridement that asks the clinician to consider if the task is within his or her standard of practice.[13]

How are BPGs Developed?

In the years that have passed since BPGs or CPGs were introduced into the healthcare system, they have permeated into every area of clinical practice. Originally, healthcare chief executive officers regarded BPGs as "the answer" to reduce

inappropriate or unnecessary variation in clinical practice.[8] Between 1990 and 1996, the Agency for Health Care Policy and Research (AHCPR), now the AHRQ, introduced 19 practice guidelines in an effort to support evidence-based methods to assess medical treatments and to set high standards for the development of guidelines.

In Canada, the International Affairs and Best Practice Guidelines Program, a signature program of the RNAO, is being funded by the Ministry of Health and Long-Term Care in Ontario to develop, implement, evaluate, disseminate, and support the uptake of both clinical and healthy work environment BPGs.[14] Though the RNAO is a professional nursing association, its guidelines are developed with interprofessional support as well as patient guidance and advice. Since 1999, the RNAO has developed and maintained (through regularly scheduled revisions) 44 clinical and healthy work environment BPGs. Translation into a range of languages including French, Italian, Spanish, Japanese, and Chinese has made these resources accessible to a range of practitioners provincially, nationally, and internationally. Additionally, the RNAO utilizes the *Appraisal of Guidelines for Research and Evaluation (AGREE II instrument)* to support a best practice approach to guideline development.[15]

The International Affairs and Best Practice Guidelines Program's goals are to:
- Improve patient care
- Reduce variation in care
- Transfer research evidence into practice
- Promote nursing knowledge base
- Assist with clinical decision-making
- Identify gaps in research
- Stop interventions that have little effect or cause harm
- Reduce cost.

Guidelines are designed to be used as recommendations to inform care decisions rather than rules for care to enable the practitioner to provide the best possible care by adopting new information and changing practice.[16] Guidelines must provide healthcare professionals with adequate notice of the boundaries of acceptable and prescribed behaviors yet not be so narrow or rigid that they create a detrimental effect on innovative and individualized patient care.[15]

Quality guideline development requires that rel-

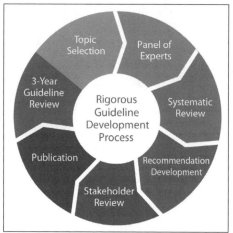

Figure 1. RNAO guideline development methodology process. Reprinted with permission from the Registered Nurses' Association of Ontario. Transforming Nursing Though Knowledge. Available at: http://www.rnao.org/Page.asp?PageID=122&ContentID=1557&SiteNodeID=158&BL_ExpandID=.

evant literature and practice patterns are reviewed and the data appraised for weight of evidence. The results are then distilled and collated into a succinct, user-friendly format. In the final stage, these guidelines are reviewed widely and modified based on feedback by experts in the field before being endorsed by a credible sponsoring body or association. At this point, the guideline is ready for dissemination to appropriate bodies leading to knowledge transfer or implementation into practice.

The final important stage in the cycle of BPGs is a feedback loop of ongoing reevaluation and refinement through gathering of new evidence as the cycle continues. Regularly scheduled reviews should include changing practice patterns, new evidence, and barriers and enablers to implementation. For example, the RNAO guidelines are revised every 3–5 years (Figure 1).[17]

According to Roberts, *attributes of a good practice guideline are validity, reliability, reproducibility, clinical applicability, clinical flexibility, clarity, interdisciplinary process, scheduled review and documentation, and simplicity*.[8]

Selecting a Best Practice Guideline for Implementation

Developing BPGs is an expensive and time-

consuming process. If one wishes to adopt an existing guideline into practice, how does one select the most rigorous yet practical one? The AGREE II instrument is the new international tool for the assessment of guidelines. The AGREE II is both valid and reliable and comprises 23 items organized into the original 6 quality domains. It helps guideline developers and users assess the methodological quality of CPGs.[18] The AGREE II instrument has 3 goals: 1) to assess the quality of CPGs, 2) to provide a methodological strategy for guideline development, and 3) to recommend what information should be reported in guidelines.

Assessment of a guideline involves evaluation of its quality (using the AGREE II tool), how up-to-date it is, and the consistency of the recommendation with the underlying evidence. Assessment also consists of the feasibility of applying recommendations. This process can result in different alternatives ranging from adopting a guideline unchanged, to adapting the format, modifying single recommendations, and producing a customized guideline based on various guidelines used as sources.[19]

The AGREE II instrument is a tool designed primarily to help guideline developers and users assess the methodological quality of CPGs.[15] The 6 quality domains include:

1. Scope and purpose: overall aim of the guideline, clinical question, and target population
2. Stakeholder involvement: extent to which the guideline represents the views of the intended users
3. Rigor of development: process used to gather and synthesize the evidence and methods to formulate the recommendations and to update them
4. Clarity and presentation: the language and format of the guideline
5. Applicability: organizational, behavioral, and cost implications of application
6. Editorial independence: independence of the recommendations and acknowledgement of possible conflict of interest from the development group.

Once the review is complete, a quality score is calculated for each of the 6 AGREE II domains. The 6 domain scores are independent and should not be aggregated into a single quality score. Reviewers are provided with the opportunity to comment on the overall quality of the guideline and whether the guideline would be recommended for use in practice.

Wimpenny and van Zelm compared 4 national pressure ulcer guidelines from Australia, Canada, the Netherlands, and the United Kingdom to identify similarities and differences in their quality and content.[20] The domain scores for each guideline show some but not total agreement among reviewers. One guideline was identified as scoring highest in a majority of AGREE II domains.

While the AGREE II tool identifies the quality of the guideline development process, it still requires practitioners to determine which guideline would be most appropriate to implement in their clinical settings. The potential for evidence overload also suggests that brevity might be best, even in algorithm or decision-tree format.

National and international bodies have made major efforts to improve the quality of guidelines, but less time has been spent understanding how guidelines can be implemented. Developing BPGs is an expensive and time-consuming process. If one wishes to adopt or modify an existing guideline, how does one select the most rigorous yet practical one? Adaptation of existing guidelines for individual facility use enhances applicability. National guidelines often lack specific details on what changes in the organization are required to apply the recommendations. Adaptation of evidence may promote a sense of ownership by those who are engaged in this process.[19]

The *ADAPTE collaboration* (www.adapte. org) is a group whose purpose is to increase the use of evidence-based guidelines. The ADAPTE process consists of 3 phases, including planning, adaptation, and development of the guideline. The planning phase outlines the tasks to be completed before adapting the guideline, including identifying necessary skills and resources and determining who should be on the panel. The panel should include end users of the guideline, such as clinicians and patients.[19]

Since 2000, the *Canadian Association of Wound Care (CAWC)* has authored best practice recommendations relating to wound bed preparation and the prevention and management of pressure ulcers, diabetic foot ulcers, and venous leg ulcers. These were not intended to be BPGs but rather a distillation of existing guidelines into a succinct practice article and bedside enabler (the *Quick Reference Guide* or *QRG*) backed by the existing articles, research, and guidelines for more in-depth information.

When it came time to update and revise the CAWC recommendations, the CAWC board recognized the quality of the RNAO guidelines and decided to create regional teams to revise the recommendations utilizing the RNAO wound-related guidelines. The updated articles and *QRGs serve as practice enablers* that help to interpret these guidelines for the multiple healthcare professionals involved in the management of chronic wounds. Each article takes the practice enabling statements and discusses their relationship to the corresponding RNAO guideline as well as additional resources from the literature to enhance and support an interprofessional approach. To further enable practice, each QRG is related to a Pathway to Assessment and Treatment, which provides an algorithm to guide clinical decision-making.

A Health Canada initiative to encourage adaptation of the RNAO guidelines stimulated the development of regional wound care guidelines in Saskatchewan. In January 2004, the Health Quality Council (HQC) and the Saskatchewan Association of Health Organizations (SAHO) convened a provincial Skin and Wound Care Action Committee to develop a strategy to ensure that patients receive consistent, high-quality skin and wound care. The results of their initiative involved a partnership between the HQC and the RNAO to adapt the RNAO guidelines to produce a regionally specific pressure ulcer guideline.[21]

The *Wound, Ostomy, and Continence Nurses Society (WOCN)* developed evidence-based guidelines using a clinically diverse panel of WOCN nurses, a topical outline with specific questions to guide the literature search for evidence, and studies reporting primary data relevant to the topic with specific diagnostic modalities and treatment therapies included in the review. The search targeted meta-analyses, randomized controlled trials, prospective and retrospective clinical trials, and systemic reviews.

In early 2003, the *Wound Healing Foundation* put out a request for proposal (RFP) for a project to formulate and publish chronic wound care guidelines. Multidisciplinary committees were set up to complete the project with the majority of the group members in agreement with the recommendations. Publically held forums on the National Institutes of Health (NIH) campus solicited input from other interested parties, societies, and industry.

The American **National Pressure Ulcer Advisory Panel (NPUAP)** and the **European Pressure Ulcer Advisory Panel (EPUAP)** collaborated to develop guidelines on the prevention and treatment of pressure ulcers. The guidelines were produced by a guideline development group along with several small working groups. The entire process of the guideline development could be followed on a designated website by stakeholders of this process.

The first step in any guideline development process is identifying the evidence. Generally, electronic databases are searched with specific predetermined inclusion criteria, such as dates of the searches, subject titles, such as pressure ulcers, pressure sores, and decubitus ulcers, and type of studies to be included, such as randomized controlled trials, meta-analyses, systematic reviews, etc. All retrieved references are then sorted by topic and placed in evidence tables. The level of evidence is then noted for each study based on a predetermined classification system set up by the guideline group. Recommendations about the body of available evidence are then identified based on the level of evidence found in the tables.

Implementing Best Practice Guidelines and Algorithms

Many BPGs have been developed and disseminated; however, their implementation across all disciplines and delivery sites remains a major challenge.

In a Minnesota study, approximately two-thirds of family physicians were unaware of the existence of the AHCPR guidelines for pressure ulcers (#3 and #15). Ninety percent of the physicians who had browsed the prevention guidelines had found them helpful, and all who read them in entirety said they were helpful.[22] A survey of Ontario family physicians showed that 78% indicated that they complied with lipid-lowering guidelines, but further questioning revealed that only 5% actually followed them.[23] Davis and Taylor-Vaisey[14] reviewed the literature on adoption of CPGs by healthcare professionals. They found that the variables affecting adoption include the qualities of the guidelines, the characteristics of the healthcare professional, the characteristics of the practice setting, incentives, regulation, and patient factors.

Davis and Taylor-Vaisey[14] also reviewed interventions aimed at the adoption of guidelines and classified them as weak (didactic, traditional continuing medical education, and mailings), moderately effective (audit and feedback, especially concurrent, targeted to specific providers and delivery by peers or opinion leaders), and relatively strong (reminder systems, academic detailing, and multiple interventions).

The first hurdle is promoting a culture or environment that supports the adoption and application of evidence-based practice. Guidelines involve change, and any change must be based on a need. Therefore, any system's change should be based on a needs assessment that identifies care gaps. The needs assessment should involve the users, recipients, educators, and appropriate administrators who may be involved in ultimate implementation. Toward this end (system change), the RNAO clinical guidelines not only identify clinical practice recommendations but also contain a recommendation section directed toward **organization and policy** (identifying the structures and resources that need to be in place to support evidence-based practice) as well as a section dedicated to the educational requirements (the knowledge and skills) required to successfully implement the guideline recommendations.[21] This approach to guideline development recognizes that the nature of nursing practice falls on a continuum from being a solo practitioner to being interdependent team members, which requires organizational structures and resources to ensure consistency in practice.

An often overlooked element in creating evidence-based practice cultures is sustainability. The **Knowledge-to-Action Cycle** identifies attention to sustaining knowledge use as a critical element of moving knowledge to action[22] (Figure 2). A study by Higuchi et al reported on a 3-year follow-up evaluation of nursing care indicators following the implementation of 2 RNAO BPGs.[23] They found that clinical guidelines provide credible resources for evaluating and improving prac-

Table 1. Barriers and bridges to best practice

Category	Barrier	Bridge
Financial Issues	• Support for programs and interdisciplinary teams • Technology • Infrastructure to support guidelines	• Clear identification of outcomes will support a cost-effective delivery of best practices • Efficiencies regarding supply/equipment acquisition and purchase
Educational Issues	• Location of existing guidelines • Dissemination of guideline-specific education and knowledge • Changing the attitudes and expectations of healthcare providers • Understanding the tools for documentation • Lack of leadership • Educational resources and time • Patients refusing evidence-based practice	• Websites specific to needs • Program leader to integrate guidelines into policies, procedures, and protocols • Regular communication to provide ongoing information (newsletter, emails, alerts) • Regularly scheduled staff and team meetings to educate, learn, provide a forum for discussion, and support change • Easy-to-read, healthcare provider-specific, and client-specific evidence-based educational material (current, simple, holistic, and easy to adapt based on client need and clinical judgment)
Practice Issues	• Clinical integration of evidence-based practice among healthcare providers • Staff skill level • Staff stress level and staff shortages	• Clinical integration of evidence-based practice among healthcare providers • Clinical pathway • User-friendly format for protocols and procedures • Interdisciplinary team (opinion leaders) to provide ongoing support to staff regarding clinical issues and change • Agency support and effective resource management • Alternative, cost-effective methods of service delivery (clinics) • Continuity of care and care providers

tice, but the changes required at the individual and system levels are frequently significant and require considerable time. Two significant contributors to guideline sustainability they identified were documentation and reminder systems, which support change at the systems level.

Challenges to implementing wound care BPGs occur across all service delivery sites (hospital, outpatient clinics, home, and long-term care). These challenges include information transfer, integration of payment sources into the dialogue to realize potential savings in overall program costs, consistency of wound management approaches among all service delivery sites, and development and maintenance of interdisciplinary care teams.

Successful implementation strategies:
• Provide educational offerings that teach concepts of the BPG
• Provide an educational offering for each new BPG
• Include a pathophysiology review during each educational offering
• Provide routine, ongoing educational offerings on BPG information.[6]

The literature is replete with barriers to guideline implementation, which can be condensed into 3 main categories.[17–20,24] No listing of barriers would be complete, however, without dis-

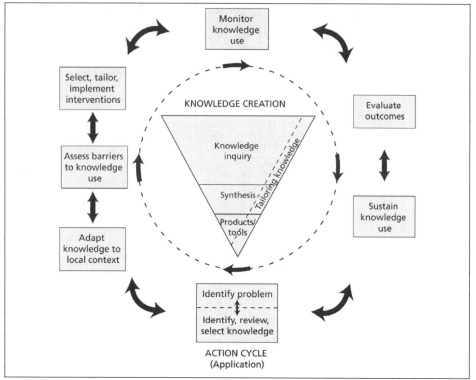

Figure 2. Knowledge-to-Action Cycle. Reprinted with permission from Graham ID, Logan J, Harrison MB, et al. Lost in knowledge translation: time for a map? *J Contin Educ Health Prof.* 2006;26(1):13–24.

cussing recommended solutions (bridges). Table 1 reviews "bridges for barriers," discussing solutions from the literature and from clinical experience.[25]

Best practice guideline implementation requires strong leadership from clinicians who understand concepts of planned change, program planning and evaluation, and research utilization. This knowledge will support the development of a program plan that enables the transformation of organizations toward best practice. In 2002, the RNAO developed a toolkit to assist organizations through a planned change process for successful implementation.[26]

Graham et al indicated that in order for guidelines to be implemented successfully, a critical initial step must be the *formal adoption of the guideline recommendations into the policy and procedure structure.*[27] This key step provides direction regarding the expectations of the organization and facilitates integration of the guideline into systems, such as the quality management process.[27]

Shiffman and colleagues developed the *Guideline Implementability Appraisal (GLIA)* to facilitate guideline implementation. The instrument is designed to systematically highlight barriers to implementation including executability, decidability, validity, flexibility, effect on process of care, measurability, novelty/innovation, and computability. The GLIA is intended to provide feedback about a guideline's ability to be implemented to the authors of the guideline and to those individuals who choose to apply the guideline within a healthcare system. The GLIA consists of 31 items, arranged into 10 dimensions, and is applied individually to each recommendation of the guideline. Evidence of content validity and preliminary support for construct validity was obtained by the authors.[28]

It is understood that if healthcare professionals are to provide best practices, they must seek valid, reproducible, useful, and relevant studies and support material that enable the growth of their practice into a best practice standard.[29] However, how does that information get into practice? Healthcare professionals also need to participate in recognized, accredited continuing educational opportunities that allow them to participate with skill and confidence as members of interprofessional wound care teams. Agencies need to provide a full scope of support for nurses seeking professional education.[30,31]

The question remains: How can we be assured that knowledge is developed, delivered, evaluated, and sustained by an educational event or program, such as described in the Knowledge-to-Action Cycle?[22]

The CAWC and the Canadian Association for Enterostomal Therapy (CAET) collaborated toward the development, evaluation, and publication of a standard for wound management education and programming that can be used by healthcare professionals and their employers to appraise existing and future investments in wound care education.[32] The *Wound CARE Instrument* contains standards obtained from literature focused on knowledge mobilization that support a collaborative and evidence-informed approach to the appraisal and recommendation process of wound management education and programming. This instrument supports decision-makers in their efforts to improve wound care knowledge, skills, and attitude and to improve the health of patients at risk for or suffering from wounds.

The Wound CARE Instrument:

1. Provides a foundation to identify the components required to plan, develop, implement, evaluate, and sustain evidence-informed wound management education and programming

2. Provides a benchmark to appraise the quality of wound management education and programming

3. Supports collaboration in the development and implementation of wound management education and programming

4. Informs decisions related to the endorsement, adoption, adaptation, purchase, or rejection of wound management education and programming

5. Improves patient care and health outcomes relating to the prevention and management of wounds.

The Wound CARE Instrument has dem-

onstrated that it is a valuable tool to aid in the appraisal and evaluation of wound management education and programming within a clinical setting. The Wound CARE Instrument is now available online and downloadable for no cost at http://www.cawc.net or http://www.caet.ca.

Are Algorithms and Best Practice Guidelines Effective?

Algorithms. Beitz and van Rijswijk published a study in which they attempted to establish content validation data for a set of wound care algorithms.[33] They tried to identify strengths and weaknesses of the algorithms in order to gain further insight into the wound care decision-making process. With this set of wound care algorithms, they identified 11 themes of difficulty in 5 areas. These 5 areas included the length of the algorithm, wound care terminology, wound assessment, wound context (patient issues), and clinical decision-making. The algorithms provided 3 positive aspects to care: a focus on goals, an ability to improve consistency, and a high content validity index of the wound assessment and care concepts. They concluded that the wound care algorithm studies were valid; however, the algorithms lacked valid and reliable wound assessment and care definitions.

Best practice guidelines. In a study of 5 client care settings, including a home care agency, the prevalence rates of pressure ulcers showed a decrease from 19% to 7.4% 4 months after the introduction of guidelines. The decrease continued to 6.7% after 8 months and 6.1% after 1 year.[34]

The response to BPGs varies. Many practitioners, especially physicians, worry that CPGs will lead to "cookbook medicine" with little room for clinical decision-making, consideration of patient and local condition variations, or innovation. Many practitioners fear that even the slightest variation from the guidelines will make them more liable to be successfully sued. Legal concerns relating to guidelines have been addressed by Goebel and Goebel who reviewed legal databases for malpractice awards for pressure ulcers.[16] The authors found that substantial savings in malpractice costs would have occurred and only 4 of 14 findings in favor of the defendant would have been reversed had guidelines been followed.

It is important to remember that in the com-

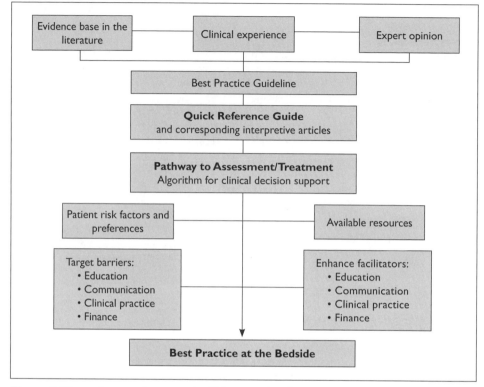

Figure 3. The pathway to best practice.[38] Reprinted with permission from Keast D, Orsted H. The pathway to best practice. *Wound Care Canada.* 2006;4(1):10.

plex wound-healing environment, interventions — even those based on guidelines — need to be regularly assessed by skilled professionals to ensure that outcomes of care are achieved. Care delivery must be based on lifestyle and client choice as well as best evidence.

Conclusion

A Health Policy Forum convened an interprofessional summit in Toronto, Canada, including patient representatives, practicing physicians (both generalists and specialists), nurses, researchers, and healthcare administrators.[35] The following 3 questions were asked:

- What goals should underlie CPG development?
- How can we improve CPGs?
- Who should participate in CPG development, use, and evaluation?

The results from the various working groups were remarkably consistent. They agreed that

CPGs should serve one central goal: providing better care for patients.

The forum made a number of recommendations regarding the production and role of CPGs that include the following:

1. Education: CPGs are an educational tool and must not be used to regulate medical practice
2. Flexibility: CPGs must be flexible enough to meet the needs of individual patients while incorporating all aspects of care
3. Multidisciplinary: The CPG process must be truly interprofessional with a focus on frontline caregivers rather than academics — the process must include all parties involved in care
4. Patient input: Patient representatives must have meaningful input at all stages of CPG development, including outcome measures used
5. Quality assurance: A standardized process for developing and evaluating CPGs should be employed with periodic or continuous re-

view processes incorporated to keep CPGs up to date

6. Accountability: The CPG process must be visible and accountable to healthcare professional and patient groups; the level of evidence used to formulate a CPG must be explicitly stated, as must potential bias

7. Outcomes orientation: CPGs should facilitate treatment choices by providing clear information about what works and what does not work — the outcomes examined should reflect patient priorities

8. Accessible: Successful strategies to encourage adoption of CPGs must be shared and materials and technologies developed to make them immediately available for consultation

9. National clearinghouse: Many participants identified the need for a central body to oversee CPG development, funding, and use. This central body would ensure that existing CPGs are regularly updated and reviewed and that implementation strategies are shared.

Marketing experts have suggested that organizations *focus on the exchange rather than on the change about to be encountered*.[36] The adoption and implementation of new tools can provide the implementers and the users support for knowledge exchange. Through expert opinion and current extensive scientific research and available evidence, guidelines define best practices that in turn support the attainment of competency and skill level. Basing a wound care program on tools that enable evidence-based practice will promote excellence in skin care, foster collegial relationships, and permit replication with other clinical populations.[37]

Guidelines and algorithms integrated into the continuum of care can provide:

- Cost-effective care delivery
- Documentation that is consistent, complete, standardized, comparable, outcome generated, and shared
- Care that will be evidence based, holistic, and patient specific.

To support the implementation of best practice at the bedside, clinicians and facilities must integrate BPGs that endorse recommendations related not only to practice but also to educational, organizational, and policy changes. Re-

gional differences related to population and resources need to be considered when program development is considered. To accomplish this, the clinician must be supported in an environment that breaks down barriers related to communication, education, practice, and resources. Barriers to best practice must be identified and modified, and bridges to best practice must be identified and enhanced. This is an active process that requires a receptive environment supported by administrators, the allocation of appropriate resources, and the cooperation of interprofessional team members. Figure 3 summarizes the entire process.

Most importantly, when it comes to best practice, you may know best practice, but are you providing it?

Practice Pearls

- Not all guidelines are created equal.
- Awareness of the best evidence does not ensure a change in practice.
- The strength of the evidence must be combined with a willingness of the environment to change practice and appropriate facilitation of the new information.
- Practice change needs to be system-wide and supported by policy.

Self-Assessment Questions

1. A guideline is a document that outlines the best available evidence for a health-related problem.
   A. True
   B. False

2. The AGREE II instrument allows the clinician to evaluate if the recommendations outlined in the guideline will work at the bedside.
   A. True
   B. False

3. Guideline recommendations are more effective if supported by agency policy and procedure.
   A. True
   B. False

Answers: 1-A, 2-B, 3-A

References

1. Leape LL. Practice guidelines and standards: an overview. *QRB Qual Rev Bull.* 1990;16(2):42–49.
2. Atkins D, Kamerow D, Eisenberg JM. Evidence-based medicine at the Agency for Health Care Policy and Research. *ACP J Club.* 1998;128(2):A12–A14.
3. US Department of Health & Human Services. Agency for Healthcare Research and Quality. What is comparative effectiveness research? Available at: http://www.effectivehealthcare.ahrq.gov/index.cfm/what-is-comparative-effectiveness-research1/. Accessed February 2010.
4. Sackett DL, Straus SE, Richardson WS, Rosenberg W, Haynes RB. *Evidence-Based Medicine: How to Practice and Teach EBM.* 2nd ed. New York, NY: Churchill Livingstone; 2000:1.
5. Kitson A, Harvey G, McCormack B. Enabling the implementation of evidence based practice: a conceptual framework. *Qual Health Care.* 1998;7(3):149–158.
6. Centre for Evidence Based Medicine. What is EBM? Available at: http://www.cebm.net/index.aspx?o=1914. Accessed February 2010.
7. Field MJ, Lohr KN. *Clinical Practice Guidelines: Directions for a New Program.* Washington, DC: National Academy Press; 1990.
8. Roberts KA. Best practices in the development of clinical practice guidelines. *J Healthc Qual.* 1998;20(6):16–32.
9. Gaines C. Concept mapping and synthesizers: instructional strategies for encoding and recalling. *J N Y State Nurses Assoc.* 1996;27(1):14–18.
10. Hadorn DC, McCormick K, Diokno A. An annotated algorithm approach to clinical guideline development. *JAMA.* 1992;267(24):3311–3314.
11. Tallon R. Critical paths for wound care. *Adv Wound Care.* 1995;8(1):26–34.
12. Tellez RD. Wound care 2000: challenges to integration across the continuum. *Home Care Provid.* 1997;2(4):192–196.
13. Registered Nurses' Association of Ontario. Assessment and management of foot ulcers for people with diabetes. Available at: http://www.rnao.org/Page.asp?PageID=924&ContentID=719. Accessed September 2010.
14. Davis DA, Taylor-Vaisey A. Translating guidelines into practice. A systematic review of theoretic concepts, practical experience and research evidence in the adoption of clinical practice guidelines. *CMAJ.* 1997;157(4):408–416.
15. Registered Nurses' Association of Ontario. Nursing best practice guidelines. Available at: http://www.rnao.org/Page.asp?PageID=861&SiteNodeID=133. Accessed September 2010.
16. Goebel RH, Goebel MR. Clinical practice guidelines for pressure ulcer prevention can prevent malpractice lawsuits in older patients. *J Wound Ostomy Continence Nurs.* 1999;26(4):175–184.
17. The AGREE Collaboration. Appraisal of guidelines research and evaluation. Available at: http://www.agreetrust.org/. Accessed September 2010.
18. Dans AL, Dans LF. Appraising a tool for guideline appraisal (the AGREE II instrument). *J Clin Epidemiol.* 2010;63(12):1281–1282.
19. Harrison MB, Légaré F, Graham ID, Fervers B. Adapting clinical practice guidelines to local context and assessing barriers to their use. *CMAJ.* 2010;182(2):E78–E84.
20. Wimpenny P, van Zelm R. Appraising and comparing pressure ulcer guidelines. *Worldviews Evid Based Nurs.* 2007;4(1):40–50.
21. Edwards N, Davies B, Ploeg J, et al. Evaluating best practice guidelines. *Can Nurse.* 2005;101(2):18–23.
22. Graham ID, Logan J, Harrison MB, et al. Lost in knowledge translation: time for a map? *J Contin Educ Health Prof.* 2006;26(1):13–24.
23. Higuchi KS, Davies BL, Edwards N, Ploeg J, Virani T. Implementation of clinical guidelines for adults with asthma and diabetes: a three-year follow-up evaluation of nursing care. *J Clin Nurs.* 2011;20(9-10):1329–1338.
24. Gander L, Delaney C. Saskatchewan Health Quality Council test drives new pressure-ulcer guidelines. *Wound Care Canada.* 2006;4(2):26–27.
25. Kimura S, Pacala JT. Pressure ulcers in adults: family physicians' knowledge, attitudes, practice preferences, and awareness of AHCPR guidelines. *J Fam Pract.* 1997;44(4):361–368.
26. Registered Nurses' Association of Ontario. Toolkit: implementation of clinical practice guidelines. Available at: http://www.rnao.org/Page.asp?PageID=924&ContentID=823. Accessed September 2010.
27. Graham ID, Harrison MB, Brouwers M, Davies BL, Dunn S. Facilitating the use of evidence in practice: evaluating and adapting clinical practice guidelines for local use by health care organizations. *J Obstet Gynecol Neonatal Nurs.* 2002;31(5):599–611.
28. Shiffman RN, Dixon J, Brandt C, et al. The Guideline Implementability Appraisal (GLIA): development of an instrument to identify obstacles to guideline implementation. *BMC Med Inform Decis Mak.* 2005;5:23.
29. Ryan S, Perrier L, Sibbald RG. Searching for evidence-based medicine in wound care: an introduction. *Ostomy Wound Manage.* 2003;49(11):67–75.
30. Best MF, Thurston NE. Measuring nurse job satisfaction. *J Nurs Adm.* 2004;34(6):283–290.
31. Gottrup F. Optimizing wound treatment through health care structuring and professional education. *Wound Repair Regen.* 2004;12(2):129–133.
32. Orsted HL, Woodbury G, Stevenson K. The Wound CARE Instrument. *International Wound Journal.* In press.
33. Beitz JM, van Rijswijk L. Using wound care algorithms: a content validation study. *J Wound Ostomy Continence Nurs.* 1999;26(5):238–249.
34. Hanson DS, Langemo D, Olson B, Hunter S, Burd C. Decreasing the prevalence of pressure ulcers using agency standards. *Home Healthc Nurse.* 1996;14(7):525–531.
35. Usher S, ed. *Health Policy Forum.* Montreal, Canada: June, 1999.
36. Landrum BJ. Marketing innovations to nurses, Part 2: marketing's role in the adoption of innovations. *J Wound Ostomy Continence Nurs.* 1998;25(5):227–232.
37. Suntken G, Starr B, Ermer-Seltun J, Hopkins L, Preftakes D. Implementation of a comprehensive skin care program across care settings using the AHCPR pressure ulcer prevention and treatment guidelines. *Ostomy Wound Manage.* 1996;42(2):20–32.
38. Keast D, Orsted H. The pathway to best practice. *Wound Care Canada.* 2006;4(1):10.

Translating Wound Care Strategies:
From Principles to Practice to Outcomes

Special Considerations in Wound Bed Preparation 2011: An Update

R. Gary Sibbald, BSc, MD, FRCPC(Med, Derm), MACP, FAAD, MEd, MAPWCA; **Laurie Goodman**, BA, RN, MHScN; **Kevin Y. Woo**, PhD, RN, FAPWCA; **Diane L. Krasner**, PhD, RN, CWCN, CWS, MAPWCA, FAAN; **Hiske Smart**, MA, RN, PG Dip(UK), IIWCC(Canada); **Gulnaz Tariq**, RN, BSN, PG Dip(Pak); **Elizabeth A. Ayello**, PhD, RN, ACNS-BC, CWON, MAPWCA, FAAN; **Robert E. Burrell**, PhD, MSc; **David H. Keast**, MD, MSc, BSc(Hon), DipEd, CCFP, FCFP; **Dieter Mayer**, MD, FEBVS, FAPWCA; **Linda Norton**, BScOT, OT Reg(ONT), MScCH; **Richard Salcido**, MD

Objectives

The reader will be challenged to:

- Treat the cause and patient-centered concerns (the whole patient) before treating the hole in the patient
- Classify wounds as healable, non-healable, and maintenance
- Assess and treat the local wound: Debridement, Infection/inflammation, Moisture balance for healable wounds
- Classify and treat bacterial damage: NERDS criteria for superficial critical colonization and STONEES criteria for deep and surrounding infection.

Background

This chapter incorporates a framework for assessing, diagnosing, and treating wounds along the continuum toward optimal healing.[1] The authors will introduce evidence-based and best clinical practice-based strategies for providing holistic and patient-centered care. It is important to treat the whole patient and not just the "hole" in the patient. The preparation and optimization of the wound bed for functional healing may not always result in complete healing, despite the clinicians' comprehensive team efforts. It is also important to recognize that some wounds may remain in the static or "stalled" phase of the wound healing trajectory.

The authors recognize that wound healing trajectories can be heterogeneous and nonuniform. They will explore several concepts to effectively manage nonhealable wounds or a new category the authors term *maintenance wounds* that are potentially healable but with existing patient or system barriers to effective treatment. These include patient adherence or competence to participate in treatment plans or systems-based errors embracing logistical issues that impede optimal healing. By reading this chapter, clinicians will

Reprinted from Sibbald RG, Goodman L, Woo KY, et al. Special considerations in wound bed preparation 2011: an update©. *Adv Skin Wound Care.* 2011;24(9):415–436; quiz 437–438. © 2011 R. Gary Sibbald. Used with permission.

Table 1. Quick reference guide wound bed preparation 2011

#	Recommendations for Wound Bed Preparation	RNAO Level of Evidence
1.	**Treat the cause** a. Determine if there is adequate blood supply to heal b. Identify the cause(s) as specifically as possible or make appropriate referrals c. Review cofactors/comorbidities (systemic disease, nutrition, medications) that may delay or inhibit healing d. Evaluate the person's ability to heal: healable, maintenance, nonhealable.	IV
2.	a. Develop an individualized plan of care b. Treat the cause(s) related to specific wound etiology/diagnosis.	IV
3.	**Patient-centered concerns** Assess and support individualized concerns a. Pain b. Activities of daily living c. Psychological well-being d. Smoking e. Access to care, financial limitations.	IV
4.	Provide education and support to the person and his or her circle of care, including referral to increase adherence (coherence) to the treatment plan.	IV
5.	**Local wound care** Assess and monitor the wound history and physical exam.	
6.	Gently cleanse wounds with low-toxicity solutions: saline, water, and acetic acid (0.5%–1.0%). Do not irrigate wounds when you cannot see where the solution is going or cannot retrieve (or aspirate) the irrigating solution.	Ib
7.	Debride: **Healable wounds** — sharp or conservative surgical, autolytic, mechanical, enzymatic, biological (medical maggots); **Non-healable and maintenance wounds** — conservative surgical or other methods of removal of nonviable slough.	IV
8.	Assess and treat the wound for superficial critical colonization/deep and surrounding infection/abnormal or persistent inflammation: **any 3 NERDS** — treat topically: Non-healing, ↑Exudate, Red, friable tissue, Debris, Smell; **any 3 STONEES** — treat systemically: ↑Size, ↑Temperature, Os, New breakdown, ↑Exudate, ↑Erythema/edema (cellulitis), Smell; **Persistent inflammation** (non-infectious): Topical and/or systemic anti-inflammatories.	IIa
9.	Select a dressing to match the appropriate wound and individual person characteristics **Healable wounds: Autolytic debridement:** Alginates, hydrogels, hydrocolloids, acrylics **Critical colonization:** Silver, iodides, PHMB, honey **Persistent inflammation:** Anti-inflammatory dressings **Moisture balance:** Foams, hydrofibers, alginates, hydrocolloids, films, acrylics **Nonhealable, maintenance wounds:** Chlorhexidine, povidone-iodine.	IV
10.	Evaluate expected rate of wound healing: Healable wounds should be 30% smaller by Week 4 to heal by Week 12. Wounds not healing at the expected rate should be reclassified or reassessed, and the plan of care revised	III-IV
11.	Use active wound therapies (skin grafts, biological agents, adjunctive therapies, etc) when other factors have been corrected and healing still does not progress (stalled wound).	Ia-IV
12.	**Provide organization support** For improved outcomes, education and evidence-informed practice must be tied to interprofessional teams and improved cost-effective patient care outcomes with the cooperation of healthcare systems.	IV

© 2000 Sibbald et al.

Table 2. Levels of evidence employed by RNAO guideline development panels[7] (2005)

Ia	Evidence obtained from meta-analysis or systematic review of randomized controlled trials.
Ib	Evidence obtained from at least one randomized controlled trial.
IIa	Evidence obtained from at least one well designed controlled study without randomization.
III	Evidence obtained from well designed, nonexperimental descriptive studies, such as comparative studies, correlation studies, and case studies.
IV	Evidence obtained from expert committee reports or opinions and/or clinical experiences of respected authorities.

comprehend and apply clinical criteria to help select and use the appropriate topical agents for superficial critical colonization versus systemic anti-infective agents for deep and surrounding tissue infection utilizing the mnemonics **NERDS** and **STONEES.** Clinicians also will be able to interpret new bedside diagnostic tests introduced in this chapter that may identify wounds stuck in the inflammatory stage.

This 2011 wound bed preparation (WBP) update also links evidence-informed practices to the evidence summarized in the recent Best Practice Guidelines of the Registered Nurses' Association of Ontario. To date, 3 best practice documents related to the treatment of wounds (pressure, venous, and diabetic) have been issued by the Registered Nurses' Association of Ontario, and the components related to local wound care have been considered for this summary along with updated literature searches. The information is organized with a quick reference guide of the key bedside assessment and treatment steps organized with the components of the WBP paradigm.

Introduction

As the population ages, acute and chronic wounds will become more frequent and prevalent, with increased chronicity. Any wound greater than 6 weeks old is considered chronic.[2] Preparing the wound bed was first described in 2000 by Sibbald et al[3] and Falanga[4] with sequential updates by Sibbald et al in 2003[5] and 2006–2007[6] and reprinted by the World Health Organization (WHO) in 2010.[6] The 2011 updated evidence-informed practice documents that link the WBP paradigm to the evidence-based literature, expert opinion, the clinical environment, and organizational context are presented. In Table 1, the 3 components of Sackett's triad have been ac-

commodated: clinical evidence and expert opinion with the need to address patient preference (patient-centered concerns). In addition, the WoundPedia Best Practice summaries (www.woundpedia.com) utilized in this update are meant to provide a practical, easy-to-follow guide or a bedside enabler for patient care. The levels of scientific evidence-based grading systems are outlined in Table 2. For more detailed information on this grading system, the reader is referred to the Registered Nurses' Association of Ontario (RNAO) Nursing Best Practice Guidelines (http://www.rnao.org) and/or the designated references.

Chronic Wounds: Nonhealable and Maintenance Wound Categories

The holistic approach to healable wound management as outlined in Table 1 stresses an accurate diagnosis and successful treatment with a team approach. (See Wound Bed Preparation Enabler 2011: Persons with Healable Chronic Wound(s).) For patient wounds that do not have the ability to heal, the approach is different. (See Wound Bed Preparation Enabler 2011: Persons with Nonhealable or Maintenance Wound(s).) These wounds with the inability to heal (*nonhealable wound*) may be due to inadequate blood supply and/or the inability to treat the cause or wound-exacerbating factors that cannot be corrected. The second category, a *maintenance wound*, is due to the patient refusing treatment of the cause (eg, will not wear compression) or a health system error or barrier (no plantar pressure redistribution is provided in the form of footwear or the patient cannot afford the device). These may change, and periodic reevaluation may be indicated (see Wound Bed Preparation Enabler 2011).

Chronic wounds are disabling and constitute

Wound Bed Preparation Enabler 2011

Wound Bed 2011	Recommendations
Treat the Cause	• Determine blood supply to heal • Identify/treat the cause (if possible) to determine healability • Review cofactors/comorbidities to create individualized plan of care
Patient Centered Concerns	• Assess, support, provide education for individualized concerns • Pain, Activities of daily living, Psychological wellbeing, Smoking, Access to care
Local Wound Care (DIM+ E)	• Cleanse, Assess characteristics & monitor local wound • Debride healable wounds (conservative for non-healable, maintenance) • Treat critical colonization, infection, persistent inflammation • Achieve moisture balance • Consider advanced therapies for healable but stalled chronic wounds
Systems	• Link improved cost-effective patient outcomes to: education, evidence-informed practice, interprofessional teams & healthcare system support

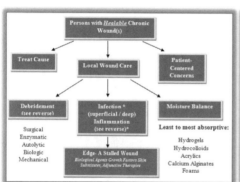

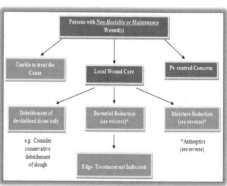

Determining the Healability of a Wound			
Wound Prognosis	**Treat the Cause**	**Blood Supply**	**Co-existing medical Conditions/ drugs**
Healable	Yes	Adequate	Not prevent healing
Maintenance	NO	Adequate	+/- prevent healing
Non-Healable	NO	Often Inadequate	May inhibit healing

Healable Wounds; Key Factors in Deciding Method of Debridement

	Surgical	Enzymatic	Autolytic	Biologic	Mechanical
Speed	1	3	5	2	4
Tissue selectivity	3	1	4	2	4
Painful wound	5	2	1	3	4
Exudate	1	4	3	5	2
Infection	1	4	5	2	3
Cost	5	2	1	3	4

**Where 1 is the most desirable and 5 is least desirable

Sibbald RG, Goodman L, Woo KY, Krasner DL, Smart H, Tariq G, Ayello EA, Burrell RE, Keast DH, Mayer D, Norton L, Salcido RS. Special Considerations in Wound Bed Preparation 2011: An Update©. *Advances Skin & Wound Care* 2011;24(9):415-435.©

Wound Bed Preparation Enabler 2011

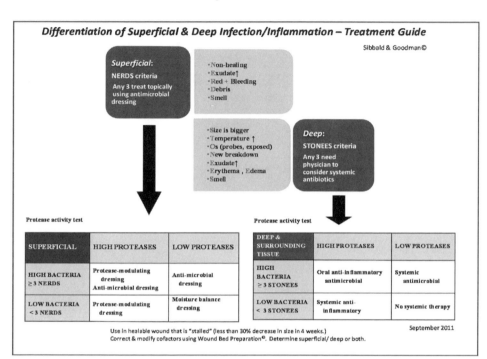

Differentiation of Superficial & Deep Infection/Inflammation – Treatment Guide

Sibbald & Goodman©

Superficial:
NERDS criteria
Any 3 treat topically using antimicrobial dressing

- Non-healing
- Exudate↑
- Red + Bleeding
- Debris
- Smell

- Size is bigger
- Temperature ↑
- Os (probes, exposed)
- New breakdown
- Exudate↑
- Erythema , Edema
- Smell

Deep:
STONEES criteria
Any 3 need physician to consider systemic antibiotics

Protease activity test

SUPERFICIAL	HIGH PROTEASES	LOW PROTEASES
HIGH BACTERIA ≥ 3 NERDS	Protease-modulating dressing Anti-microbial dressing	Anti-microbial dressing
LOW BACTERIA < 3 NERDS	Protease-modulating dressing	Moisture balance dressing

Protease activity test

DEEP & SURROUNDING TISSUE	HIGH PROTEASES	LOW PROTEASES
HIGH BACTERIA > 3 STONEES	Oral anti-inflammatory antimicrobial	Systemic antimicrobial
LOW BACTERIA < 3 STONEES	Systemic anti-inflammatory	No systemic therapy

Use in healable wound that is "stalled" (less than 30% decrease in size in 4 weeks.)
Correct & modify cofactors using Wound Bed Preparation©. Determine superficial/ deep or both.

September 2011

Newer Antiseptics

Agent	Effects
Acetic Acid (0.5% to 5%) *Hypochlorous Acid*	• Low pH • Effective against pseudomonas • May select out staph aureus • May cause stinging
Chlorhexidene 2% alcohol solution or 0.5% aqueous solution *PHMB derivatives*	• Active against gram negative and gram positive organisms • Low toxicity to tissue • Water based formulations best
Povidone iodine 10% aqueous solution delivers 0.9% iodine at wound bed *Cadexomer Iodine Inadine (Not USA)*	• Broad spectrum of activity, gram negative, gram positive, anaerobes, fungi and viruses • Activity decreased in the presence of pus or exudate • Toxic with prolonged use over large areas
Crystal violet – Methylene Blue *Hydrofera Blue*	• Broad spectrum antimicrobial activity • Lower tissue toxicity with slow release form • Can be used with enzymatic agents to prevent secondary bacterial infection

Antiseptic Agents for use in Non-Healable wounds where cytotoxicity is less important than anti-microbial action

GOOD AGENT	EFFECTS
Chlorhexidine (PHMB)	Low toxicity
Povidone Iodine- Betadine	Broad spectrum
Acetic Acid	Pseudomonas
BAD AGENT	EFFECTS
Dyes-Scarlet red, Proflavine	Select out Gm neg.
Na Hypochlorite-Dakins, Eusol	Toxic = bleach
Hydrogen Peroxide	Action = Fizz
Quaternary Ammonia- Cetrimide	Very high toxicity

Sibbald RG, Goodman L, Woo KY, Krasner DL, Smart H, Tariq G, Ayello EA, Burrell RE, Keast DH, Mayer D, Norton L, Salcido RS. Special Considerations in Wound Bed Preparation 2011: An Update©. *Advances Skin & Wound Care* 2011;24(9):415-435.©

Table 3. Arterial status is related to vascular results

ABPI	Toe Pressure, mmHg	Toe Brachial Index	Ankle Doppler Waveform	TcPO2, mmHg	Diagnosis
> 0.8	> 80	> 0.6	Normal/triphasic	> 40	No relevant arterial disease
> 0.5	> 50	> 0.4	Biphasic/monophasic	30–39	Some arterial disease: Modify compression
> 0.4	> 30	> 0.2	Biphasic/monophasic	20–29	Arterial disease predominates
< 0.4	< 30	< 0.2	Monophasic	< 20	High risk for limb ischemia

Modified (with permission) from Browne and Sibbald[14] and Sibbald et al.[15]

a significant burden on patients' activities of daily living (ADLs) and the healthcare system. Of persons with diabetes, 2% to 3% develop a foot ulcer annually, whereas the lifetime risk of a person with diabetes developing a foot ulcer is as high as 25%.[8] It is estimated that venous leg ulcers (VLUs) affect 1% of the adult population and 3.6% of people older than 65 years.[9] As our society continues to age, the problem of pressure ulcers (PUs) is growing. Each of these common types of chronic wound will require accurate and concise diagnosis and appropriate treatment as part of holistic care.

Local wound care also may be difficult to optimize. Chronic wounds are often recalcitrant to healing, and they may not follow the expected trajectory that estimates a wound should be 30% smaller (surface area) at Week 4 to heal in 12 weeks.[10,11] If all 5 components of WBP have been corrected (cause, patient-centered concerns, and the 3 components of local wound care) and a healable wound is stalled, reevaluation of the current diagnosis and treatment plan is necessary to be sure each component has been idealized before considering active local advanced therapies (edge effect). This update will clarify the system outlined above, dividing chronic wounds into healable, maintenance, and nonhealable categories. The authors will develop the clinical parameters around critical colonization with any 3 or more of the 5 NERDS mnemonic criteria for topical therapy or any 3 or more of the 7 STONEES mnemonic criteria associated with the deep and surrounding skin infection for systemic antimicrobial agents.

The updated WBP 2011 quick reference guide is intended for all wound healing practitioners from basic to intermediate or advanced levels ideally organized in transdisciplinary teams. To clarify the rationale for the evidence-informed practices, the authors discuss each item individually with reference to key supporting literature and enablers for practice where indicated.

Identify and Treat the Cause(s) of the Wound

1A: Determine if there is adequate blood supply to heal. This is often important, especially for ulcers on the leg or foot. It is important to inspect the foot and lower leg for signs of arterial compromise (dependent rubor, pallor on elevation, and loss of hair on the foot or toes), as well as palpate for a plantar pulse (dorsalis pedis or posterior tibial). Practitioners need to remember that a small percentage of patients may have an anomalous or anatomical variance resulting in absence of the dorsalis pedis artery. A palpable pulse indicates a foot arterial pressure of 80 mmHg or higher. The authors record a pulse as present or absent. However, a palpable pulse may not always exclude an arterial etiology. Although a foot pulse might be palpable, the nonhealing wound might be situated in a different angiosome that has to be revascularized in order to induce healing (angiosome model).[12] Doppler examination of the ankle brachial pressure index (ABPI) is indicated if the pulse is not palpable or to assess the appropriateness of high or modified compression bandaging for venous ulcers (Table 3).

The audible Doppler signals also may be useful diagnostically: a triphasic normal sound, a biphasic sound indicative of some arterial compromise, and the monophasic or absent signal with advanced ischemia. Complete segmental lower leg arterial Doppler examinations are needed if there is a possibility of a proximal lesion or arterial restriction or blockage that is amendable through surgical bypass or endovascular dilatation. If blood supply is inadequate or cannot be immediately determined, dressing selection should be based on a maintenance wound program with moisture reduction and bacterial reduction until further assessments are performed.

Toe pressures are useful because about 80% of people with diabetes and 20% of the nondiabetic population have calcified large leg arterial vessels that are nonpliable and stiff, leading to falsely high ABPI levels often greater than 1.3.[13] When ABPI levels are this high, no conclusions can be drawn about the quality of limb perfusion without further investigation. In Table 3, the arterial status is co-related to the vascular testing results.

1B: Identify the cause(s) as specifically as possible or make appropriate referrals. A comprehensive wound assessment is required to determine the cause of the wound. In order to achieve this, a holistic approach to the patient assessment is needed. An interprofessional team approach will facilitate a comprehensive review of the whole patient, the environmental factors, and the wound. In a recent community, comprehensive, interprofessional assessment of leg and foot ulcer patients, more than 60% of diagnoses were changed or made more specific, leading to the implementation of best practices, thus facilitating the optimization of WBP and improving healing rates of chronic wounds.[16]

1C: Review cofactors/comorbidities (systemic disease, nutrition, medications) that may delay or inhibit healing. Wound healing can be delayed or interrupted in persons with coexisting systemic diseases and the multiple comorbidities associated with chronic wounds. In the case of diabetes, excess glycosylation of hemoglobin due to poor diabetic glucose control can result in a prolonged inflammatory phase in addition to decreased neutrophil and macrophage phagocytosis of bacteria. Furthermore, diabetes affects the erythrocytes' ability to deliver oxygen

to the wound, a fundamental step in collagen synthesis and tissue proliferation[17] along with numerous other important factors in wound healing. An original investigation by Markuson et al[18] demonstrated that individuals with lower hemoglobin A1c (HgbA1c) levels had improved and shorter healing times. This translated to a cost reduction because the closed wounds had decreased risk of infection compared with the ulcers that were still in the healing phase.

A detailed review and clinical analysis of patient cofactors and comorbidities that may influence healing should be carried out in a systems-based approach. Systemic diseases, such as diabetes or autoimmune disease, may interfere with the stages of wound healing and stall or prevent healing.

A low protein intake or relative deficiency can prevent the production of granulation tissue that will contribute to a stalled healing environment for the wound. A given albumin measurement in a patient implies nutritional status over a few months, and these levels are a gross indicator of long-term nutritional deficit. Albumin levels measure the large reservoir of amino acids that serve as the fundamental building block for wound healing. Several other patient stressors can influence albumin levels.[19] Normal serum albumin levels are 3.4 to 5.4 g/dL,[20] and levels of 2.0 to 3.4 g/dL are associated with potential delayed healing, and the wound may need to be treated as a maintenance wound until the levels are corrected. Prealbumin (transthyretin) is a more sensitive indicator of protein deficiency, reflecting levels over 18 to 21 days. Transferrin is often thought of as an indirect measurement of nutrition; however, levels elevate in response to infection or inflammation. Therefore, results can be misleading in persons with a chronic wound.[21] Cost and access to transferrin level testing may be a challenge in some practice settings. Published literature attributes recumbent positioning of patients with a direct decrease in serum liver proteins, such as albumin, prealbumin, and transferrin.[22,23] Therefore, in utilizing the "whole patient" concept, we should optimize activity and mobilization.

Individualized patient medicine reconciliation should take place as part of any wound management protocol. Several medications that may alter the healing processes on the cellular level need to be identified. Some medications important to note

Table 4. Determining the healability of a wound

Wound Prognosis	Treat the Cause	Blood Supply	Coexisting Medical Conditions/Drugs	No. of Wounds + Ability of Wound to Heal[a]
Healable	Yes	Adequate	Not prevent healing	121 (69.9%)[a]
Maintenance	No[a]	Adequate	± Prevent healing	43 (24.9%)[a]
Nonhealable including Skin Changes at Life's End (SCALE)	No	Usually inadequate	May inhibit healing	9 (5.2%)[a]

Modified from Sibbald, Krasner, Lutz SCALE document 2010.
[a]Results from comprehensive interprofessional assessment of leg and foot ulcers.[16]

in the assessment of a wound are high doses of systemic steroids, immunosuppressive drugs, and antimetabolite cancer chemotherapy. Vitamin E intake of more than the recommended 100 IU daily can impair healing[24] because of its oxygen-scavenging property at the tissue level that is opposite to the oxygen-sparing property of vitamin C.

1D: Evaluate the person's ability to heal: healable, maintenance, nonhealable. Categorizing a wound according to its ability to heal (healability) assists the clinician in determining an accurate diagnosis along with a realistic individualized treatment approach. Adequate tissue perfusion is necessary for a healable wound. As outlined above, decreased vasculature will increase the risk of infection and decrease healability. In order to be classified as a healable wound, the wound should have several attributes, including an adequate blood supply; the cause of the wound must be corrected; and existing cofactors, conditions, or medications that could potentially delay healing must be optimized or ideally corrected. A maintenance wound is a wound that may be healable, but either healthcare system factors or patient-related issues are preventing the wound from healing. A nonhealable wound is a wound that does not have adequate blood supply to support healing or the cause cannot be corrected. In nonhealable wounds, moist interactive healing is contraindicated and debridement should be on a conservative basis only (expert opinion for SCALE document).

Woo et al[25] (Table 4) assessed patients with lower leg and foot ulcers. The healability percentages of consecutive consenting home care patients with leg and foot ulcers from Toronto and Mississauga (Ontario, Canada) districts have

been tabulated in the final column of Table 4. The results indicated that most subjects had a demonstrated ability to correct the cause and achieve adequate circulation for healing (69.9%). Determining if a patient is healable, nonhealable (5.2%), or maintenance (24.9%) allows the clinician to identify and address specific individualized challenges, particularly for the nonhealable and maintenance wound patients. Along with the patient's input, the clinician is able to tailor the nonhealable or maintenance care plan, facilitating responsible use of available resources along with realistic treatment goals. In general, advanced active therapies are not indicated for maintenance or nonhealable wounds.

When a healable wound does not progress at the expected rate, a chronic and stalled wound results. These wounds are more prevalent in older adults and are attributed to the aged skin and comorbidities, such as neuropathy, coexisting arterial compromise, edema, unrelieved pressure, inadequate protein intake, coexisting malignancy, and some medications. Persistent inflammation may be the cause of a stalled wound and in some cases may not be correctable. The presence of multiple comorbidities in some older adult patients implies that healing is not a realistic endpoint.[26] For nonhealable or maintenance wounds, pain and quality of life may be indicated as the primary goals of care. Palliative wound care often includes nonhealable wounds, but patients undergoing palliative care may have maintenance or even healable wounds.

Frequently, skin changes at life's end may be associated with individual risk factors and comorbidities. In 2009, an 18-member international expert panel explored the issues and research literature surrounding end-of-life skin and wound

Table 5. Types of wounds and treatment

Type of Wound	Treatment of the Cause in a Healable Wound
Venous ulcers	• Compression therapy wraps for healing and stockings for maintenance • High compression in absence of arterial disease if Ankle Brachial Pressure Index > 0.8 (ABPI or ABI) • Modified compression for mixed vascular disease with ABPI 0.65–0.8 (extreme caution 0.5–0.65)
Arterial ulcers	• Revascularization where possible • Angioplasty, stents, or bypass (grafting or synthetic)
Pressure ulcers	• Pressure redistribution to reduce pressure, friction, and shear forces • Optimize mobility • Incontinence and moisture management
Diabetic foot ulcers	V = Confirm adequate vascular supply I = Infection treatment P = Plantar pressure redistribution according to local provisions S = Sharp surgical serial debridement

care, including the Kennedy Terminal Ulcer (case series evidence)[27] and the concept of skin compromise.[28] The panel developed a consensus document entitled "Skin Changes At Life's End" (SCALE).[29] A modified Delphi process with 52 international distinguished reviewers was utilized to reach consensus on the document. The 10 final consensus statements have clarified the authors' views on skin and wound conditions at the end of life.

Of the 10 SCALE consensus statements, statement 1 is key: "Physiologic changes that occur as a result of the dying process may affect the skin and soft tissues and may manifest as observable (objective) changes in skin color, turgor, or integrity, or as subjective symptoms, such as localized pain. These changes can be unavoidable and may occur with the application of appropriate interventions that meet or exceed the standard of care."[29] The panel explored the work by Kennedy,[27] where the phenomenon of PUs that occur in the sacral area of dying patients was observed in a long-term care facility. Kennedy's work[27] was the first modern descriptive research to discuss this issue that was depicted in 1877 by Jean-Martin Charcot and termed the decubitus ominosus.

In an observational study that took place in a large teaching hospital 10-bed palliative care unit, the staff reported that 5% of the patients had skin changes of reddish-purple discoloration ranging from 2 hours to 6 days prior to death. These areas of intact skin rapidly became full-thickness PUs.[30]

The staff turned patients hourly. Within minutes of the prior skin assessment, skin changes that were reddish-purple and found over various areas of the body appeared shortly before death. This study provides observational data on some of the unavoidable skin changes at life's end.

2A: Develop an individualized plan of care. Following the wound assessment as described above, an individualized wound care plan of care should be developed by the interprofessional team. The plan must be tailored to the individual, taking into consideration his or her unique biopsychosocial needs, including:

• Risk factors
• Comorbidities
• Quality-of-life issues
• Support systems/circle of care
• Access to care
• Personal preferences.

As discussed by Sackett et al,[31] individualized patient preference must be honored and reflected in the wound care plan. Sackett et al[31] recognized 3 dimensions of equal importance: best available scientific evidence, clinical expertise, and patient preference. This model of evidence-based medicine has been one of the most important healthcare trends in the past 20 years. Interprofessional, individualized patient-centered care must drive the care process.[32]

The wound care plan of care should be as follows:

• In writing and part of the permanent healthcare record

- Routinely evaluated and updated
- Updated with any significant change in the individual's health status.

2B: Treat the cause(s) related to specific wound etiology/diagnosis. Once an accurate type of wound is established, the treatment can be planned and implemented (Table 5).

For example, in a person with a venous ulcer, compression therapy is contraindicated when the ABPI is 0.5 or less, and a vascular consult is required for limb preservation.[33] Under the care of an expert wound care team, modified compression therapy for patients with ABPIs between 0.5 and 0.8 is beneficial and assists perfusion by increasing pulsatile flow,[34] thereby decreasing venous pressure and facilitating the arterial-venous gradient.[35]

Importance of Holistic Interprofessional Coordinated and Collaborative Care

Accurate wound diagnosis and development of successful treatment plans can be a challenging undertaking, given the complexity of chronic wounds. A holistic interprofessional approach is required. Each member of the team possesses a unique professional skill set and knowledge base that should contribute to the individualized plan of care. Implemented treatment plans that do not yield wound healing rates at the expected trajectory require a timely referral to an interprofessional team that can reevaluate the diagnosis and causative factors. Redefining the treatment goals with the input from the patient, family, and healthcare provider is essential as well.

2C: Modify (if possible) systemic factors/other cofactors that may impair healing: medications, nutrition, hemoglobin, blood pressure, creatinine, congestive heart failure (CHF), liver function tests (LFTs), and so on. A good example of systemic factors that affect wound healing is the hemoglobin level. Because hemoglobin carries the oxygen that is essential for new tissue building, hemoglobin levels should be optimized. Potential negative influences for adequate hemoglobin are common in patients living with other chronic illnesses, such as renal disease and sickle cell and other anemias, to name a few.

Persons with cardiopulmonary disease, cardiovascular disease (including congestive heart failure), and related conditions have diminished extremity tissue perfusion as a result of reduced ejection fractions. In particular, heart failure and associated decreased tissue perfusion to the periphery results in edema accumulation in the lower extremities, creating higher risk for lower leg wound formation or delayed healing in existing wounds. In many cases, an internal medicine or subspecialty referral can optimize heart function and manage fluid balance and edema reduction. The offending co-contributors and cofactors that impede wound healing should be adjusted and corrected. Improving as many factors as possible may contribute to overall improvement of the patient's quality of life, reducing pain, improving mobility, and facilitating improved wound outcomes.

A patient with a chronic wound may require a thorough nutritional assessment by a registered dietitian to address any underlying and correctable nutritional deficits. Proteins have a fundamental role throughout the wound healing cycle, influencing the function of leukocytes, phagocytes, monocytes, lymphocytes, and macrophages, all integral to a normal healing trajectory.[36,37] A multinational European, prospective, randomized, controlled, double-blind trial studied the effects of specific oral nutritional supplementation in nonmalnourished patients specific to PU healing. The provision of a high-protein, micronutrient-enriched and arginine supplement resulted in improved healing rates and less wound care intensity for the care providers.[38]

Medications that may inhibit or delay wound healing should be reviewed, including the benefit, risk, and dose of each medication. Refer to section 1C for more detail.

Address and Treat Individualized Concerns

3. Assess and support individualized concerns. 3A: Pain. McCaffery[39] has stated that pain is what the patient says it is. Every person experiences pain differently. Clinicians cannot treat pain that they do not know patients are experiencing. Pain measurement is subjective. However, the universally accepted measurement techniques are the visual analog scale (the patient places an "x" at the appropriate point on a 10-cm line with no pain at one end and worst possible pain at the other end), the Faces Pain Scale (various levels of happy and sad faces), and the numerical rating

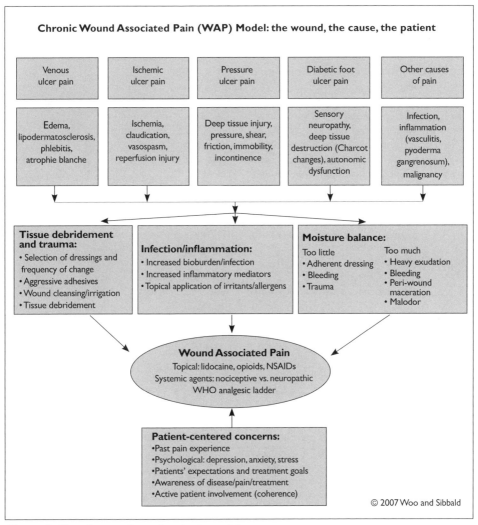

Figure 1. Chronic wound-associated pain model.

scale. The numerical rating scale asks if the patient has any pain on a 0- to 10-point scale with the anchors that 0 is no pain, 5 is the pain associated with a bee sting, and 10 would be the amount of pain experienced by slamming the car door on your thumb. Even in patients who cannot respond verbally, such as those with dementia, pain still needs to be assessed. There are pain scales for these patients that rely on nonverbal clues, such as facial grimaces and pupil dilatation. (Assessment of pain for people with dementia can be found at www.hartfordign.org.) Pain levels should be

recorded before dressing change, during dressing change, and after dressing reapplication.

Krasner has defined wound-associated pain at dressing change (intermittent and recurrent) versus incident pain from debridement or the persistent pain between dressing changes. Woo et al[40] carried the Krasner concept further and demonstrated that anxiety and other patient-related factors could intensify the pain experience. The Wound Associated Pain model of Woo and Sibbald (Figure 1) defines pain from the cause of the wound as often being persistent or present between dressing changes and distinguishes this pain from the pain associated with local wound care components (dressing change, debridement, infection, lack of moisture balance). All of these factors can be modified by patient-centered concerns, including previous pain experience, anxiety, depression, mobility, awareness of or lack of comfort with the setting, and the procedure or treatment plan. Pain is an under-recognized and under-treated component of chronic wound care that has been demonstrated to be more important to patients than healthcare professionals. Causes of pain at dressing change include the dressing material adhering to the wound base, skin stripping from strong adhesives, and aggressive trauma from cleansing technique (eg, scrubbing with gauze).

Many patients also express chronic persistent pain between dressing changes even at rest. A systematized approach should examine other systemic and disease factors that may play a role in precipitating and sustaining persistent wound-related pain. Common systemic factors are bacterial damage from superficial critical colonization or deep and surrounding compartment infections; deep structural damage (eg, acute Charcot foot in patients with diabetes); abnormal inflammatory conditions (eg, vasculitis, pyoderma gangrenosum); and periwound contact irritant skin damage from enzyme-rich wound exudate.

The impact of chronic unrelenting pain can be devastating, eroding the individual's quality of life and constituting a significant amount of stress. Increased levels of stress have been demonstrated to lower pain threshold and decrease tolerance. The result is a vicious cycle of pain, stress/anxiety, anticipation of pain, and worsening of pain. Increased stress also activates the hypothalamus-pituitary-adrenal axis, producing hormones that modulate the immune system, compromising normal wound healing. Medications including non-narcotics for moderate pain and narcotic analgesics for moderate to severe pain are required to treat pain as outlined below. A consult from a pain and symptom management team may be considered. Comprehensive management should also include careful selection of atraumatic dressings, prevention of local trauma, treatment of infection, patient empowerment, stress reduction, and patient education.

The medical treatment of wound-associated pain and other components of pain management

are outlined in the World Union of Wound Healing Societies documents.[40,41] In general, wound-associated pain is both nociceptive- and stimulus-dependent (gnawing, aching, tender, throbbing) versus neuropathic or non–stimulus-dependent or spontaneous pain (burning, stinging, shooting, stabbing). Nociceptive pain is treated with the World Health Organization (WHO) pain ladder medication starting with aspirin and nonsteroidal anti-inflammatory drugs and then progressing to weak and strong narcotics.[42] Short-acting agents are often used to determine the dose of longer acting agents, and then the short-acting agents may be used for breakthrough. The neuropathic pain often responds to tricyclic agents, particularly second-generation agents high in antinoradrenaline activity (nortriptyline and desipramine are often better than amitriptyline), and to alternate agents gabapentin and pregabalin or other antiepileptic agents in nonresponders. Neuropathic pain occurs even with the loss of protective sensation and can awaken persons with neuropathy at night with lightning-like flashes of pain.

3B: Activities of daily living. Living with a chronic leg ulcer and ADLs has the largest body of evidence, mainly using qualitative methodology, compared with other ulcer etiologies. Patients reported numerous negative influences on their ability to carry out ADLs, including, pain, odor, mobility, finances, and aspects of living.[43] Depression and anxiety were reported in as many as 68% of the subjects. Another recent study highlighted the dominant impact of social isolation in patients suffering from chronic leg ulcers.[44] One study compared patients living with diabetic foot ulcers (DFUs) with those with amputations following foot ulcers and concluded that a higher quality of life was reported in those who underwent lower-limb amputations.[45] Assessing the unique individual's concerns can be a time-consuming but necessary piece in addressing the patient's holistic needs. This highlights the emotional burden of living with a chronic wound.

3C: Psychosocial well-being. Psychosocial well-being is the dimension of quality of life that most people equate with the quality piece.[46] It includes the individual's psychological perspectives on his or her wound and overall life. It reflects the person's ability to socialize and interact with others.

There are many wound care interventions that can address and support a person's wound-related psychosocial issues. For example:

- If wound odor is an issue, charcoal or other odor-reducing dressings can be utilized.
- Dressing routines can be modified to accommodate individualized hygiene practices. For showers Mondays-Wednesdays-Fridays, dressing changes can be coordinated to Mondays-Wednesdays-Fridays right after the shower.

3D: Smoking. Cigarette smoking is a leading preventable health problem causing damage to the endothelial function of arteries throughout the body,[47] contributing to the development of vascular disease of both arterial and venous origin. The direct cutaneous effect of smoking is stated clearly by Rayner.[48] Cutaneous blood flow decreases as much as 40% to produce ischemia and impair healing.[49] Smoking a single cigarette creates a vasoconstrictive effect for up to 90 minutes, while smoking a packet results in tissue hypoxia that lasts an entire day.[50]

Delayed wound healing for individuals who use tobacco is attributed to resultant tissue hypoxia.[51] Smoking disrupts the normal healing process at many levels, decreasing cell proliferation and migration across the wound bed.[52–54] Cigarettes contain more than 4,000 substances, including carbon monoxide, nicotine, and cyanide derivatives,[55] and each substance can potentially negatively influence wound healing. Useful patient smoking cessation strategies, including the pharmacological, behavioral, and effectiveness of these programs, are outlined by Ahn et al.[55] Offering patients these strategies to quit smoking and improve tissue oxygenation may enhance healing.

3E: Access to care/financial limitations. Living with a wound can be a challenge for many patients who may have limited financial resources or access to care. Patients living with chronic illnesses compounded by a wound may have difficulties with transportation for medical appointments, and many are unemployed or on limited incomes. Depending on where the patient lives, there are differing resources available. Healthcare professionals should advocate for required patient resources. When a wound is determined to be maintenance or nonhealing, the healthcare team, along with the patient, can individualize the care

plan to be most efficient for both the patient and the system.

4. Provide education and support to the person and his or her circle of care (including referral) to increase adherence (coherence) to the treatment plan. One strategy to provide support and education to a patient is by developing a therapeutic relationship.[56] Trust implies sharing of information and communication, and open dialogue allows patients and those in their circle of care to understand that each person involved has a meaningful contribution. Active participation by the patient in the development of an individualized plan of care provides reassurance to the patient that the team is working with them to achieve the best possible outcome. This helps to enhance adherence to the agreed upon treatment plan, as there is trust. An additional concept in team dynamics is unit cohesion or the process of "sticking together" for the accomplishment of a mission or task. If the patient provides substantive input into the treatment plan, there is a greater chance that the patient will adhere (cohere) to a given plan. By way of example, patient participation, such as removing the dressing at dressing change, should be encouraged as clinically appropriate. People in the patient's circle of care, such as family, caregivers, and healthcare professionals, should also be part of the plan, including implementation and reevaluation. Communication is paramount between healthcare sectors and professionals when managing chronic wounds. Once an expert team has determined that a wound is maintenance or nonhealable, it is important that this be communicated to prevent unnecessary investigations or interventions that may have already been unsuccessful. Healthcare professionals should review and educate the patient and family after determining their current knowledge gaps and teach the patient to report important signs that could indicate a deterioration of the wound. Strategies to improve adherence have been reported in a comprehensive review by Osterberg and Blaschke.[57]

Local Wound Care

5. Assess and monitor the wound history and physical examination. Documentation of a detailed patient and wound assessment is a legal requirement from both an organizational and professional standards perspective. Specific details about the wound history and physical will facilitate communication within the patient's circle of care. This includes the type of wound and history and the patient-centered plan of care and targeted patient-specific goals.[58] The details of the wound assessment should be communicated to other professionals when referrals are made. If a wound is healable, nonhealable, or maintenance, an individualized care plan is made to identify specific interventions and outcomes that the patient and interprofessional team agree upon and modify based on a new holistic interprofessional assessment. One example is the mnemonic MEASURE,[59] which describes the wound location plus MEASURE:

- Measure size (longest length with the widest width at right angles)
- Exudate amount (none, scant, moderate, heavy) and characteristics (serous, sanguinous, pustular, or combinations)
- Appearance (base: necrotic [black], fibrin [firm yellow], slough [soft yellow], or granulation tissue [pink and healthy vs red and friable = easy bleeding, unhealthy])
- Suffering (pain)
- Undermining (measure in centimeters and use hands of clock to document: 12 o'clock, 6 o'clock, and so on)
- Reevaluate
- Edge (hyperkeratotic, macerated, normal).

Using a framework allows consistent documentation of a wound. When a framework is used to assess a wound over time, clinicians can identify if a wound is improving, stalled, or deteriorating.

There are several new electronic technologies available for wound assessment, but they may be costly for clinicians and healthcare systems. Novel camera systems accurately calculate length, width, depth, and surface of exposed wound areas. Limitations include undermined areas or sinuses that are not measureable using this technology, requiring supplementation by visual clinical inspection and probing. Wound assessment devices markedly differ from computer-based documentation systems that capture multiple data points and assessments about wound parameters inputted by skilled clinicians.

6. Gently cleanse wounds with low-toxicity solutions: saline, water, and acetic acid (0.5%–1.0%). Do not irrigate wounds when you cannot see where the solution is going and cannot retrieve (or aspirate) the irrigating solution. The standard of care for wound cleansing is to use those solutions that are gentle and least cytotoxic to the wound as possible: saline, water, and acetic acid (0.5%–1.0%). Research has shown that certain solutions can be cytotoxic to healing cells, such as fibroblasts, *in vitro*.[60]

In the analysis of Cochrane Reviews prior to 2008, the authors concluded, "There is not strong evidence that cleansing wounds per se increases healing or reduces infection." The Cochrane Collaboration updated evidence reviews on wound cleansing for PUs and concluded that "there is no good trial evidence to support use of any particular wound cleansing solution or technique for pressure ulcers."[61] A specific type of solution for wound cleansing in adults was an additional evidence review. The authors concluded that there is no evidence to indicate that using tap water to cleanse an acute wound increased infection rates. In addition, there is no strong evidence demonstrating that cleansing of wounds at all decreases infection or promotes healing.[62] Expert opinion recommends that caution should be considered in the use of tap water for immunocompromised individuals, especially the use of nonpotable water, which may be a problem in developing countries.

Avoiding cytotoxic solutions, such as Dakin's and povidone-iodine, to cleanse healable wounds or using them for only limited periods is reasonably prudent practice. However, there is a place for these agents in the management of maintenance or nonhealable wounds to potentially control bioburden and odor. In these cases, the reduction in bioburden and moisture reduction outweighs the small potential for tissue toxicity.

Wound irrigation has also been the subject of controversy and disagreement between health professionals. In general, the authors recommend that clinicians should not irrigate wounds when they cannot see where the solution is being instilled into the dead space at the base of the wound or if they cannot retrieve the irrigating solution. More research on wound cleansing is needed. (See Wound Bed Preparation Enabler 2011 for antiseptic solutions and their utility for wound care.)

7. **Debride: Healable wounds — sharp or conservative surgical, autolytic, mechanical, enzymatic, biological (medical maggots); nonhealable and maintenance — conservative surgical or other methods of removal of nonviable slough**. The wound bed is optimally prepared by aggressive and regular debridement of any firm eschar or soft slough if the wound is healable. A firm eschar serves as a proinflammatory stimulus inhibiting healing, whereas the slough acts as a culture media for bacterial proliferation and should be removed.[63] Debridement may also promote healing by removing senescent cells that are deficient in cellular activities and biofilms that contain the bacterial colonies.[64]

Sharp debridement is the most expeditious method but may not always be feasible because of pain, bleeding potential, cost, professional/system regulations, and the lack of clinician expertise. Cardinal et al[65] conducted a retrospective review on 366 persons with VLUs and 310 persons with DFUs over 12 weeks, observing wound surface area changes and closure rates. Interestingly, VLUs had a significantly higher median wound surface area reduction with surgical debridement (when clinically indicated due to the presence of debris) versus no surgical debridement (34%, $P = .019$). Centers with more frequent debridement were associated with higher rates of wound closure ($P = .007$ VLUs, $P = .015$ DFUs). The debridement frequency did not statistically correlate to higher rates of wound closure. There was some minor evidence of a positive benefit of serial debridement in DFUs (odds ratio, 2.35; $P = .069$).

Alternatively, autolytic debridement is most accepted by keeping a moist wound environment to enhance the activities of phagocytic cells and endogenous enzymes on nonviable tissues. *Mechanical debridement with saline wet-to-dry dressings contributes to local trauma and pain. In the United States, the Centers for Medicare & Medicaid Services, in its Tag F314 guidance, cautions that there should be limited use of wet-to-dry dressings.* Emerging technology using ultrasonic devices also has been demonstrative of WBP without the incumbent painful and traumatic scraping and cutting associated with sharp and mechanical debridement. When using enzymatic debridement, clinicians should ensure that the cleansing solutions and type of dressing used to cover the wound do not interfere with or cancel out the action of the enzyme.

Select the appropriate method of wound debridement considering the patient, the wound characteristics, and the skill and knowledge of the clinician, along with the available resources. In summary, the different methods of debridement have distinct features in terms of pain potential, cost, healthcare professional time and skill level required, resources used, and wound characteristics. (See Wound Bed Preparation Enabler 2011: Key Factors in Deciding Method of Debridement.)

8. **Assess and treat the wound for superficial critical colonization/deep infection/abnormal persistent inflammation (mnemonic STONEES) or persistent inflammation:** For any 3 NERDS (**N**onhealing, ↑**E**xudate, **R**ed, friable tissue, **D**ebris, **S**mell), treat topically. For any 3 STONEES (↑**S**ize, ↑**T**emperature, **O**s, **N**ew breakdown, ↑**E**xudate, ↑**E**rythema/edema (cellulitis), **S**mell), treat systemically. For persistent inflammation (non-infectious), treat with topical and/or systemic anti-inflammatories. (See Wound Bed Preparation Enabler 2011.)

Chronic wounds containing bacteria and/or the presence of bacteria obtained from a surface swab do not define or portend infection. In fact, the mean number of bacterial species per chronic ulcer has been found to range from 1.6 to 4.4.[66] Critical to wound healing is achieving an appropriate bacterial balance and understanding the differences between contamination or colonization or frank bacterial damage with surface critical colonization or surrounding/deep infection. The risk of infection is determined by the number and nature of invading bacteria as well as host resistance as outlined in the following equation:

Infection = number of organisms x organism virulence

Host Resistance

Host resistance is the most important factor, and it refers to the host immune response to resist bacterial invasion and prevent bacterial damage.[67] In addition, adequate blood supply is needed for the wound to heal, as a decreased or inadequate blood supply favors bacterial proliferation and damage that may prevent or delay healing. Infection is more prevalent in certain disease conditions. For example, individuals with diabetes have at least a 10-fold greater risk of being hospitalized for soft tissue and bone infections of the foot than nondiabetic individuals.[68] Local factors inhibiting healing may include a large wound size, the presence of foreign bodies (prosthetic joints, a thread, or remnants of gauze or a retained suture), and an untreated deeper infection, such as osteomyelitis.[69] External contamination of the wound bed by microorganisms can occur from the ambient environment, dressings, the patient's secretions and hands, and the hands of healthcare providers (alcohol hand rinses are more effective in reducing hand bacteria than washing with soap and water).

By using this superficial and deep-surrounding tissue separation, the clinician can identify wounds with increased bacterial burden that may respond to topical antimicrobials and deep infection that usually requires the use of systemic antimicrobial agents. The mnemonics NERDS and STONEES represent the initials of the signs to categorize the 2 levels of bacterial damage or infection. This concept was introduced[70] in 2006 and validated[71] in 2009. Three or more of these signs should be sought for the diagnosis in each level. If increased exudate and odor are present, additional signs are needed to determine if the damage is superficial, deep, or both.

There are now at least 5 classes of antimicrobial dressings and some miscellaneous products for use in chronic wounds with critical colonization as defined by any 3 of the NERDS criteria:
- Silver dressings combined with alginates, foams, hydrofibers, and hydrogels
- Honey dressings in a calcium alginate wafer and hydrogel
- Iodine in a cadexomer carbohydrate or polyethylene glycol slow-release formulation (not available in the United States)
- PHMB (polyhexamethylene biguanide) derivative of chlorhexidine in a foam or gauze packing
- Miscellaneous antimicrobial dressings often with a paucity of clinical studies to support their use.

The treatment of critical colonization often takes 2 to 4 weeks in a healable wound where the cause has been corrected and patient-centered concerns have been addressed. There is some, but limited, evidence to show the benefit of these dressings if the wound is in bacterial balance. Antibacterial dressings are not needed for the re-epithelization stage of wound healing, unless they also provide anti-inflammatory activity.[72,73] They also are not efficacious in the treatment of deep and surrounding tissue infection that requires the use of systemic agents. Studies that do not select the proper subpopulation (eg, healable critically colonized wounds without deep infection) or measure complete wound healing have failed to demonstrate any benefit from these dressings.[74]

The use of antimicrobial dressings should be reviewed at frequent and regular intervals every 1 to 2 weeks and discontinued if critical colonization has been corrected or if they do not demonstrate a beneficial effect after 2 to 4 weeks. There is currently a great tendency to overuse antimicrobial dressings, creating a cost-inefficient use of these useful devices. The conflicting evidence and misuse of these dressings have led some European healthcare systems to completely delist silver products.

Silver Dressings

The effectiveness of silver-releasing dressings in the management of nonhealing (stalled) chronic wounds was reviewed by a meta-analysis.[75] In comparison to alternative antimicrobials, silver dressings significantly:
- Improved the wound healing rate (95% confidence interval [CI], 0.16–0.39, $P < .001$)
- Reduced odor (95% CI, 0.24–0.52, $P < .001$) and pain-related symptoms (95% CI, 0.18–0.47, $P < .001$)
- Decreased wound exudate (95% CI, 0.17–0.44, $P < .001$)
- Had a prolonged dressing wear time (95% CI, 0.19–0.48, $P = .028$) when compared with alternative wound management approaches.

Silver's broad spectrum of antimicrobial activity can be used in critically colonized chronic wounds that have the ability to heal. Silver must be ionized to exert an antimicrobial effect. Ionized silver requires an aqueous or water environment and should not be used in a maintenance or nonhealable wound where the desired outcome is the combination of moisture reduction and bacterial reduction. Silver should not be in close proximity to any oil-based products (eg, petrolatum, zinc oxide) where the oil molecules may interfere with the ionization of the silver. Products that produce a continuous supply of ionized silver are likely to be more efficacious, and higher levels of silver release are often necessary to treat microorganisms, such as pseudomonas, in a complete environment, such as a wound. Pseudomonas requires a higher silver level for silver to work than most other bacterial organisms. Silver resistance is uncommon because there are at least 3 antimicrobial mechanisms with silver targeting and combining with membranes, cytoplasmic organelles, and DNA.

The amount of silver released from these dressings is a fraction of the silver released from silver sulfadiazine (SSD) cream formulations. Serum silver levels even from high-release silver dressings are in the 1–5 micromolar range. Modern silver dressings seldom exceed normal range unless large surface areas are treated over prolonged time or the patient has a large skin surface area to total weight. Silver dressings can cause temporary periwound staining but do not leave permanent silver deposits in the dermis (argyria or blue discoloration of the skin). The silver in the dressing should be combined with the appropriate moisture balance format matched to the wound to control exudate and prevent maceration but facilitate the delivery of ionized silver to the wound surface.

Honey, Iodine, and PHMB

The Cochrane Collaboration conducted a systematic review of the honey literature and concluded that honey, as a topical treatment for superficial and partial-thickness burns, may improve healing times compared with some conventional dressings. Jull et al[76] conducted a multicenter, randomized controlled trial on VLUs with compression comparing honey to usual care. There were 187 patients in the honey group and 181 patients in the usual-care group with no difference between the 2 groups for total wound healing at 12 weeks.

In clinical practice, honey dressings may be useful for thick eschar that often continuously reforms when treated with other dressings. Some of this action may be due to the antibacterial and hyperosmolar characteristics of the honey. Scoring the wound with a blade to help break down the eschar may facilitate the process.

There are 10 trials with cadexomer iodine, and some of these trials are old, with venous ulcers treated topically without compression. In a randomized controlled trial comparing cadexomer iodine with standard care with both groups receiving compression, the daily or weekly healing rates favored cadexomer iodine.[77]

In a pilot study of PHMB foam compared with foam alone, the PHMB dressing resulted in decreased pain and no change in wound size.[78]

Evaluating Evidence of Antimicrobials *in vitro* and Animal Models: The Literature

Beware of *in-vitro* testing of antimicrobial dressings because the results often do not correlate with clinical activity. Although the studies may demonstrate statistical significance, clinical significance is the parameter of interest; moreover, the strength of evidence for the majority of these *in-vitro* studies is low. When evaluating topical antimicrobial agents for wound treatment, appropriate tests must be used. For instance, the *in-vitro* evaluation of an antimicrobial agent, such as silver, can be performed with a multitude of tests, but of these, only the logarithmic reduction or decimal reduction time test conducted in serum has been shown to predict clinical outcomes.[79,80] *In-vivo* antimicrobial assays, such as the Walker Mason modified model (rodent) or the Wright model (porcine), also can be used with success to determine antimicrobial efficacy.[81] Similarly, the evaluation of the efficacy of topical agents on wound healing can be evaluated *in vitro* (cellular culture or tissue explant models) or *in vivo* (rodent or porcine wound healing models). However, the only model that predicts a clinical outcome is the porcine model of wound healing.[82]

A recent Cochrane Review explored antibiotic and antiseptic use for persons with VLUs. The authors concluded that there is no evidence for routine use of systemic antibiotics[83] when treating the cause of VLUs.

9. Select a dressing to match the appropriate wound and individual person characteristics:
- Healable wounds: Autolytic debridement: Alginates, hydrogels, hydrocolloids, acrylics
- Critical colonization: Silver, iodides, PHMB, honey
- Persistent inflammation: Anti-inflammatory dressings

Table 6. Modern classes of dressings

Class	Description	Tissue Debridement	Infection	Moisture Balance	Indications/ Contraindications
1. Films/ membranes	Semipermeable adhesive sheet; impermeable to water molecules and bacteria	+	-	-	Moisture vapor transmission rate varies from film to film. Should not be used on draining or infected wounds.[a] Create occlusive barrier against infection.
2. Nonadherent	Sheets of low adherence to tissue; Nonmedicated tulles	-	-	-	Allow drainage to seep through pores to secondary dressings. Facilitate application of topical.
3. Hydrogels	Polymers with high water content Available in gels, solid sheets, or impregnated gauze	++	-/+	++	Should not be used on draining wounds. Solid sheets should not be used on infected wounds.
4. Hydrocolloids	May contain gelatin, sodium carboxymethylcellulose, polysaccharides and/or pectin; sheet dressings are occlusive with polyurethane film outer layer	+++	-/+	++	Should be used with care on fragile skin. Should stay in place for several days. Should not be used on heavily draining or infected wounds.[a] Create occlusive barrier to protect the wound from outside contamination. Odor may accompany dressing change and should not be confused with infection.
5. Acrylics	Clear acrylic pad enclosed between 2 layers of transparent adhesive film	+++	-/+	++	Use on low to moderately draining wounds where dressing may stay in place for extended time. May observe wound without changing.
6. Calcium alginates	Sheets or fibrous ropes of calcium sodium alginate (seaweed derivative); have hemostatic capabilities	++	+	+++	Should not be used on dry wounds. Low tensile strength — avoid packing into narrow deep sinuses. Bioabsorbable.
7. Composite dressings	Multilayered, combination dressings to increase absorbency and autolysis	+	-	+++	Use on wounds where dressings may stay in place for several days[a]

[a]Use with caution if critical colonization is suspected; - no activity; + minimal activity; ++ moderate activity; +++ strong activity.
Adapted from Canadian Association of Wound Care, Revised.

- Moisture balance: Foams, hydrofibers, alginates, hydrocolloids, films, acrylics
- Nonhealable, maintenance wounds: Chlorhexidine, povidone–iodine

Whenever patients and healthcare professionals are developing a treatment plan for patients with wounds, dressing selection is an important primary focus. Once healable, nonhealable, or maintenance is determined, appropriate holistic interprofessional interventions that address cofactors can be optimized. The dressing selection should be the last part of the process because if the healability is not accurately assessed or other cofactors are unmanaged, then the wound will

Table 6. Modern classes of dressings *continued*

Class	Description	Tissue Debridement	Infection	Moisture Balance	Indications/ Contraindications
8. Foams	Nonadhesive or adhesive polyurethane foam; may have occlusive backing; sheets or cavity packing; some have fluid lock	-	-	+++	Use on moderately to heavily draining wounds. Occlusive foams should not be used on heavily draining or infected wounds.[a]
9. Charcoal	Contains odor-absorbing charcoal within product	-	-	+	Some charcoal products are inactivated by moisture. Ensure dressing edges are sealed.
10. Hypertonic	Sheet, ribbon, or gel impregnated with sodium concentrate	+	+	++	Gauze ribbon should not be used on dry wounds. May be painful on sensitive tissue. Gel may be used on dry wounds.
11. Hydrophilic fibers	Sheet or packing strip of sodium carboxymethylcellulose; converts to a solid gel when activated by moisture (fluid lock)	+	-	+++	Best for moderate amount of exudate. Should not be used on dry wounds. Low tensile strength — avoid packing into the narrow deep sinus.
12. Antimicrobials	Silver, iodides, PHMB, honey aniline dyes with vehicle for delivery: sheets, gels, alginates, foams, or paste	+	+++	+	Broad spectrum against bacteria. Should not be used on patients with known hypersensitivities to any product components.
13. Other devices	Negative pressure wound therapy applies localized negative pressure to the surface and margins of wound	-	+	+++	This negative pressure-distributing dressing actively removes fluid from wound and promotes wound edge approximation. Advanced skill required for patient selection for this therapy.
14. Biologics	Living human fibroblasts provided in sheets at ambient or frozen temperature; extracellular matrix; collagen-containing preparations; hyaluronic acid; platelet-derived growth factor	-	-	-	Should not be used on wounds with infection, sinus tracts, or excessive exudate or on patients known to have hypersensitivity to any of the product components. Cultural issues related to source. Advanced skill required for patient selection for this therapy.

[a]Use with caution if critical colonization is suspected; - no activity; + minimal activity; ++ moderate activity; +++ strong activity.
Adapted from Canadian Association of Wound Care, Revised.

not heal. Dressing choice needs to consider unit costs and clinical effectiveness. Kerstein et al[84] explored cost-effectiveness for venous ulcers and PUs and concluded that the purchase price of the dressing should not be the only indicator. Normal saline gauze dressings (least expensive for product) were found to be the most expensive when nursing time and patient feedback were taken into account (Table 6).

Persistent Inflammation

Chronic wounds may be stalled in the inflammatory stage. These wounds demonstrate markedly increased activity of inflammatory cells and

Table 7. Summary of advanced therapy options

Substantiated Advanced Therapies	Indication	RCT or Meta-analysis Available	Results
OASIS	VLU DNFU	Yes[91] Yes[92]	Complete healing Complete healing equal to PDGF
Growth factors (PDGF)	DNFU	Yes[93,94]	Complete healing
Apligraf (epidermal cells, dermal fibroblasts, bovine collagen)	DNFU VLU	Yes[95-97] Yes[98]	Complete healing Complete healing
Dermagraft (fibroblasts)	DNFU	Yes[99-101]	Complete healing
Hyperbaric oxygen therapy	DNFU	Yes[102]	Prevent amputation
Electrical stimulation	PU	Yes[103]	Complete healing
Therapeutic ultrasound	VLU DNFU	Yes[104] Yes[105]	Faster healing Complete healing
Negative-pressure wound therapy	Postsurgical wounds	Yes[106]	Complete healing
Promogran	VLU	Yes[107,108]	Decrease wound size

Abbreviations: DNFU, diabetic neurotrophic foot ulcer; PDGF, platelet-derived growth factor; PU, pressure ulcer; RCT, randomized controlled trial.
© 2006 Woo and Sibbald.

associated mediators, such as matrix metalloproteinases (MMPs) and elastase.[85] Wound healing is stalled because degradation of extracellular matrix and growth factors occurs more rapidly than their synthesis, hindering the wound from progressing toward the proliferative phase and ultimately re-epithelization. Harding et al[86] reported that the longer a wound remains in the inflammatory phase, the more cellular defects are detected with potential delayed healing. Recently, there has been a renewal of interest in wound diagnostic testing that will result in tests for increased MMPs that will be available soon for bedside testing. There are wound dressings with oxidized reduced collagen and cellulose that can trap MMPs, and these dressings can be combined with antimicrobials, such as silver. These specialized dressings can be combined antimicrobials, depending on the presence of the mnemonic NERDS (superficial antibacterial dressing criteria) or mnemonic STONEES (systemic antibiotic criteria) and where the presence of increased inflammation also can be treated topically or systemically.

Appropriate moisture is required to facilitate the action of growth factors and cytokines and the mi-

gration of cells, including fibroblasts and keratinocytes. Moisture balance is a delicate process. Excessive moisture can potentially cause damage to the surrounding skin of a wound, leading to maceration and potential breakdown.[87] Conversely, inadequate moisture in the wound environment can impede cellular activities and promote eschar formation, resulting in poor wound healing. A moisture-balanced wound environment is maintained primarily by modern dressings with occlusive, semiocclusive, absorptive, hydrating, and hemostatic characteristics, depending on the drainage and other wound bed properties.

10. Evaluate expected rate of wound healing: Healable wounds should be 30% smaller by Week 4 to heal by Week 12. Wounds not healing at the expected rate should be reclassified or reassessed and the plan of care revised. It is noted that a 20% to 40% reduction in 2 and 4 weeks is likely to be a reliable predictor of healing.[88,89] Sheehan et al[90] noted a 50% reduction at Week 4 was a good predictor for persons with DFUs. One measure of healing is the clinical observation of the edge of the wound. If the wound edge is not migrating after appropriate WBP (debridement, bacterial balance, moisture balance) and healing is stalled, then advanced therapies should be considered. The first step prior to initiating the edge-effect therapies is a reassessment of the patient to rule out other causes and cofactors. Clinicians need to remember that wound healing is not always the primary outcome. Consider other wound-related outcomes, such as reduced pain, reduced bacterial load, reduced dressing changes, or an improved quality of life.

11. Use active wound therapies (eg, skin grafts, biological agents, adjunctive therapies) when other factors have been corrected and healing still does not progress (stalled wound). A nonhealing wound may have a cliff-like edge between the upper epithelium and the lower granulation in comparison to a healing wound with tapered edges like the shore of a sandy beach. Several edge-effect therapies support the addition of missing components: growth factors, fibroblasts, epithelial cells, or matrix components. If all the factors are corrected in a healable wound, active adjunctive therapies may be considered (Table 7).

Provide Organization Support

12. For improved outcomes, education and evidence-informed practice must be tied to interprofessional teams and improved cost-effective patient care outcomes with the cooperation of healthcare systems. When a patient has a wound, it is important that the team provide education to the patient and his or her circle of care to involve everyone in the treatment plan. Healthcare professionals may assume that patients know more about their wounds than their current understanding. One study surveyed persons with DFUs and their self-foot-care behaviors. Healthcare providers conducted a detailed foot assessment and provided education on each visit. Results indicated that the knowledge base is often less than expected by the healthcare professional and leads to treatment gaps.[109] Behavior of healthcare providers changed during the course of the study, resulting in an increased chance that the patient's socks were removed, leading to a thorough examination and patient education.

Importance of Holistic Interprofessional Coordinated and Collaborative Care

Accurate wound diagnosis and development of successful treatment plans can be a challenging undertaking, given the complexity of chronic wounds. A holistic interprofessional approach to care requires that each member of the team has a unique professional knowledge that contributes to the individualized plan of care. The management of patients with DFUs utilizing a team approach and primary healing outcomes can be associated with relatively low costs related to a visit with an interprofessional team, antibiotics, and plantar pressure downloading in the community setting.[110] When healing occurs following an amputation, multiple hospital admissions and extended length of hospital stay are tabulated, with the cost for healing being significantly higher. Implemented treatment plans that do not yield wound healing rates at the expected trajectory require a timely referral to an interprofessional team that can reevaluate the diagnosis and causative factors. Redefining the treatment goals with the input from the patient, family, and healthcare provider is essential. Given the geographical and system differences, the ideal full complement of an interprofessional expert team may not always be accessible. Therefore, it is important to realize that only 2 disciplines working collaboratively with the patient and/or family may be successful.

Clinicians must distinguish between interdisciplinary networks with 2 members of the same profession (such as 2 nurses or assistants versus a nurse practitioner who may have a similar role to a physician on an interprofessional team), compared with the physician and nurse of an interprofessional team. For chronic wound care, the physician and nurse are best supplemented with a member of the allied healthcare team (eg, occupational therapist, physical therapist, foot care specialist, dietitian, social worker).

Many patients with chronic stalled wounds are complex, older adults who reside with multiple comorbidities, requiring lengthy assessment and coordination of the treatment interventions. This necessitates the healthcare system policy maker to support interprofessional clinician teams to provide the best possible evidence-informed practice.

Conclusion

The concept of WBP includes the treatment of the whole patient (treat the cause and patient-centered concerns). The approach to the local wound bed has 4 components starting with the mnemonic DIM: Debridement, Infection/prolonged Inflammation control, and Moisture balance, before the mnemonic DIME that includes the advanced Edge-effect therapies for wounds with the ability to heal.

In addition, this chapter has introduced the concept of healable, nonhealable, and maintenance wounds along with the integration of clinical criteria for superficial critical colonization (mnemonic NERDS) and topical antimicrobial dressings versus deep and surrounding tissue infections (mnemonic STONEES) requiring systemic agents. Bacterial damage needs to be distinguished from persistent inflammation with soon to be available bedside matrix metalloproteases (MMPs) testing. The ultimate treatment process should include the leadership of an interprofessional wound management team, and patient participation is paramount for the best achievable outcome.

After reading this chapter, clinicians can distinguish between healable, nonhealable, and maintenance wounds and design the appropriate management plans.

Self-Assessment Questions

1. Identify all options for a maintenance wound:
   A. A healable wound but patient adherence factors prevent healing
   B. A nonhealable wound
   C. A healable wound but health system factors prevent healing
   D. A stalled chronic wound
   E. A and C

2. When is/are the potential time/times to experience the greatest wound-related pain?
   A. Autolytic debridement
   B. Dressing removal
   C. Saline cleansing
   D. B and C

3. Topical silver's antibacterial action may be related to:
   A. DNA binding
   B. Cell membrane damage
   C. Cytoplasmic organelle function
   D. Ionized form of silver
   E. All of the above

Answers: 1–E, 2–D, 3–E

Practice Pearls

- Assess and treat the whole patient and not just the hole in the patient (treat the cause, patient-centered concerns).
- Determine healability of the wound: healable, nonhealable, maintenance.
- Evaluate local wound care: Debridement, Infection and inflammation, Moisture balance (DIM).
- Identify wounds that are not 30% smaller by Week 4 for reassessment or Edge effect (advanced therapies).

References

1. Sibbald RG, Williamson D, Orsted HL, et al. Preparing the wound bed: debridement, bacterial balance and moisture balance. *Ostomy Wound Manage.* 2000;46(11):14–35.
2. Bowler PG, Davies BJ. The microbiology of acute and chronic wounds. *WOUNDS.* 1999;11:72–99.
3. Sibbald RG, Orsted H, Schultz G, et al. Preparing the wound bed 2003: focus on infection and inflammation. *Ostomy Wound Manage.* 2003;49(11):24–51.
4. Falanga V. Classifications for wound-bed preparation and stimulation of chronic wounds. *Wound Repair Regen.* 2000;8:347–352.
5. Schultz GS, Sibbald RG, Falanga V, et al. Wound bed preparation: a systematic approach to wound management. *Wound Repair Regen.* 2003;11(Suppl 1):S1–S28.
6. Sibbald RG, Orsted HL, Coutts PM, et al. Best practice recommendations for preparing the wound bed: update 2006. *Adv Skin Wound Care.* 2007;20:390–405.
7. Registered Nurses' Association of Ontario. Assessment and Management of Stage I to IV Pressure Ulcers (Revised). Toronto, ON, Canada: Registered Nurses' Association of Ontario; 2007.
8. Brem H, Sheehan P, Rosenberg H, et al. Evidence-based protocol for diabetic foot ulcers. *J Plast Reconstr Surg.* 2006;117:193S–209S.
9. London NJ, Donnelly R. ABC of arterial and venous disease. Ulcerated lower limb. *BMJ.* 2000;320:1589–1591.
10. Falanga V, Sabolinski M. A bilayered living skin construct (APLIGRAF) accelerates complete closure of hard-to-heal venous ulcers. *Wound Repair Regen.* 1999;7:201–207.
11. Margolis DJ, Allen-Taylor L, Hoffstad O, et al. The accuracy of venous leg ulcer prognostic models in a wound care system. *Wound Repair Regen.* 2004;12:163–168.
12. Attinger CE, Evans KK, Bulan E, Blume P, Cooper P. An-

giosomes of the foot and ankle and clinical implications for limb salvage: reconstruction, incisions and revascularization. *Plast Reconstr Surg.* 2006;117(suppl):261S.

13. Sibbald RG, Alvi A, Norton L, et al. Compression therapies. In: Krasner DL, Rodeheaver GT, Sibbald RG, eds. *Chronic Wound Care: A Clinical Source Book for Healthcare Professionals.* 4th ed. Malvern, PA: HMP Communications; 2007:481–488.

14. Browne AC, Sibbald RG. The diabetic neuropathic ulcer: An overview. *Ostomy Wound Manage.* 1999;45(suppl 1A):6S–20S.

15. Sibbald RG, Alavi A, Norton L, Browne AC, Coutts P. Compression therapies. In: Krasner DL, Rodeheaver GT, Sibbald RG, eds. *Chronic Wound Care: A Clinical Source Book for Healthcare Professionals.* 4th ed. Malvern, PA: HMP Communications; 2007:481–488.

16. Woo K, Lo C, Alavi A, et al. An audit of leg and foot ulcer care in an Ontario community care access centre. *Wound Care Canada.* 2007;5(suppl 1):S17–S27.

17. Marston WA. Risk factors associated with healing chronic diabetic foot ulcers: the importance of hyperglycemia. *Ostomy Wound Manage.* 2006;52(3):26–8,30,32.

18. Markuson M, Hanson D, Anderson J, et al. The relationship between hemoglobin A(1c) values and healing time for lower extremity ulcers in individuals with diabetes. *Adv Skin Wound Care.* 2009;22:365–372.

19. Zagoren AJ, Johnson DR, Amick N. Nutritional assessment and intervention in the adult with a chronic wound. In: Krasner DL, Rodever GT, Sibbald RG, eds. *Chronic Wound Care: A Clinical Source Book for Healthcare Professionals.* 4th ed. Malvern, PA: HMP Communications; 2007:127–136.

20. Albumin-serum. MedlinePlus Medical Encyclopedia. NIH. Available at: http://www.nlm.nih.gov/medlineplus/ency/article/003480.htm. Accessed July 11, 2011.

21. Hess CT. *Clinical Guide to Wound Care.* 5th ed. Philadelphia, PA: Lippincott Williams & Wilkins; 2005:34.

22. Lacy JA. Albumin overview: use as a nutritional marker and as a therapeutic intervention. *Crit Care Nurse.* 1991;11:46–49.

23. Doweiko JP, Nompleggia DJ. Role of albumin in human physiology and pathophysiology. *JPEN J Parenter Enteral Nutr.* 1991;15:207–211.

24. Stotts NA, Wipke-Telvis DD, Hopf HW. Cofactors in impaired wound healing. In: Krasner DL, Rodeheaver GT, Sibbald RG, eds. *Chronic Wound Care: A Clinical Source Book for Healthcare Professionals.* 4th ed. Malvern, PA: HMP Communications; 2007:215–220.

25. Woo K, Alavi A, Botros M, et al. A transprofessional comprehensive assessment model for persons with lower extremity leg and foot ulcers. *Wound Care Canada.* 2007;5(suppl 1):S35–S47.

26. Enoch S, Price P. Cellular, molecular and biochemical differences in the pathophysiology of healing between acute wounds, chronic wounds and wounds in the aged. World Wide Wounds, 2004. Available at: http://www.worldwidewounds.com/2004/august/Enoch/PathophysiologyOf-Healing.html. Accessed July 11, 2011.

27. Kennedy KL. The prevalence of pressure ulcers in an intermediate care facility. *Decubitus.* 1989;2:44–45.

28. Langemo DK, Brown G. Skin fails too: acute, chron-

ic and end-stage skin failure. *Adv Skin Wound Care.* 2006;19:206–211.

29. Sibbald RG, Krasner DL, Lutz JB, et al. The SCALE Expert Panel: Skin Changes at Life's End. Final Consensus Document. October 1, 2009. Available at: http://www.gaymar.com/webapp/wcs/stores/servlet/ProductDisplay?catalogId=10001&storeId=10053&partNumber=CONDOCS& langId=-1&parentCategoryId=11652&currentTopCategory=11652. Accessed July 11, 2011.

30. Brennan MR, Trombley K. Kennedy terminal ulcers: a palliative care unit's experience over a 12 month period of time. *WCET.* 2010;30:20–22.

31. Sackett DL, Strauss SE, Richardson WS, et al. *Evidence-Based Medicine: How to Practice and Teach EBM.* 2nd ed. Edinburgh, Scotland: Churchill Livingstone; 2000.

32. Krasner DL, Rodeheaver GT, Sibbald RG. Interprofessional wound caring. In: Krasner DL, Rodeheaver GT, Sibbald RG, eds. *Chronic Wound Care: A Clinical Source Book for Healthcare Professionals.* 4th ed. Malvern, PA: HMP Communications; 2007:3–9.

33. Mosti G, Vattaliano V, Polignano R, et al. Compression therapy in the treatment of leg ulcers. *Acta Vulnol.* 2009;7:1–12.

34. Mayrovitz HN. Compression-induced pulsatile blood-flow changes in human legs. *Clin Physiol.* 1998;18:117–124.

35. Delis KT, Nicolaides AN. Effect of intermittent pneumatic compression of foot and calf on walking distance, hemodynamics and quality of life in patients with arterial claudication: a prospective randomized controlled study with 1-year follow-up. *Ann Surg.* 2005;241:431–441.

36. Harris CL, Fraser C. Malnutrition in the institutionalized elderly: the effects on wound healing. *Ostomy Wound Manage.* 2004;50(10):54–63.

37. Sussman C. Wound healing biology and chronic wound healing. In: Sussman C, Bates-Jensen B, eds. *Wound Care: A Collaborative Practice Manual for Physical Therapists and Nurses.* Gaithersburg, MD: Aspen Publication; 1998:49–82.

38. Van Anholt RD, Sobotka L, Meijer EP, et al. Specific nutritional support accelerates pressure ulcer healing and reduces wound care intensity in non-malnourished patients. *Nutrition.* 2010;26:867–872.

39. McCaffery M. Nursing practice theories related to cognition, bodily pain and main environment interactions. Los Angeles, CA: University of California Los Angeles; 1968.

40. Woo K, Sibbald G, Fogh K, et al. Assessment and management of persistent (chronic) and total wound pain. *Int Wound J.* 2008;5:205–215.

41. WUWHS guidelines for wound healing policy. Available at: http://www.wuwhs.com. Accessed August 5, 2011.

42. World Health Organization (WHO) pain relief ladder. 2005. Available at: www.who.int/cancer/palliative/painladder/en/. Accessed July 11, 2011.

43. Phillips T, Stanton B, Provan A, et al. A study of the impact of leg ulcers on quality of life: financial, social, and psychological implications. *J Am Acad Dermatol.* 1994;31:49–53.

44. Persoon A, Heinen MM, van der Vleuten CJ, et al. Leg ulcers: a review of their impact on daily life. *J Clin Nurs.* 2004;13:341–354.

45. Carrington AL, Mawdsley SK, Morley M, et al. Psycho-

logical status of diabetic people with or without lower limb disability. *Diabetes Res Clin Pract.* 1996;32:19–25.

46. Price P. Health-related quality of life. In: Krasner DL, Rodeheaver GT, Sibbald RG, eds. *Chronic Wound Care: A Clinical Source Book for Healthcare Professionals.* 4th ed. Malvern, PA: HMP Communications; 2007:79–83.

47. Chalon S, Moreno H, Benowitz NL, et al. Nicotine impairs endothelium-dependent dilation in human veins *in vivo. Clin Pharmacol Ther.* 2000;67:391–397.

48. Rayner R. Effects of cigarette smoking on cutaneous wound healing. *Prim Intent.* 2006;14:100–102,104.

49. Sorensen LT. Smoking and wound healing. *Eur Wound Manage Assoc J.* 2003;3:13–15.

50. Smith JB, Smith SB. Cutaneous manifestations of smoking. *eMedicine.* 2004.

51. Ninikoski J. Oxygen and wound healing. *Clin Plast Surg.* 1977;4:361–373.

52. Arrendondo J, Hall LL, Ndoye A, et al. Central role of fibroblast alpha3 nicotinic acetylcholine receptor in mediating cutaneous effects of nicotine. *Lab Invest.* 2003;83:207–225.

53. Snyder HB, Caughman G, Lewis J, Billman MA, Schuster G. Nicotine modulation of *in vitro* human gingival fibroblast beta1 integrin expression. *J Periodontol.* 2002;73:505–510.

54. Wong LS, Green HM, Feugate JE, Yadav M, Nothnagel EA, Martins-Green M. Effects of "second-hand" smoke on structure and function of fibroblasts, cells that are critical for tissue repair and remodelling. *BMC Cell Biol.* 2004;5:13.

55. Ahn C, Mulligan P, Salcido RS. Smoking-the bane of wound healing: biomedical interventions and social influences. *Adv Skin Wound Care.* 2008;21:227–236.

56. Establishing Therapeutic Relationships. Registered Nurses' Association of Ontario Best Practice Guideline; 2007. Available at: http://www.rnao.org/Page.asp?PageID=861&SiteNodeID=133. Accessed July 11, 2011.

57. Osterberg L, Blaschke T. Adherence to medication. *N Engl J Med.* 2005;353:487–497.

58. Wild T, Rahbarnia A, Kellner M, et al. Basics of nutrition and wound healing. *Nutrition.* 2010;26:862–866.

59. Keast DH, Bowering CK, Evans AW, et al. MEASURE: a proposed assessment framework for developing best practice recommendations for wound assessment. *Wound Repair Regen.* 2004;12:S1–S17.

60. Rodeheaver GT, Ratliff CR. Wound cleansing, wound irrigation, wound disinfection. In: Krasner DL, Rodeheaver GT, Sibbald RG, eds. *Chronic Wound Care: A Clinical Source Book for Healthcare Professionals.* 4th ed. Malvern, PA: HMP Communications; 2007:331–342.

61. Moore ZEH, Cowman S. Wound cleansing for pressure ulcers. *Cochrane Database Syst Rev.* 2005;(4):CD004983.

62. Fernandez R, Griffiths R. Water for wound cleansing. *Cochrane Database Syst Rev.* 2008;(1):CD003861.

63. National Collaborating Centre for Women's and Children's Health. Surgical site infection: prevention and treatment of surgical site infection. London: NICE; 2008. (NICE guideline CG74). Available at: http://www.nice.org.uk/nicemedia/live/11743/42378/42378.pdf. Accessed July 11, 2011.

64. Hurlow J, Bowler PG. Clinical experience with wound

65. Cardinal M, Eisenbud DE, Armstrong DG, et al. Serial surgical debridement: a retrospective study on clinical outcomes in chronic lower extremity wounds. *Wound Repair Regen.* 2009;17:306–311.

66. Landis S, Ryan S, Woo K, Sibbald RG. Infections in chronic wounds. In: Krasner DL, Rodeheaver GT, Sibbald RG, eds. *Chronic Wound Care: A Clinical Source Book for Healthcare Professionals.* 4th ed. Malvern, PA: HMP Communications; 2007:299–221.

67. Sibbald RG, Woo K, Ayello EA. Increased bacterial burden and infection: the story of the NERDS and STONES. *Adv Skin Wound Care.* 2006;19:447–461.

68. Lavery LA, Armstrong DG, Wunderlich RP, et al. Risk factors for foot infections in individuals with diabetes. *Diabetes Care.* 2006;29:1288–1293.

69. Gardner SE, Frantz RA, Doebbeling BN. The validity of the clinical signs and symptoms used to identify localized chronic wound infection. *Wound Repair Regen.* 2001;9:178–186.

70. Sibbald RG, Woo K, Ayello EA. Increased bacterial burden and infection: the story of the NERDS and STONES. *Adv Skin Wound Care.* 2006;19:447–461.

71. Woo K, Sibbald RG. A cross-sectional validation study of using NERDS and STONEES to assess bacterial burden. *Ostomy Wound Manage.* 2009;55(8):40–48.

72. Demling RH, DeSanti L. The rate of re-epithelialization across meshed skin grafts is increased with exposure to silver. *Burns.* 2002;28:264–266.

73. Nadworney PL, Wang JF, Tredget EE, Burrell RE. Anti-inflammatory activity of nanocrystalline silver in a porcine contact dermatitis model. *Nanomedicine: Nanotechnology, Biology and Medicine.* 2008;4:241–251.

74. Vermeulen H, van Hattem JM, Storm-Versloot MN, et al. Topical silver for treating infected wounds. *Cochrane Database Syst Rev.* 2007;(1):CD005486.

75. Lo SF, Chang CJ, Hu WY, et al. The effectiveness of silver-releasing dressings in the management of non-healing chronic wounds: a meta-analysis. *J Clin Nurs.* 2009;18:716–728.

76. Jull A, Walker N, Rogers A, et al. Honey for leg ulcers: the HALT trial. *Br J Surg.* 2008;95:175–182.

77. O'Meara S, Al-Kurdi D, Ologun Y, et al. Antibiotics and antiseptics for venous leg ulcers. *Cochrane Database Syst Rev.* 2010;(1):CD003557.

78. Sibbald RG, Coutts P, Woo K. Reduction of bacterial burden and pain in chronic wounds using a new poly-hexamethylene biguanide antimicrobial foam dressing: clinical trial results. *Adv Skin Wound Care.* 2011;24:79–84.

79. Spacciapoli P, Buxton D, Rothstein D, et al. Antimicrobial activity of silver nitrate against periodontal pathogens. *J Periodontal Res.* 2001;36:108–113.

80. Nadworny PL, Burrell RE. A review of assessment techniques for silver technology in wound care. Part 1: *in vitro* methods for assessing antimicrobial activity. *J Wound Technol.* 2008;2:6–13.

81. Burrell RE, Heggers JP, Davis GJ, et al. Efficacy of silver-coated dressings as bacterial barriers in a rodent burn sepsis model. *WOUNDS.* 1999;11(4):64–71.

82. Nadworny PL, Burrell RE. A review of assessment tech-

niques for silver technology in wound care. Part II: tissue culture and *in vivo* methods for determining antimicrobial and anti-inflammatory activity. *J Wound Technol.* 2008;2:14–22.

83. O'Meara S, Al-Kurdi D, Ologun Y, et al. Antibiotics and antiseptics for venous leg ulcers. *Cochrane Database Syst Rev.* 2010;(1):CD003557.

84. Kerstein MD, Gemmen E, van Rijswijk L, et al. Cost and cost-effectiveness of venous and pressure ulcer protocols of care. *Dis Manage Health Outcomes.* 2001;651–663.

85. Trengove NJ, Stacey MC, MacAuley S, et al. Analysis of the acute and chronic wound environments: the role of proteases and their inhibitors. *Wound Repair Regen.* 1999;7:422–452.

86. Harding KG, Moore K, Phillips TJ. Wound chronicity and fibroblast senescence: implications for treatment. *Int Wound J.* 2005;2:364–368.

87. Basketter D, Gilpin G, Kuhn M, et al. Patch tests versus use tests in skin irritation risk assessment. *Contact Dermatitis.* 1998;39:252–256.

88. Falanga V. Wound healing and its impairment in the diabetic foot. *Lancet.* 2005;366:1736–1743.

89. Margolis DJ, Allen-Taylor L, Hoffstad O, et al. The accuracy of venous leg ulcer prognostic models in a wound care system. *Wound Repair Regen.* 2004;12:163–168.

90. Sheehan P, Jones P, Caselli A, et al. Percent change in wound area of diabetic foot ulcers over a 4-week period is a robust predictor of complete healing in a 12-week prospective trial. *Diabetes Care.* 2003;26:1879–1882.

91. Niezgoda JA, Van Gils CC, Frykberg RG, et al. Randomized clinical trial comparing OASIS Wound Matrix to Regranex Gel for diabetic ulcers. *Adv Skin Wound Care.* 2005;18:258–266.

92. Arevalo JM, Lorente JA. Skin coverage with Biobrane biomaterial for the treatment of patients with toxic epidermal necrolysis. *J Burn Care Rehabil.* 1999;20:406–410.

93. Smiell JM, Wieman TJ, Steed DL, et al. Efficacy and safety of becaplermin (recombinant human platelet-derived growth factor-BB) in patients with nonhealing, lower extremity diabetic ulcers: a combined analysis of four randomized studies. *Wound Repair Regen.* 1999;7:335–346.

94. Steed DL. Clinical evaluation of recombinant human platelet-derived growth factor for the treatment of lower extremity ulcers. *Plast Reconstr Surg.* 2006;117:143S–51S.

95. Dinh TL, Veves A. The efficacy of Apligraf in the treatment of diabetic foot ulcers. *Plast Reconstr Surg.* 2006;117:152S–59S.

96. Veves A, Falanga V, Armstrong DG, et al. Graftskin, a human skin equivalent, is effective in the management of noninfected neuropathic diabetic foot ulcers: a prospective randomized multicenter clinical trial. *Diabetes Care.* 2001;24:290–295.

97. Redekop WK, Stolk EA, Kok E, et al. Diabetic foot ulcers and amputations: estimates of health utility for use in cost-effectiveness analyses of new treatments. *Diabetes Metab.* 2004;30:549–556.

98. Falanga V, Margolis D, Alvarez O, et al. Rapid healing of venous ulcers and lack of clinical rejection with an allogeneic cultured human skin equivalent. Human Skin Equivalent Investigators Group. *Arch Dermatol.* 1998;134:293–300.

99. Newton DJ, Khan F, Belch JJ, et al. Blood flow changes in diabetic foot ulcers treated with dermal replacement therapy. *J Foot Ankle Surg.* 2002;41:233–237.

100. Hanft JR, Surperant MS. Healing of chronic foot ulcers in diabetic patients treated with a human fibroblast-derived dermis. *J Foot Ankle Surg.* 2002;41:291–299.

101. Marston WA, Hanft J, Norwood P, et al. The efficacy and safety of Dermagraft in improving the healing of chronic diabetic foot ulcers: results of a prospective randomised trial. *Diabetes Care.* 2003;26:1701–1705.

102. Roeckl-Wiedmann I, Bennett M, Kranke P. Systematic review of hyperbaric oxygen in the management of chronic wounds. *Br J Surg.* 2005;92:24–32.

103. Akai M, Kawashima N, Kimura T, et al. Electrical stimulation as an adjunct to spinal fusion: a meta-analysis of controlled clinical trials. *Bioelectromagnetics.* 2002;23:496–504.

104. Flemming K, Cullum N. Therapeutic ultrasound for venous leg ulcers. *Cochrane Database Syst Rev.* 2000;(4):CD00180.

105. Baba-Akbari SA, Flemming K, Cullum NA, et al. Therapeutic ultrasound for pressure ulcers. *Cochrane Database Syst Rev.* 2006;(3):CD001275.

106. Armstrong DG, Lavery LA, Diabetic Foot Study Consortium. Negative pressure wound therapy after partial diabetic foot amputation: a multicentre, randomized controlled trial. *Lancet.* 2005;366:1704–1710.

107. Vin F, Teot L, Meaume S. The healing properties of Promogran in venous leg ulcers. *J Wound Care.* 2002;11:335–341.

108. Wollina U, Schmidt WD, Kronert C, et al. Some effects of a topical collagen-based matrix on the microcirculation and wound healing in patients with chronic venous leg ulcers: preliminary observations. *Int J Low Extrem Wounds.* 2005;4:214–224.

109. Litzelman DK, Slemenda CW, Langefeld CD, et al. Reduction of lower extremity clinical abnormalities in patients with non-insulin-dependent diabetes mellitus. A randomized, controlled trial. *Ann Intern Med.* 1993;119:36–41.

110. Apelqvist J, Ragnarson-Tennvall G, Larsson J, Persson U. Diabetic foot ulcers in a multidisciplinary setting. An economic analysis of primary healing and healing with amputation. *J Intern Med.* 1994;235:463–471.

Cofactors in Impaired Wound Healing

Nancy A. Stotts, RN, EdD;
Deidre D. Wipke-Tevis, RN, PhD;
Harriet W. Hopf, MD

Objectives

The reader will be challenged to:
- Examine the major cofactors associated with impaired healing in chronic wounds
- Analyze the wound healing impairment caused by various cofactors
- Assess the mechanisms by which the major factors impair healing.

Introduction

Healing of chronic wounds is a complex process that requires the interaction of many factors for normal repair. Healing is the restoration of structure and function after tissue injury. In acute wounds, healing progresses in an established sequence and in a broad but accepted timeframe.[1] When this sequence or timeframe is interrupted or altered for any reason, the result is a chronic wound. The rate of healing in such wounds is slower and not as predictable. Impairment in healing is manifest as a delay in the rate of healing and/or the development of wound-related complications.

Many factors are associated with impaired healing of chronic wounds. These factors vary to some extent by the nature of the wound. A complete list of the factors related to impaired healing across all populations would be long and not very meaningful. There are, however, factors related to healing that cross the various wound populations. Assessing these factors will allow the practitioner to screen patients and address the major and most common factors known to impair healing in chronic wounds. Thus, this chapter describes the major factors in impaired healing of chronic wounds, the effect of each factor on wound healing, and the mechanism by which each is thought to lead to impairment. Common factors that impair wound healing include *old age, insufficient oxygenation/perfusion, malnutrition, increased bacterial levels, old wound tissue, excess pressure, psychophysiological stress, concomitant conditions*, and *adverse effects of therapy* (Table 1). Identification of these factors is critical

Stotts NA, Wipke-Tevis DD, Hopf HW. Cofactors in impaired wound healing. In: Krasner DL, Rodeheaver GT, Sibbald RG, Woo KY, eds. *Chronic Wound Care: A Clinical Source Book for Healthcare Professionals.* Vol 1. 5th ed. Malvern, PA: HMP Communications, 2012:199–206.

Table 1. Cofactors in impaired healing

Old age

Insufficient oxygenation/perfusion

Malnutrition

Increased bioburden

Old wound tissue

Excess pressure

Psychophysiological stress

Concomitant conditions

Adverse effects of therapy

to healing of chronic wounds, as correction of impediments to healing generally leads to healing. Conversely, if an impediment is not recognized and corrected, the wound is unlikely to heal.

Age

Age has been associated with impaired healing, as there are differences in healing in the fetus, child, adult, and the elderly. Fetal wound healing occurs without an inflammatory response.[2] Wound healing and contraction occur more rapidly in childhood than in adulthood. As adulthood progresses, dermal vascularity decreases, collagen density decreases, the basement membrane flattens, fragmentation of elastin occurs, and the number of mast cells decreases. As people age, the entire healing process occurs more slowly, including the inflammatory response.[3]

Although the elderly experience these physiological changes, their rate of healing remains within a normal range or only slightly delayed in the absence of chronic disease.[4] Yet the elderly are more likely to have chronic illnesses, such as cardiovascular disease, pulmonary disease, and diabetes, and because of this association, age is often noted as a cofactor in impaired healing. Differentiating which dimensions of impaired healing in the elderly are due to concomitant disease and which are due to aging is the subject of ongoing research.

Low Oxygen and Perfusion

Low oxygen levels and *decreased perfusion* are often related to impaired healing, as well as increased risk of infection. Oxygen is needed for collagen formation; the rate and quality of collagen are decreased when sufficient oxygen is not present. Angiogenesis (replacement of injured blood vessels) and epithelization are similarly impaired in hypoxic wounds. In addition, hypoxia inhibits resistance to infection. When neutrophils and macrophages ingest foreign material and microorganisms, more oxygen is consumed than during their resting state. Lack of sufficient oxygen slows leukocyte activity, decreases superoxide release and, therefore, bacterial killing, and often is associated with wound infection.[5,6]

Although **hemoglobin** carries much of the oxygen content in the blood, dissolved oxygen is most important for wound healing, because wounds depend on diffusion from relatively scarce capillaries for oxygenation. Thus, anemia does not result in impaired healing unless the anemia is severe (hematocrit < 18%). Wound oxygen tension is not decreased when subjects are anemic as long as the subjects have adequate circulating intravascular volume.[7] Cardiac output increases to compensate for the decreased oxygen content, and that, combined with decreased viscosity, increases wound blood flow sufficiently to increase wound temperature by 1.5°C to 2°C and to maintain normal wound oxygen. Clinical studies have confirmed and extended these early findings: levels of hydroxyproline, a major component of collagen, are not decreased in subjects with anemia.[8,9] Data indicate that anemia is not a cofactor in impaired healing unless the anemia is sufficient to impair cardiac output or the patient does not have sufficient circulating volume.

Smoking tobacco clearly impairs wound healing via several mechanisms. The triad of nicotine, carbon monoxide, and hydrogen cyanide from smoking are thought to interact to produce deleterious effects.[10] Nicotine acts as a potent vasoconstrictor, increases platelet adhesiveness, and enhances the risk of microvascular thrombosis and ischemia. Carbon monoxide binds with hemoglobin and aggravates the situation, reduces available sites for oxygen carrying, and lowers oxygen saturation. Hydrogen cyanide inhibits the enzyme systems necessary for oxidative metabolism and the cellular transport of oxygen. Thus, a major adverse effect of smoking is the creation or worsening of wound hypoxia.[11]

Hypovolemia (ie, the lack of adequate intravascular volume) has also been associated with impaired healing.[12,13] With hypovolemia, circulating volume is insufficient to transport oxygen and nutrients to the tissues; if the state is prolonged, cellular activities needed for healing are diminished. Unfortunately, even supplemental oxygen does not increase tissue oxygen levels when tissues are hypoperfused.[12] Hypovolemia that is clinically obvious (eg, hypoxemia, thirst, decreased urine output, or hypotension) is treated with supplemental fluid. A more difficult situation occurs when subclinical hypovolemia or underhydration is present. Subclinical hypovolemia is defined as the presence of decreased intravascular volume with no overt clinical signs and symptoms. Subclinical hypovolemia can be detected by measuring capillary refill time at the forehead (< 3 sec) or prepatellar knee (< 5 sec) or by measuring cutaneous (skin) oxygen levels, a more precise, though more complex and expensive, method.

Subclinical hypovolemia has been well documented in the surgical population. In examining the effects of various levels of inspired oxygen on tissue and wound oxygenation, researchers found tissue hypoxia in a subset of the study sample.[12] Treatment with a bolus of fluid resolved the hypoxia, and the authors concluded that subclinical hypovolemia had been present. It is important to note that no signs or symptoms were present that would have allowed the clinician to diagnose the hypovolemia. Follow-up studies showed that fluid titration based on subcutaneous oxygen levels led to higher tissue oxygen levels and greater quantities of hydroxyproline being synthesized in surgical patients in the early postoperative period than when fluid was administered based on a traditional fluid formula.[13] In the chronic wound population, subclinical hypovolemia has been identified in pilot work with elderly nursing home residents with pressure ulcers.[14] Fluid administration for subclinical hypovolemia, however, has potential deleterious effects. Although inadequate hydration is much more common than fluid overload, care must be taken to maximize intravascular volume without causing fluid overload. Vasoconstriction caused by pain, psychophysiologic stress, or cold cannot be overcome by fluid administration. Thus, cold and vasoconstricted patients are at higher risk of fluid overload. Conversely, patients who are warm and well perfused will tolerate high volumes of fluid

infusion, resulting in higher tissue oxygen levels and lower infection rates.[5]

Malnutrition

Either *inadequate intake of nutrients* or *pre-existing malnutrition* has the potential to delay healing or result in infection. While most wounds heal regardless of nutritional status, severe protein-calorie malnutrition or specific nutritional deficits that are symptomatic can impair healing.[15] Providing adequate nutrition to all persons with injuries should be a therapeutic goal so that wound healing can occur within an optimal environment.[5]

Most wound healing abnormalities are associated with protein-calorie malnutrition rather than depletion of a single nutrient.[16] Nonetheless, *inadequate quantities of specific nutrients* can impact healing. Deficiencies of protein result in decreased fibroblast proliferation, reduced proteoglycan and collagen synthesis, decreased angiogenesis, and disrupted collagen remodeling. Protein requirements increase with healing. Provision of arginine and glutamine supplements (nonessential amino acids) has produced mixed results. Of these, arginine has shown the most significant wound healing effects, specifically increasing the inflammatory response in patients with diabetes.[16] Recent intake rather than remote intake of nutrients is more important in supporting collagen deposition and healing.

With *insufficient carbohydrate intake*, body protein is catabolized for energy. Protein, thus, is diverted from repair to provide the glucose needed for cellular maintenance. This adaptation process is especially important in fighting infection, as leukocytes require glucose for phagocytosis. *Fat inadequacy* is seen only in prolonged starvation or severe hypermetabolic states, and deficiencies of the fat-soluble vitamins (A, D, E, and K) may develop in these situations. Lack of vitamin A can result in an inadequate inflammatory response, while an excess of it may cause an excess inflammatory response; both impair healing.[16] *Thiamine (B1) deficiency* results in decreased collagen formation, while pantothenic acid (B5) deficiency results in decreased tensile strength and fewer fibroblasts. Inadequate vitamin C may result in lysis of collagen exceeding synthesis, meaning new wounds may have delayed collagen formation, and old wounds may break-down. Levels of vitamin E in excess of the recom-mended 100 IU daily may result in retardation of healing and fibrosis.

Zinc, *iron*, *copper*, and *manganese* are needed in small quantities for normal collagen formation. Data strongly suggest that zinc deficiencies im-pair healing, and repletion in states of deficiency returns healing to its normal rate. Supplementing those with normal zinc levels has not been shown to augment healing. Zinc deficiencies are seen in the elderly as well as those with chronic metabol-ic stress, excessive wound drainage, and persistent diarrhea. Regarding copper, impaired healing has been seen with decreased copper stores, although somewhat more rarely. Iron deficiency is primar-ily a problem in infants and may impair collagen formation. Severe iron deficiency also results in impaired healing because of its role in hydroxyl-ation of proline and lysine to make collagen. Of these mineral deficiencies, iron deficiency is most often detected and treated.[16]

Most studies that examine nutrition and chronic wounds address the pressure ulcer pop-ulation.[17] Review articles indicate that research has not demonstrated a cause-and-effect rela-tionship between nutritional status or intake and the development or healing of pressure ulcers. Nonetheless, provision of adequate nutrition, es-pecially protein, is important in optimizing host status to tissue tolerance and healing of existing ulcers. Additionally, data indicate that nutritional deficiencies are present in a portion of venous ulcer patients.[18] Further work is needed to con-firm these findings.

Bioburden

Bioburden, the metabolic load imposed by bacteria on tissue, is often a cofactor in impaired healing.[19,20] Wounds that have impaired healing are more susceptible to infection, and infected or heavily contaminated wounds demonstrate im-paired healing. *All wound surfaces are contami-nated* with bacteria, yet it is rare that the organ-isms on the wound surface cause the infection. Nonetheless, contamination is important, because the organisms compete with new tissue for nu-trients and oxygen, and their byproducts are del-eterious to the normal physiological balance of the healing wound. Overall, contamination pre-

disposes the patient to delayed healing and sets up an environment for infection to develop.

Wound infection is present when microorgan-isms invade tissue. Diagnosis usually is based on clinical signs, ie, the presence of pus, warmth, pain, erythema, and induration. In immunocompro-mised persons and those with neuropathy, often the only sign of infection is a change in sensation around the wound. Also, in some chronic wounds, poorly granulating tissue may be a sign of infec-tion.[20] Wound infection in the elderly presents as decreased cognitive function or functional status, requiring the provider to investigate to find the source of the problem.[14]

Wound culture is performed to identify the specific organism(s) and identify an antibiotic to which the organism(s) is(are) sensitive. **Qualita-tive** wound cultures are not useful in diagnosing wound infection, because all wounds are con-taminated to some degree. **Quantitative** culture (either of a tissue biopsy or a carefully obtained swab) may be more reliable but is not available at most hospitals. A wound that contains $\geq 10^5$ organisms per gram of tissue is unlikely to heal without treatment because of excessive bacterial burden. The exception to this criterion is with beta hemolytic streptococcus where fewer organ-isms (10^3 organisms per gram of tissue) are re-quired to produce infection.[19,20]

Host resistance and the local environment are important in determining whether a contami-nated wound becomes infected. Normal, healthy tissue is resistant to microorganisms. In fact, con-tamination by a small number ($\leq 10^2$) of organ-isms per gram of tissue will activate leukocytes and has been seen as a factor that supports rather than impairs healing.[14]

Local environmental factors that contribute to bacterial proliferation and the development of impaired healing include the presence of devital-ized tissue, dirt in the wound, an abscess distant from the site of the injury, and a hematoma or large wound space.[20] Super-infection from con-tamination, regardless of whether from stool, urine, or another wound site, is also associated with infection in pressure ulcers.[17]

Old Tissue

Old tissue is a factor recently recognized as an impediment to healing. In studies of recombinant growth factors, debridement of old tissue from chronic wounds was shown to enhance healing.[21] This supports clinical experience that radical debridement of tissue is essential to effective treatment of chronic wounds. While the exact mechanism by which old tissue impairs healing is not entirely understood, debridement involves removal of senescent fibroblasts, inflammatory cells, and old scar tissue, implicating these factors in the impairment. It is not clear, however, exactly when tissue converts to "old" tissue; further research should clarify this issue.

Excess Pressure

Pressure, *shear*, and *friction* are cofactors in all types of chronic wounds. They are most often associated with *pressure ulcers*[17] but also are significant factors in the majority of chronic wounds. Little documentation exists to support this triad as contributing to chronic wounds, but clinical experience supports these as important factors in impaired healing. In the *venous ulcer population*, this problem is seen in the shear and friction that occur when compression stockings or bandages are utilized. Friable epithelial tissue may be disrupted under the stocking or bandage, especially along the previously intact skin of the shin, over the bony prominences of the ankle, and around the edge of the ulcer. Shear and friction occur most often during stocking application or removal and with ambulation. Clinically, this problem is most often seen in the elderly who have limited strength and manual dexterity. Often, coexisting arterial disease is present in the patient with venous ulcers. Inappropriate application of compression stockings and/or bandages may result in additional damage due to ischemia.

In persons with *neuropathic ulcers*, it is well accepted that excess pressure that is not perceived and that continues beyond tissue tolerance causes damage and prevents repair.[5] In the pressure ulcer population, data show that low pressures for long periods of time or high pressures for short periods produce pressure ulcers.[17] Controversy exists over what level of pressure causes vessel occlusion that leads to ischemia and necrosis.

Psychophysiological Stress

Stress has been identified as a potential cofactor in impaired healing. The proposed mechanism is through stimulation of the sympathetic nervous system, with the outflow of vasoactive substances and subsequent vasoconstriction. Increased cortisol levels also have been implicated, as steroids are known to impair wound healing. The major stressors that have been investigated in this category are *psychological stress*, *pain*, and *noise*. Stress has been linked with pressure ulcer development in patients transferred from acute care to long-term care, using cortisol as an objective measure of stress. Although the numbers are small, and the ulcers are not severe, data show that subjects with higher cortisol levels developed ulcers, while subjects with lower cortisol levels did not develop ulcers. Relaxation and guided imagery also are related to healing in persons with wounds. Stress, measured with cortisol levels, and inflammation were reduced with relaxation and imagery. These data suggest that available therapies might be used to decrease the sympathetic nervous system response to stress and thus support healing in persons with wounds.[22] Further research is needed to establish the direct effect on healing.

Intuitively, *pain* is thought to be an important issue in the development and healing of chronic wounds. For example, a recent large database study found that the presence of pain upon admission to a nursing home was associated with pressure ulcer development within the first 6 months after admission. Data do not indicate, however, if pain is a cofactor in healing impairment.[23] Pain reduction using transcutaneous electrical nerve stimulation (TENS) and music has been shown to be effective in reducing pain in persons with open wounds.[22] Unfortunately, healing was not an outcome measure when evaluating these treatments. It would seem logical that a reduction in pain would mitigate vasoconstriction thus increasing wound perfusion and supporting wound healing. Whether this is true remains to be established.

Noise is another stressor that results in a systemic cardiovascular response that may affect repair. Noise has been shown to increase epinephrine levels and later *in-vitro* leukocyte function. In addition, intermittent noise has been shown to decrease healing in an animal model.[22] However, studies have not specifically addressed this issue in the chronic wound patient population.

Concomitant Conditions

A myriad of concomitant conditions is associated with impaired healing. Major conditions include *peripheral vascular disease, diabetes mellitus, pulmonary disease, cardiac disease, conditions that result in immunocompromise*,[4,5] and *specific treatments*, including *surgery*.[24]

Persons with *vascular disease* are at risk for impaired healing. In arterial disease, the cause is accepted as tissue hypoxia due to arteriosclerotic disease. In venous disease, back pressure from venous hypertension and edema is thought to contribute to impaired healing. *Persons with diabetes* mellitus are at risk for impaired healing. Glucose control is essential for normal healing, and high glucose levels are often seen in diabetes, especially during periods of physiological stress and repair. High glucose levels result in impaired leukocyte function and increased risk of infection. Diabetes also appears to reduce growth factors and growth factor receptors in wounds. Lack of sensation is a serious problem in the more advanced states of diabetes where Charcot foot and neuropathy occur. When persons lack normal protective sensation, initial damage may occur without the person being aware of it. In addition, an existing wound may be exacerbated by excess pressure and mechanical or thermal damage in persons who lack sensation.[4] Unfortunately, it is common to see persons with multiple concomitant conditions, such as a person with a venous leg ulcer and coexistent arterial disease and diabetes.

Immunocompromised patients include persons who are HIV-positive, those with cancer, the malnourished, those receiving immunosuppressive agents, and the aged. Persons who are immunocompromised are unable to mount an adequate inflammatory response or the response is delayed. With immunocompromise, all phases of healing are delayed, and patients may be at risk for infection or wound disruption.[22]

Adverse Effects of Treatment

Iatrogenic effects of therapy also may result in impaired healing. Thus, treatment for pathologies may be a cofactor in healing impairment. Examples of such treatments are *radiation therapy, chemotherapy, steroid therapy*, and *anti-inflammatory drugs*.[22]

Radiation disrupts cell mitosis at the time of the treatment and has ongoing effects for the individual's life. These include obliterative arteritis and fibrosis that result in woody, hypoxic skin that does not heal well after injury. The dose and dose rate, along with the patient's genetics, determine the extent of damage and the speed at which it occurs. Bone marrow is the organ most sensitive to radiation exposure. The effects of radiation are seen immediately in terms of the number and various circulating cell types. Recovery depends on the dose of radiation and the half-life of the various cells.

Chemotherapy is designed to interrupt the cell cycle. It affects cells while they are dividing. This is accomplished in most anticancer drugs by damaging DNA or preventing DNA repair. Hormonal anticancer agents prevent binding of hormones, while others antagonize receptors to inhibit tumor growth. The primary effects of chemotherapy on healing are experienced during the treatment period and immediately after treatment.

A newly introduced form of cancer treatment is the use of *antiangiogenic agents (eg, bevacizumab)*, which block new blood vessel formation around the tumor by binding to a particular growth factor. Although these agents have the potential to impair wound healing, the pathway for wound angiogenesis and tumor angiogenesis appears to be somewhat different, and these agents have not caused the wound healing problems many anticipated.[25]

Steroids impair all phases of healing by suppressing the inflammatory response, reducing immunocompetent lymphocytes, decreasing antibody production, and diminishing antigen processing. Clinical signs of inflammation are suppressed. If steroids are administered at the time of injury, their impact is greater than if they are administered several days after injury because of their effect on the inflammatory response that accompanies the initial injury. When the initial inflammatory response is decreased, all subsequent phases of healing are delayed, and the risk of infection is increased. Other medications, such as nonsteroidal anti-inflammatory agents, phenylbutazone, and vitamin E, disrupt the normal healing process. Their effects are primarily anti-inflammatory and, thus, are seen early after injury.[5]

Conclusion

Healing in individuals with chronic wounds is a complex process. One cannot simply dress the wound and expect healing to occur. It is important to assess the individual for the presence of each of the potential cofactors described in this chapter. Typically, evaluation of cofactors for impairment is integrated into the initial history and physical and should be an integral part of the ongoing holistic patient assessment. Early identification of the cofactors for impaired healing allows the practitioner to make a differential diagnosis, initiate appropriate referrals, and develop a comprehensive plan of care. Management of local and systemic cofactors that impact repair will mitigate their adverse effects and facilitate healing of chronic wounds.

Practice Pearls

- A thorough history is the basis for determining factors present that may impair healing.
- It is important to assess the scientific evidence for the manifestation of specific factors on healing for patients with wounds.
- Current scientific knowledge about the mechanisms by which specific cofactors impair healing should be utilized when evaluating patients with wounds.

Self-Assessment Questions

1. Factors associated with impaired healing are:
   A. Warm temperature and low perfusion
   B. Warm temperature and high perfusion
   C. Cold temperature and high perfusion
   D. Cold temperature and low perfusion

2. Factors that contribute to impairment in healing due to infection are:
   A. Albumin of 4.5 g/dL
   B. Abscess distant from the wound
   C. 10^3 organisms per gram of tissue
   D. Healthy tissue

3. Anemia is a risk factor for impaired healing when:
   A. People are smokers
   B. Diabetes mellitus is present

C. Intravascular volume is low
D. Chemotherapy is utilized

Answers: 1-D, 2-B, 3-C

References

1. Lazarus GS, Cooper DM, Knighton DR, et al. Definitions and guidelines for assessment of wounds and evaluation of healing. *Arch Dermatol.* 1994;130(4):489–493.
2. Yang GP, Lim IJ, Phan TT, Lorenz HP, Longaker MT. From scarless fetal wounds to keloids: molecular studies in wound healing. *Wound Repair Regen.* 2003;11(6):411–418.
3. Gosain A, DiPietro LA. Aging and wound healing. *World J Surg.* 2004;28(3):321–326.
4. Enoch S, Price P. Cellular, molecular and biochemical differences in the pathophysiology of healing between acute wounds, chronic wounds and wounds in the aged. Available at: http://www.Worldwidewounds.com/2004/august/Enouch/pathophysiology-Of-Healing.html. Accessed April 23, 2006.
5. Ueno C, Hunt TK, Hopf HW. Using physiology to improve surgical wound outcomes. *Plast Reconstr Surg.* 2006;117(7 Suppl):59S–71S.
6. Hunt TK, Hopf H, Hussain Z. Physiology of wound healing. *Adv Skin Wound Care.* 2000;13(2 Suppl):6–11.
7. Hopf HW, Viele M, Watson JJ, et al. Subcutaneous perfusion and oxygen during acute severe isovolemic hemodilution in healthy volunteers. *Arch Surg.* 2000;135(12):1443–1449.
8. Jonsson K, Jensen JA, Goodson WH 3rd, et al. Tissue oxygenation, anemia, and perfusion in relation to wound healing in surgical patients. *Ann Surg.* 1991;214(5):605–613.
9. Hopf HW, Hunt TK. Does — and if so, to what extent — normovolemic dilutional anemia influence postoperative wound healing? *Chirurgische Gastroenterologie.* 1992;8:148–150.
10. Sorensen LT, Hemmingsen U, Kallehave F, et al. Risk factors for tissue and wound complications in gastrointestinal surgery. *Ann Surg.* 2005;241(4):654–658.
11. Jensen JA, Goodson WH, Hopf HW, Hunt TK. Cigarette smoking decreases tissue oxygen. *Arch Surg.* 1991;126(9):1131–1134.
12. Chang N, Goodson WH 3rd, Gottrup F, Hunt TK. Direct measurement of wound and tissue oxygen tension in postoperative patients. *Ann Surg.* 1983;197(4):470–478.
13. Hartmann M, Jonsson K, Zederfeldt B. Effect of tissue perfusion and oxygenation on accumulation of collagen in healing wounds. Randomized study in patients after major abdominal operations. *Eur J Surg.* 1992;158(10):521–526.
14. Stotts NA, Hopf HW. Facilitating positive outcomes in older adults with wounds. *Nurs Clin North Am.* 2005;40(2):267–279.
15. Albina JE. Nutrition in wound healing. *JPEN J Parenter Enteral Nutr.* 1994;18(4):367–376.
16. Arnold M, Barbul A. Nutrition and wound healing. *Plast Reconstr Surg.* 2006;117(7 Suppl):42S–58S.
17. Thomas DR. Prevention and treatment of pressure ul-

cers. *J Am Med Dir Assoc.* 2006;7(1):46–59.

18.   Wipke-Tevis DD, Stotts NA. Nutritional risk, status, and intake of individuals with venous ulcers: a pilot study. *J Vasc Nurs.* 1996;14(2):27–33.

19.   Healy   B,   Freedman   A.   Infections.   *BMJ.* 2006;332(7545):838–841.

20.   Frantz RA. Identifying infection in chronic wounds. *Nursing.* 2005;35(7):73.

21.   Attinger CE, Janis JE, Steinberg J, et al. Clinical approach to wounds: debridement and wound bed preparation including the use of dressings and wound-healing adjuvants. *Plast Reconstr Surg.* 2006;117(7 Suppl):72S–109S.

22.   Stotts NA. Impaired wound healing. In: Carrieri-Kohlman VK, Lindsey AM, West CM, eds. *Pathophysiological Phenomena in Nursing: Human Responses to Illness.* 3rd ed. Philadelphia, PA: WB Saunders; 2003:331–347.

23.   Newland PK, Wipke-Tevis DD, Williams DA, Rantz MJ, Petroski GF. Impact of pain on outcomes in long-term care residents with and without multiple sclerosis. *J Am Geriatr Soc.* 2005;53(9):1490–1496.

24.   Khuri SF, Henderson WG, DePalma RG, et al; for the Participants in the VA National Surgical Quality Improvement Program. Determinants of long-term survival after major surgery and the adverse effect of postoperative complications. *Ann Surg.* 2005;242(3):326–343.

25.   Zondor SD, Medina PJ. Bevacizumab: an angiogenesis inhibitor with efficacy in colorectal and other malignancies. *Ann Pharmacother.* 2004;38(7-8):1258–1264.

Dermatological Aspects of Wound Care

R. Gary Sibbald, BSc, MD, FRCPC(Med, Derm), MACP, FAAD,
MEd, MAPWCA; **Afsaneh Alavi**, MD, FRCPC(Derm);
Gordon Sussman, MD, FRCPC(Allergy and Immunology), FACP,
FAAAAI; **Elizabeth A. Ayello**, PhD, RN, ACNS-BC, CWON,
MAPWCA, FAAN; **Laurie Goodman**, RN, BA, MHScN

Objectives

The reader will be challenged to:

- Analyze the normal functions of the skin and disorders that can compromise the cutaneous barrier
- Identify and avoid common contact allergens (including latex) involved in the treatment of chronic skin ulcers and surrounding skin
- Implement an evidence-informed approach to the treatment of the dermatological aspects of wound care in clinical practice, including the assessment and treatment of peristomal skin conditions.

Introduction

The skin is an important organ with various functions. The cutaneous surface offers a barrier from infection and provides thermal insulation, protection from the environment, and an external seal for prevention of fluid and electrolyte loss.[1-4]

The skin is composed of 2 distinct layers, the epidermis and the dermis, which are separated by the dermal-epidermal junction. The epidermis (Plate 8, page 318) is the outermost layer of the skin. When the basal layer of epidermal cells divides, one cell stays behind for further division. The other epidermal cell migrates from its attachment to the basal layer through the granular layer to the surface stratum corneum. At the level of the stratum corneum, the cell dies and forms keratin on the skin surface. The epidermis is also the home for pigment cells (melanocytes) and immune processing cells (the Langerhans cells). There are no blood vessels in the epidermis, which relies entirely on the underlying dermis for nutrient supply. The epidermis also forms appendages that protrude into the dermis in the form of hair follicles and sweat glands.

The dermis attaches to the anchoring fibrils of collagen in the basement membrane zone. The superficial dermis consists of extracellular matrix (collagen, elastin, and ground substances), a network of blood vessels, and dermal fibroblast cells. The superficial dermis lies between regularly spaced epidermal ridges (rete pegs). Fibroblasts are responsible for producing the dermal collagen backbone and the elastin that gives the skin flexibility. The fibroblast-secreted ground sub-

Sibbald RG, Alavi A, Sussman G, Ayello EA, Goodman L. Dermatological aspects of wound care. In: Krasner DL, Rodeheaver GT, Sibbald RG, Woo KY, eds. *Chronic Wound Care: A Clinical Source Book for Healthcare Professionals.* Vol 1. 5th ed. Malvern, PA: HMP Communications; 2012:207–222.

Table 1. Composition of topical formulations[8]

Base	Composition
Lotion	Powder in water
Cream	Oil in water
Ointment	Water in oil
Paste	Powder in ointment
Gel	Particles in lattice

stance includes fibronectin and hyaluronic acid to promote nutrient and cellular traffic through the skin. The deep dermis is positioned over the subcutaneous fat with larger vascular networks and collagen fibers to provide tensile strength. The subcutaneous fat has a large storage capacity of energy and a protective function.

The Skin in Disease

A break in the cutaneous barrier can result in several changes on the skin surface. A loss of the surface epidermis with an epidermal base is called *erosion*. A loss of the entire epidermis with a dermal or deeper base is correctly termed an *ulcer*. A *skin tear* is a wound caused by shear, friction, and/or blunt force, resulting in separation of skin layers.[5] A thin linear crack in the skin with a dermal base is a *fissure*. Dry keratin on the surface of the skin represents *scale*. An exudation of fluid from the dermis or deeper tissue forms a *crust* when it dries on the surface. Crusts may be formed from blood (sanguineous), serum (serous), or pus (pustular). The crusts often contain more than one component, eg, serosanguineous (serum and blood). Clear blisters can be small *vesicles* (less than 1 cm diameter) or large *bullae* (greater than 1 cm diameter). *Pustules* (pus-filled vesicles) can be at the surface of a hair follicle (follicular pustule or folliculitis) or centered on a non-hair-bearing surface. The use of the precise terminology and appropriate documentation will facilitate the correct diagnosis and appropriate treatment.

Skin Hydration and Lubrication

The stratum corneum requires a 10% moisture content to stay intact; otherwise, a surface similar to a cracked pavement develops (eczema crackle).[6] The surface layer contains several water-binding substances (humectants) that are referred to as the natural moisturizing factor. Some of these components include glycerine, urea, lactic acid, and alpha hydroxy acids.[7]

Moisturizers delay transepidermal water loss (TEWL) from a damaged skin barrier, soothe the skin, and fill the irregularities on the stratum corneum.[8] The emollient moisturizers make the skin smooth and soft, but humectant moisturizers increase the water content of the epidermis and stratum corneum. Examples of moisturizers in these different categories include humectants, such as glycerin, urea, and propylene glycol. Topically applied humectants draw the water from the dermis to the epidermis. The water applied to the skin rapidly evaporates, but when a humectant is applied to a hydrated skin, the skin retains the water more efficiently. Humectants are more effective if they are applied to damp skin after a bath or shower before the skin is dried. Humectants are especially capable of filling irregularities of the skin and allowing smoothness of the skin.[9]

If humectant creams are applied to open or inflamed (red) areas, they may sting or burn. The stinging is transient due to hydroscopic properties and does not indicate a true allergy. Cracks or open skin can be covered with film-forming liquid acrylates prior to the application of humectants. In the presence of neuropathy, stinging with humectants may not be an issue.

Emollient moisturizers allow the skin surface to feel smooth to the touch. Different emollient bases are available, including silicone and dimethicone, various oils, propylene glycol, and acetyl stearate.

Lubrication needs to be distinguished from hydration. Skin lubrication is the result of coating the skin surface with an oily covering (petrolatum and emollient creams) that prevents water loss. A cream has a continuous water phase with suspended oil. When the water evaporates, a small amount of oil is left behind. An ointment has a continuous oil phase with a small amount of water. Oils will leave a more complete protective film behind, but ointments are often less cosmetically acceptable and may cause folliculitis (Table 1).

Periwound skin has the potential to macerate or break down.[10] Periwound dermatitis may be endogenous (related to stasis and swelling) or

exogenous (related to different topical preparations including cleansers, barriers, topical creams
and ointments, dressings, bandages, and hosiery).
Wound exudate may contain cellular debris and
enzymes that are corrosive for the periwound
skin. Topical creams and ointments may contain
potential allergens, and if the patient with open
skin (ulcers, ostomies) absorbs the allergen, the
patient can be easily sensitized. *A substance administered orally, intravenously, or intramuscularly
is relatively hidden from the immune system and
sensitization is less frequent.* Lanolin alcohols
(wool wax), perfumes, and natural substances
(aloe, lemon, or lime) are all common topical
allergens and should be avoided, especially in
patients with ulcers. We may be unknowingly
prescribing or recommending allergens to our
patients. The frequency of positive patch test results found in patients with leg ulcers[11] has ranged
from 40% to 82%. There is a direct relationship
between duration of leg ulcers and the number
of multiple positive allergens. The interpretation
of this data means that a long duration of ulceration provides more opportunity for exposure
and sensitization to different allergens. Clinicians
should avoid common allergens in patients with
leg ulcers.[12]

Protectants and Barriers

When open surfaces are exudative or draining,
the skin margins often become over-hydrated or
macerated. The periwound skin needs protection from exudate by using absorbent dressings
along with periwound skin protectants and barriers. Over-hydrated stratum corneum takes on
a soft, white, spongy texture, and these changes
can trigger wound enlargement or infection. Increased skin pH raises the risk of bacterial growth.
When a wound is over-hydrated, switching to a
dressing with a higher level of absorbency, eg, a
calcium alginate, hydrofiber, or foam dressing, can
achieve wound moisture balance. Petrolatum is
a good protectant for the surrounding skin, but
it requires a secondary dressing before adhesive
tapes can be applied. Petrolatum may inhibit adhesion of primary dressings and cause irritation
and folliculitis. Zinc oxide paste/ointment provides a stiffer periwound protectant (Plate 9, page
318). It is important to remember that the underlying skin cannot be visualized with the applica-

tion of zinc oxide and that zinc or petrolatum
preparations interfere with the formation of silver
ions. Do not use zinc preparations in combination with silver dressings.

To stiffen zinc oxide ointment, use simple talc
with no additives on a cotton ball and dab the
surface to the required consistency. (This procedure avoids clumping of the powder if it is just
sprinkled on.) The zinc oxide paste/ointment
does not need to be removed between dressing
changes, but the healthcare provider may simply
fill in the gaps or apply additional zinc oxide over
the residual material. Application of petrolatum
or oil may facilitate removal if it is too thick or
hardens on the skin.

Skin barriers (not to be confused with petrolatum and zinc oxide ointment) will allow adhesives to form a seal around ulcers by providing a protective film on the skin. They will allow
adhesion of primary and secondary dressings,
especially in ostomy patients. Many skin barriers
contain acrylates, and some patients may develop
contact allergies or irritation. Barriers containing
acrylates (eg, Cavilon™ No Sting, 3M, Saint Paul,
Minnesota) and Skin-Prep™ (Smith & Nephew,
Largo, Florida) allow visualization of underlying
skin, and adhesive dressings may be applied directly over the barrier film. The results of a systematic review identified evidence with a high
methodological standard to recommend barrier
films for the prevention of irritant contact dermatitis and also good quality evidence against
the use of barrier creams containing aluminum
chlorhydrate in the prevention of irritant contact
dermatitis.[13]

Contact Dermatitis

Externally applied preparations or wound fluids can cause contact dermatitis. About 80% of
contact dermatitis is of an irritant subtype and
20% is of an allergic etiology. Irritation is often
due to excess local wound fluid. Soaps, scrubs,
and topical antiseptics also can act as irritants with
the threshold for irritancy varying from one individual to another.

Allergic contact dermatitis and irritant contact dermatitis may look identical, especially in
chronic form; therefore, the patch test is a gold
standard to diagnose allergic contact dermatitis.
Clinically, contact irritant dermatitis presents

Table 2. Chronic leg ulcer patient series:[16–24] patch tests and frequent sensitizers (updated 2012)

Reference	No. of Patients	Frequency of Contact Sensitivity	Wool Alcohols	Balsam of Peru	Fragrance	Cetylsterol Alcohol	Other	Neomycin	Framycetin	Other
Cameron, 1997	52	52%	✓				Parabens	✓	✓	
Fräki et al, 1979	192	69%	✓	✓						
Dooms-Goossens et al, 1979	163	63%	✓	✓			Benzocaine Parabens	✓		
Malten and Kuiper, 1973	100	69%	✓	✓	✓				✓	
Kulozik et al, 1988	59	51%	✓						✓	✓
Wilson et al, 1991	81	67%	✓			✓			✓	Gentamycin
Gallenkemper et al, 1998	36	78%	✓	✓	✓	✓	Colophony Propylene glycol	✓		Chloramphenicol
Renner and Wollina, 2002	85	28%	✓	✓	✓	✓	Parabens Benzocaine Colophony	✓		
Barbaud et al, 2009	423	73%	✓	✓	✓	✓	Antiseptics Povidone-iodine Colophony	✓		Corticosteroids Gentamycin

as scaly red papules (elevated spot, < 1 cm) or plaques (elevated spot, > 1 cm), sometimes with an accompanying folliculitis. The margins are often indiscreet, and itching or burning irritation is mild to moderate (Plate 10, page 318). Reactions usually occur within 48 hours and may be present with the first exposure. Contact allergic dermatitis[14,15] is often bright red and inflamed with discrete margins (Plate 11, page 318). It is moderately to severely itchy and may have associated burning and even pain. Severe cases need to be distinguished from infections, such as cellulitis. The Langerhans cells resident in the skin process the allergen. The cells become activated and can migrate to the regional lymph node, recruiting sensitized lymphocytes, and produce a generalized dermatitis at sites distant from the original contact allergen exposure site. Vesicles (small fluid-filled blisters) are common, and the onset of reactions may be delayed for days or even weeks.

The initial or sensitization exposure must occur before subsequent exposures elicit the allergic response. Cameron[16] reported that local dressings and topical applications sensitize 51%–78% of leg ulcer patients and many other patients with chronic wounds. This sensitization may often go unrecognized. Table 2 contains a modified and updated list of common allergens in previously published series.[16–24] Individuals with chronic leg ulcers experienced polysensitization to multiple allergens, and in some individuals, more than 3 positive patch tests were identified.[24]

Contact allergy is a delayed hypersensitivity response activated by T lymphocytes. It is differentiated from the IgE antibody-mediated respiratory allergens elucidated by immediate prick testing on the forearm. The immediate immunoglobulin E test is related to asthma, but contact allergic dermatitis is a Type 4 delayed hypersensitivity reaction as exemplified by a tuberculin test that is read 48

Table 3. Common allergens in patients with chronic wounds (modified from Cameron[16])

Ingredient	Exposure
1. Lanolin (wool alcohols)	Common in some bath oils, moisturizing creams, and ointments as well as tulle dressings
2. Perfumes and fragrances (balsam of Peru)	An additive for cosmetic appeal to many over-the-counter preparations (eg, bath oils, moisturizers, and baby products)
3. Cetyl sterol alcohol	A (vehicle/base) component of many over-the-counter and medicated creams, ointments, and paste bandages
4. Topical antibiotics • Neomycin • Framycetin	Topical antibiotics are present in powder, cream, ointment, and tulle gauze preparations as well as some combination products with topical steroids
5. Preservatives • Quaternium 15 • Parabens • Chlorocresol	Preservatives prevent bacterial contamination in creams but are not required in ointment formulations
6. • Rosin (colophony) • Gum rosin (turpentine) • Wood rosin (pine wood) • Pentolyn H (synthetic derivative)	A component of some adhesive-backed bandages (eg, hydrocolloids); previous exposure may include yellow bar soap, tapes (insulating, Scotch), epilating wax, and rosin bags
7. Rubber • Latex rubber • Rubber accelerators (Mercapto/Carba/Thiuram mixes)	An increasing problem from some ostomy appliances, elastic bandages, and stockings, as well as latex gloves

hours after testing. If a Type 4 contact allergic reaction is suspected, there are 2 important tests: the usage test and the patch test. The usage test or ROAT (Repeated Open Application Test) is performed by applying creams and ointments to normal skin on the forearm just below the elbow crease. An area the size of a silver dollar is used, and the medication is applied twice a day for 5 days. If visible redness is noted, a contact allergy must be suspected. The ingredients of the cream or ointment should be scanned and known allergens tested with the appropriate patch tests. For ostomy appliances and wound dressings, a small half-inch piece is applied to the appropriate site on the opposite side of the abdomen, leg, arm, or normal skin (Plate 12, page 318). It is important not to patch test a patient with unknown chemicals and always refer to the product material safety information.

If the potential tested products are dry, allergens should be moistened with water and occluded with hypoallergenic tape for 48 to 72 hours.

In a study of 100 patients with leg ulcers performed in Canada, a lower sensitization rate (46%) in comparison with the previous studies was reported, and this could be related to the consistent clinical practice of avoiding common contact allergens (Table 3). The 4 main allergen groups identified by Smart et al[26] were fragrances, lanolin, antimicrobials, and rubber-related substances. The common allergens identified in the Canadian leg ulcer study[26] and 2 other studies, the Mayo Clinic (1998–2000) and the North American Contact Dermatitis Group (NACDG),[27] are outlined in Table 4. The difference in the relative frequency of allergen may reflect the potential exposures (Table 5). Wound care has integrated evidence-based knowledge, expert opinion, and patient preference into practice for best standard of care.

Cream, Ointment, and Dressing Allergens

Wool alcohol (wool fat/wool grease/wool wax or lanolin) was identified as a common allergen in a contact dermatitis series of leg ulcer patients.[16-22] The wool fatty acids and esters are ubiquitous in topical lubricants and as tulle-type wound dress-

Table 4. Comparison of positive reaction rates (%) to each allergen in 3 groups: Mayo Clinic patients, North American Contact Dermatitis Group (NACDG), and Canadian leg ulcer group[26,27]

Allergen	Mayo Clinic (%)	NACDG (%)	Canadian Study (%)
Wood tar mix	10.9	10.4	21
Wool wax alcohols (lanolin alcohol)	2.4	1.6	11
Balsam of Peru	12.3	11.3	10
Colophony	2.5	2.5	9
Bacitracin	9.2	8.7	8
P-phenylendiamine	4.9	4.9	8
Carba mix	4.8	5.2	6
Potassium dichromate	5.8	9.8	6
Nickel sulfate hexahydrate	16.2	14.1	5
Neomycin sulfate	11.5	11.2	4
Thimerosal	10.8	9.3	4

Table 5. Canadian series: frequency of positive patch test response in patients with leg ulcers[26]

Rank	Allergen and #	% of +ve	Group
1	Wood tar mix	21.0%	Fragrance
2	Wood wax alcohols (lanolin alcohol)	11.0%	Lanolin
3	Balsam of Peru	10.0%	Fragrance
4	Colophony	9.0%	Fragrance
5	Bacitracin	8.0%	Antibacterial
5	Benzalkonium chloride	8.0%	Antiseptic
5	P-phenylendiamine	8.0%	Rubber
8	Amerchol (lanolin/paraffin)	7.0%	Lanolin/preservative
8	Fusidic acid sodium salt	7.0%	Antibacterial
8	Polymyxin B sulfate	7.0%	Antibacterial
8	Benzoyl peroxide	7.0%	Acne/ulcer medications/dental plastic
12	Cetyl stearyl alcohol	6.0%	Lanolin
12	Carba mix	6.0%	Rubber
12	Potassium dichromate	6.0%	Alloys
15	Nickelsulfate hexahydrate	5.0%	Alloys
16	Neomycin sulfate	4.0%	Antibacterial
16	Thimerosol	4.0%	Preservative
16	Propolis	4.0%	Cosmetics

ings. Purified lanolin preparations may reduce its allergenicity, but this also probably reduces lanolin's usefulness as an emollient.[28] Although lanolin sensitivity is low in non–eczematous skin, it is a moderate sensitizer in persons with atopic manifestations (including atopic eczema, hayfever, and/or asthma) and a potent sensitizer in persons with stasis eczema and leg ulcers.[28–31] Breit and Bandmann[32] detected a high lanolin allergy rate of 13.2% in 326 cases of leg eczema. ***Lanolin and***

CHRONIC WOUND CARE, 5th Edition

wool alcohol products should be avoided in all patients with chronic wounds.

Fragrances are ever-present in skin care products as well as perfumes, colognes, hair care, laundry detergent, dentifrices, and cleaning products. Balsam of Peru is a natural substance obtained from fir trees and can be used as a screen for fragrance allergies. The Balsam of Peru patch test elicited a positive response in approximately 50% of cases.[26] If Balsam of Peru and fragrance mix patch tests are combined, 75% of perfume allergies can be detected.[26] The remaining allergens can be detected with open usage tests (ROAT) or by applying the commercial product under a closed patch test. The confusing label of an unscented product may contain small amounts of a masking fragrance; thus, clinicians should look for products labeled fragrance free.

Balsam of Peru may cross-react with rosin (colophony),[33] and the latter may be a component of adhesive tapes, bandages, and dressings. Specifically, contact dermatitis to hydrocolloid dressings has been linked to the colophony-related adhesive pentaerythritol ester (Pentalyn H).[34] The Chinese medicine Tiger Balm also has a similar structure and potential cross-reactivity to Balsam of Peru.[33]

Bases and other components in creams, ointments, and hydrogels also may act as allergens. In one series, propylene glycol, a component of some hydrogels, showed a positive allergic reaction in 3 out of 36 patients.[20] Cetyl sterol alcohol (emulsifier, stabilizer, and preservative) is a common additive to creams. This allergy is almost unique to patients with leg ulcers where local irritation or absorption is maximized.[35] Parabens are preservatives commonly used in creams. Parabens can be avoided, as they are not present in ointments, but they seldom cause allergic sensitivity.[35] Ointments do not need preservatives to prevent bacterial contamination. Other preservatives, particularly those that release formaldehyde[35] (eg, quaternium 15), are more likely to cause significant reactions.

Local anesthetic agents, particularly products from the ester group, are also common allergens. Benzocaine[36] is a highly sensitizing ester local anesthetic present in many over-the-counter cream preparations. The allergic sensitization can be avoided by using amide group anesthetic agents, such as xylocaine and prilocaine (combined in EMLA® [Eutectic Mixture of Lidocaine and Prilocaine], AstraZeneca, Wilmington, Delaware) or pramoxine (a miscellaneous group agent often in over-the-counter hemorrhoid creams). Any cream or ointment can be placed in the refrigerator and the subsequent cooling sensation produced with application is a useful antipruritic. The cooling sensation replaces itch, as part of the Melzac and Wall gate control theory of pain and related neural signals. Menthol added in small amounts (1/4% to 1/2%) to creams produces a cooling anti-itch effect through surface evaporation, but the evaporation is not as efficient in ointment vehicles.

Topical antibacterial agents are useful for increased bacterial burden on the wound surface but are not accepted as desirable therapeutic agents by all wound care practitioners. There are 3 general rules when they are used:

1. Do not use common topical sensitizers.
2. Do not use agents topically that are used systemically.
3. Reevaluate therapy frequently if the desired response is not achieved in 2–4 weeks.

Neomycin is a potent sensitizer[37,38] with 2 distinct allergens (neosamine sugars A, B, and C and a deoxystreptamine backbone). Sixty percent of medication-related allergies are due to the neosamine sugars, and the neosamine B sugar is shared with framycetin.[37,38] The second allergen is the deoxystreptamine backbone (40% of medication-related allergies) that is also present in gentamicin, amikacin, tobramycin,[39] and the other aminoglycoside antibiotic agents.

Other Forms of Eczema

Topical steroids are the mainstay of treatment for eczema (Table 6).[40,41] They are available in lotion (powder in water or alcohol), creams, and ointments.

Lotions are too drying for many forms of chronic eczema with scale predominating. The potency of the topical corticosteroid falls into 5 groups (weak, moderate, potent, very potent, and extremely potent). On the palms and soles, topical steroids with 6–9 times the potency of hydrocortisone (potent to very potent) are generally necessary and they are usually applied twice a day. Patients should be told that every time they scratch or rub an involved area, the eczema will last for 3 more days. In order to achieve a greater anti-itch effect, topical steroid creams can often be kept in

Table 6. Topical steroids

A. Relative Potency	Generic Name	Trade Name	Concentration %	Available In
X1	1. Weak Hydrocortisone	Cortate Emo Cort	1.0 0.5	C, O C, L
X3	2. Moderate Desonide Hydrocortisone 17-valerate Mometasone furoate Triamcinolone acetonide	Tridesilon Westcort Elocom Aristocort Kenalog	0.05 0.2 0.025, 0.1 0.025, 0.1	C, 0 C C, O, L C, O C, O, L
X6	3. Potent Betamethasone 17-valerate Betamethasone dipropionate Flucocinolone acetonide	Betnovate Celestoderm Valisone Diprosone Synalar Synamol	0.05, 0.1 0.05, 0.1 0.1 0.05 0.01, 0.025	C, O C, O L C, O, L C, O, L
X9	4. Very potent Desoximetasone Flucocinonide Halcinonide	Topicort Lidemol Lidex Topsyn Gel Halog	0.025 0.05 0.01, 0.05 0.05 0.025, 0.1	C C C, O G C, O, L
X12	5. Extremely potent Betamethasone dipropionate Clobetasol 17-propionate Halobetasol propionate	Diprolene Dermovate (CAN) Temovate (US) Ultravate	0.5 0.05 0.5	C, O, L C, O, L C, O
Key: C = Cream	O = Ointment	L = Lotion	G = Gel	
B. Relative Absorption	Forearm	1.0 (X)	Plantar foot	0.14 X
	Scalp	3.5 X	Forehead	6.0 X
	Cheeks	13.0 X	Scrotum	42.0 X
relative potency x relative absorption = effective concentration				

the refrigerator to produce a cooling effect when applied. Alternatively, menthol or camphor is added to the topical steroid cream or lotion preparation for the cooling and anti-itch effects. As the patient's dermatitis improves, the topical steroid should gradually be decreased in potency and/or lubricating or hydrating creams substituted for alternate applications. Single to twice-daily applications usually suffice. The quantity of topical steroid necessary to cover 1 fingertip is referred to as a FingerTip Unit (1 FTU = 0.5 g). When severe eczema covers the lower leg, 3 FTU of potent topical steroid should be applied daily for a few days. As the eczema resolves, the amount of corticosteroid should be gradually reduced. Red areas require some topical corticosteroid application, but dry areas can be treated with over-the-counter emollients alone. One application of cream for an adult to cover the entire body would require about 50 g of cream or the equivalent of 100 FTU.

In contrast to the palms and soles, the face and body folds have increased absorption; therefore, only weak to moderate topical steroids should be used in these locations. The relative strength of a steroid can be multiplied by the relative local absorption to obtain the effective concentration applied (Table 6).[42] Absorption of topical steroids has been reported to vary not only among individuals but also by age (very young and very old have thinner skin hence more absorption) or in the presence of a defective epidermal barrier. The penetration of topical steroids is 2–10 times greater in damaged compared to healthy skin. Eczematous skin, ointment bases, and occlusion will all further increase the relative absorption of topical steroids.

Contact hypersensitivity to topical steroids has been increasingly reported. In a multicenter study, the positive identification of allergy to corticosteroids was reported to range from 0.2% to 6% of all tested patients. Because the use of topical corticosteroids is increasing and they are often prescribed for longer periods of time, it is expected that this sensitization rate will increase. All of the topical steroids belong to 4 classes (A, B, C, D) with Class C steroids, including betamethasone, being less likely to cross-react with other steroid classes. Fluorinated steroids have lower risk of hypersensitivity than non-fluorinated steroids, including hydrocortisone.[43]

When allergy to topical steroids is suspected, allergy to vehicles and preservatives, including benzyl alcohol (fragrance), imidazolinyl urea (formaldehyde releaser), lanolin, propylene glycol, and paraben, should be ruled out. Corticosteroid sensitization can be confirmed with the ROAT or usage test, but the definitive test is the patch test.[43]

Other Treatments

Eczema may become secondarily impetiginized or infected. Oral antibiotics with anti-inflammatory action, including tetracyclines (especially the high anti-inflammatory action and methicillin-resistant *Staphylococcus aureus* [MRSA] susceptibility of doxycycline), trimethoprim, clindamycin, erythromycin, and metronidazole, are useful in controlling eczema, persistent inflammation, and bacterial burden. If a topical antibacterial is used, it should be used for

short periods of time (eg, 2 weeks) to control crusting or secondary superficial infection and then reevaluated for efficacy to justify continued usage. Topical antibiotics should not be sensitizing, and they should not be the same as those used systemically (with metronidazole an exception as an anti-inflammatory, low-sensitizing potential in a gel that only treats anaerobes). Resistant organisms will emerge from topical application, making the systemic agent ineffective. For severe itch, systemic antihistamines are useful; the non-sedating antihistamine preparations can be used in the daytime, while sedating preparations can be used at night. Oral steroids are occasionally necessary to control severe exacerbation when all other measures fail. Alitretinoin is an oral retinoid that has been successfully used in the treatment of refractory hand eczema.[44] The cost effectiveness of alitretinoin, a new oral retinoid, or vitamin A derivative (related to 13 cis retinoic acid or the disease-modifying agent for acne) in the treatment of recalcitrant hand dermatitis has been demonstrated in several studies.[44]

Latex Allergy (Natural Rubber)

Latex allergy requires special attention because of its increasing frequency and risk to both patients and healthcare providers.[45] The most common reaction seen to natural rubber latex (NRL) is an irritant contact dermatitis.

More than 80% of natural rubber allergies are due to contact allergic dermatitis from residual chemicals used to convert natural rubber into long polymerized rubber molecules. These residual rubber acetylators include chemicals that attach rubber molecules to long polymer strands (thiurams, mercaptobenzothiazole, and carbonates). Testing is by patch tests and usage tests to specific products.

As previously mentioned, contact allergic dermatitis is a Type 4 delayed hypersensitivity response mediated by T lymphocytes and tested with patch tests read 48 and 96 hours later.[40] Type 1 reactions are mediated by IgE antibodies and can cause contact urticaria, respiratory conditions, such as hayfever and asthma, and immediate rubber allergies. Immediate NRL allergy hypersensitivity can cause urticaria, wheezing, and anaphylaxis.[46] These reactions are often triggered by aerosolized NRL allergic exposure

Table 7. Potential sources of latex allergy

Exposure—Medical	Exposure—House-hold/Personal
1. Gloves	1. Gloves
2. Endotracheal tube	2. Condoms
3. Pharyngeal airway	3. Diaphragms
4. Face mask/bag	4. Contraceptive sponge
5. Ventilator (hose/bellows)	5. Swim goggles/cup/mask
6. Blood pressure cuff	6. Rubber plants
7. Catheters	7. Balloons/balls
8. Penrose drain	8. Rubber toy
9. Syringe	9. Pacifiers
	10. Elastic (clothing)
	11. Crutches (pads)

students.[51] There were 1,000 systemic reactions to latex reported between 1988 and 1992, of which 15 (mostly healthcare providers) were fatal. These fatalities were associated with barium enema tips that have since been removed from the market. Potential sources of medical and household personal exposure to latex are listed in Table 7.

Children with spina bifida have multiple catheterizations with latex tips and multiple surgical procedures. Their high incidence of latex allergy[52] is reported to be between 28% and 67%. Healthcare workers with atopy had a 24% incidence of latex allergy in one study, and some of these individuals did not experience a clinically recognized reaction.[50] Generally, healthcare workers without atopy had a 7%–10% incidence of latex allergy, and the non-atopic general population had a less than 1% (1/800 patients preoperative) incidence. About half of the latex allergy-tested and -identified cases were asymptomatic, and there was a definite but rare progression from localized Type 4 contact dermatitis reactions to a generalized Type 1 IgE mediated anaphylaxis.

The plant kingdom has many shared antigens that can act as co-allergens. Latex cross-reacts with a number of fruits and vegetables including banana, chestnut, kiwi, passion fruit, potato, and tomato.[53,54] Intraoperative unexpected anaphylactic reactions also may be a clue to latex allergy[55] (anaphylaxis, angioedema, urticaria, or hypotension).[56]

If a latex prick test or Reagin Antigen Stimulation Test (RAST) is positive and the patient is symptomatic for latex allergy, latex exposure must be avoided. Only non-latex gloves (synthetic polymer, vinyl) should be used, and all medical procedures and environments should be latex-free. If the latex prick test and/or Immuno Cap is negative and only dermatitis has occurred, patch tests should be performed to the rubber allergens (acetylators). A negative patch test would suggest a contact irritant rather than an allergic reaction. Latex levels in NRL sterile gloves, non-sterile gloves, and powdered exam gloves have decreased from 639 µg/g to 2.4 µg/g (0.38% of prior levels). A latex-free environment for sensitive individuals requires no latex gloves and no direct latex contact. With the cooperation of industry and the use of low-protein-low-allergen powder-free gloves, the incidence of new onset latex allergy has significantly declined. Latex sensitivity

that may be present in the operating room, dental sites, and the intensive care unit. The immediate prick test to NRL extract contains rubber epitopes and should be performed by allergy specialists familiar with the technique in a safe environment.[45,46] An *in-vitro* test, the Immuno Cap Specific IgE assay, can detect about 75% of allergic reactions. If the specific Immuno Cap is negative and the commercial prick test antigen is not available, a moistened finger of a latex glove can be applied, followed by a whole glove if the initial testing is negative. However, it is not always reliable because of variable latex allergen protein levels in the testing material.

Type 1 reactions to latex have increased with the increased use of latex gloves for universal precautions. Because of the need for 11 billion latex gloves in the United States in 1992, a lot of raw unrefined latex with an increased allergic potential was produced.[45] Currently, there are much lower usage levels and a more refined product that may be less likely to produce allergic reactions is available. Powdered gloves are particularly efficient at aerosolizing latex particles bound to the powder when the gloves are donned and more likely to sensitize healthcare providers.[47,48] Respiratory exposure with inhalation is a particular risk with multiple exposures, especially with powdered latex gloves, as experienced in healthcare providers,[49] housekeeping workers,[50] and dental

Table 8. Periwound skin protectants [modified from Sibbald RG, Campbell K, Coutts P, Queen D. Intact skin — an integrity not to be lost. *Ostomy Wound Manage.* 2003;49(6):27–41.]

Letter	Type	Advantages	Disadvantages
L	Liquid film Forming acrylate eg, no sting, skin prep	• Transparent surface that resists removal • Low incidence of reactions	• Cost • Lack of availability on some institutional formularies
O	Ointments • Petrolatum • Zinc oxide	• Relatively inexpensive and easy to apply	• Petrolatum liquifies with heat • Ointment vehicle may interfere with the ionization of silver products • Zinc oxide ointment does not allow visualization of underlying wound margin
W	Windowed adhesive Dressing (hydrocolloid, film, acrylate, silicone)	• Provides a good seal around the wound edge • Some products facilitate visibility of the wound margins	• Reactions to the adhesive can occur • If seal is compromised, moisture may accumulate under the dressing
E	External collection devices and negative pressure therapy (NPT)	• External pouching may help in difficult locations where an external seal is difficult (eg, perirectal area) • Negative pressure therapy may help to divert harmful wound fluid	• Devices need to be monitored for external seal • NPT may be noisy and interfere with activities of daily living • These devices do not replace a search for the cause of the excessive exudate and the need to correct the cause

needs to be closely monitored and latex products avoided, particularly for healthcare professionals (especially with atopy), persons with spinal-cord injuries, and individuals undergoing multiple surgical procedures.

Tinea and Candida Infections

Tinea is a dermatophyte fungus infection of the skin and nails.[57] The individuals most susceptible to fungal infection include men, the elderly, immunocompromised patients, persons with diabetes, and individuals with chronic moisture on the palms, soles, toe webs, or skin folds. A powdery white scale that is accentuated in the natural skin surface markings characterizes fungal infection of the palms and soles and must be distinguished from anhidrosis or dryness associated with neuropathy. The fine scale of a fungus infection, unlike the dryness of neuropathy, involves the side of the foot in an area that would be covered by a moccasin. In addition, there may be maceration of the fourth and fifth toe web spaces (moist occlusion) with a moist or macerated scale that spreads proximally to the other toe webs. The nails start their involvement distally with linear yellow streaks that subsequently spread proximally. Fungal infections start asymmetrically and spread to involve the opposite foot or hand(s).

The diagnosis of tinea is confirmed by scraping the scale from the plantar aspect of the foot or sampling the affected nail clippings with subungal debris onto the non-shiny surface of black paper or other paper. Laboratory testing (eg, potassium hydroxide, KOH) using direct microscopic examination for the presence of fungal filaments or culture of the characteristic fungal colonies is recommended. Nails require clipping of the abnormal segment and removing soft sub-debris for similar processing. Sampling of skin or nails for microscopic fungal examination and fungal culture may need to be repeated up to 3 times to rule out fungus if the clinical picture is suspicious.

Topical antifungal agents are used predominantly for skin involvement, and they have improved over the last 3 decades.[58,59] Undecylenic acid powders are used for prophylaxis but not active treatment. Tolnaftate is approximately 40% effective and only treats dermatophyte fungus and not yeast. Ciclopirox cream or lotion treats less than 60% of infections, and the newer imidazole agents are effective topically in 70%–80% of involved individuals, treating both dermatophyte (tinea) and yeast (candida) infections. The topical imidazole agents include clotrimazole, miconazole, ketoconazole, and econazole.

Periwound Dermatitis

Periwound dermatitis is a challenge in the treatment of chronic wounds, and it may present as a stalled or enlarging, persistent skin ulcer. There are different ways to protect the periwound skin of an ulcer, including wound margin applications of film-forming liquid acrylates, petrolatum, zinc oxide ointment, and windowed adhesive dressings, including hydrocolloids and films. Negative pressure wound therapy and external collection devices, such as pouching, also are helpful ways to protect periwound skin. For simplicity in everyday practice, Sibbald et al[60] have proposed combining these concepts into the simple mnemonic LOWE (Table 8).

Special Problems for People with Ostomies

Besides the usual physiological functions of the skin (protection, immunological surveillance, metabolism, sensation, thermoregulation, and communication for social and sexual function), peristomal skin has one unique function: to maintain contact with the ostomy skin barrier. Peristomal skin damage is one of the most challenging aspects of living with an ostomy.[61] Woo and colleagues have created a mnemonic, MINDS, to help clinicians remember and be mindful of potential causes of peristomal skin problems.[62] MINDS stands for:

- Mechanical trauma from the ostomy equipment and skin stripping
- Infection (bacterial and fungal)
- Noxious chemicals and irritants, including strong alkaline feces or urine
- Diseases of the skin that are common in persons with ostomies, eg, pyoderma gangrenosum, psoriasis
- Skin allergens.[63]

People with ostomies may develop contact allergy and contact irritant reactions under ostomy pouches. Product allergy testing of the ostomy pouch and other supplies on the opposite side of the abdomen can confirm reactions. Contact irritation can be due to leakage of stoma contents due to poor positioning or retraction of the stoma. Treatment may include use of topical steroids in powder, spray, or lotion form. Products should not interfere with adherence of the skin barrier or appliance, so preparations that have a greasy consistency usually are not used.[62] Peristomal ulcers could be due to pyoderma gangrenosum, infection, or malignancy.

Specific diagnoses and treatment for peristomal disorders can include the following:

- For candidiasis, clinicians can consider the use of nystatin or clotrimazole powder under the appliance along with the previously mentioned antifungal azole creams for the peri-appliance surrounding skin
- For folliculitis that may be caused by a staphylococcal infection or acne type of inflammation of the hair follicle under the appliance, infection or inflammation of the hair follicle can be treated with topical clindamycin or other lotions
- Mucosal seeding often can be treated with electrocautery destruction
- Pseudo-verrucous lesions need to be checked for alkaline urine leakage — treatment includes the correction of the seal and acidification of the urine; the differential includes contact dermatitis of the skin (irritant and allergic) or urine infections
- Avoid pyoderma gangrenosum in susceptible individuals by utilizing a flat, not concave appliance to help avoid local trauma
- Suture granulomas require the removal of retained suture
- Irritant/allergic contact dermatitis requires the removal of the irritant or contact allergen
- Peristomal varices may be present and the clinician should question the patient or have a high index of suspicion of esophageal varices with chronic liver disease or previous esophageal bleeding.

Other peristomal skin complications include moisture-associated skin damage (MASD) as a result of inflammation and erosion of the skin caused by prolonged exposure to various sources of moisture.[64] MASD may result from urine, stool, perspiration, and external water sources (bathing and swimming) and/or wound drainage. Routine assessments, prevention strategies, and timely treatment help minimize damage from MASD.

Patients with peristomal complications often overlook the early signs. Specifically, dermal irritation around the stoma followed by pouch leakage is often not seen as problematic enough to warrant reporting to their healthcare professionals. One study identified that 34% of individuals presented with skin-related problems within 3 weeks of stoma surgery.[65] This repeating theme of patients' willingness to "tolerate" the new abnormal skin development and not report it is concerning. Patient education should include the importance of reporting early skin changes, and clinicians need to create a plan to address the presenting issue. Herlufsen et al[66] reported that up to 80% of peristomal complications are not reported by patients. Many times patients continued to cope independently, leading to a cascade of problems. In another study of 410 participants with peristomal leakage, 56% admitted to not seeking help and only 6% consistently elicited help from their clinician support system.[66]

The assessment of peristomal complications should aim to identify the causative factor or source of the irritant. A detailed assessment allows the patient and healthcare professional to work together to develop a mutually agreed upon corrective treatment plan. Assessment should include:

- Description and measurement of the extent of irritated skin
- Details of current and recent products used
- Record of stool volume output, emptying practices, and wear times
- Nutritional or diet review in relation to output
- Activities, including water sports
- Medications and medical conditions
- Prevention of further peristomal damage.

Allergic contact dermatitis (ACD) may be from potential allergens in stoma appliances and locally applied materials. Recently, a retrospective review (medical records over 10 years, 2000–2010) of 10 peristomal dermatitis patients who underwent patch testing revealed that patch testing was a valuable method to identify the source of allergens.[67] Each of the 10 patients with peristomal dermatitis had at least one positive patch test reaction. The researchers summarized that patch testing is a valuable tool in the management of stoma patients when allergic contact dermatitis is suspected. These researchers suggest that patch testing should include both a large standard patch test series as well as testing of the patient's own ostomy products and accessories being used.[67] This brings into focus the value of interprofessional involvement for optimal management of stoma patients, specifically a dermatology consult. It is important to involve the interprofessional team early and to include patient-centered education as part of any ostomy program.[61]

There are 2 ostomy tools that clinicians can use in practice so that a common language of peristomal skin disorders can be communicated among the interdisciplinary team members.[62] The Ostomy Skin Tool has 2 sections: one that calculates a score to describe the peristomal skin condition (Discoloration, Erosion, and Tissue overgrowth or DET) and another that is a diagnostic guide to categorize peristomal skin disorders and guide treatment protocols.[67] The DET score is derived from direct clinical observation and is obtained by evaluating the peristomal skin discoloration, erosion, and tissue overgrowth.[68] The other tool was created to proactively identify peristomal skin types (healthy, normal; thin, fragile, sensitive; dry, flaky; oily, sweaty) and needs to guide selection of appropriate skin barriers and pouches prior to skin problems.[69] Clinicians enter descriptors regarding the skin type and the skin barrier change frequency to guide skin barrier selection. These tools are available commercially. The Ostomy Skin Tool is available from Coloplast,[60,63,67,68,70,71] and the skin barrier selector is available from Hollister.[61,72,73]

Conclusion

Intact skin is the body's best defense against fluid and electrolyte loss as well as infection or external trauma that may impair healing. The early recognition, accurate documentation, diagnosis, and treatment of cutaneous disorders can prevent skin breakdown and ulcer-related complications that delay the wound healing process. Topical applications should be appropriate to maintain hydration but avoid maceration. Allergens should be avoided, and adverse reactions require a precise diagnosis to avoid future exposures.

Practice Pearls

- Do not use common topical sensitizers or agents topically that are used systemically.
- Apply proper moisturizer (humectant or lubrication) to keep skin free from dehydration, manifested clinically with xerosis and fissuring.
- Assess the advantages and disadvantages of strategies to protect peri-ulcer and peristomal skin.
- Identify potential allergens with the ROAT or patch tests.
- Examine the skin and perform appropriate diagnostic tests for an accurate diagnosis and management.
- Reevaluate therapy frequently if desired results are not achieved within 2–4 weeks.

Self-Assessment Questions

1. Which of the following is/are most appropriate for periwound protection in a patient with a leg ulcer and moderate exudate that is being dressed with a silver dressing?
   A. A film-forming liquid acrylate
   B. Windowed hydrocolloids
   C. Zinc oxide cream
   D. Negative pressure therapy
   E. Petrolatum ointment

2. Which of the following are correct for the therapeutic use of topical antibiotics?
   A. Do not use common sensitizers
   B. Do not use topical agents that are used systemically
   C. A and B
   D. None of the above

3. Which of the following is NOT a common sensitizer in patients with leg ulcers?
   A. Neomycin
   B. Pentalyn H
   C. Parabens
   D. Lanolin

4. What individual group is MOST at risk of developing a latex allergy?
   A. Healthcare professionals
   B. Individuals with spina bifida
   C. Bartenders
   D. Custodians or janitors

Answers: 1–A, 2–C, 3–C, 4–B

References

1. Ebling FJG, Eady RAJ, Leigh IM. Anatomy and organization of human skin. In: Champion RH, Burton JL, Ebling FJG, eds. *Textbook of Dermatology.* 5th ed. Oxford, UK: Blackwell Scientific Publications; 1992:49–125.

2. Ebling FJG. Functions of the skin. In: Champion RH, Burton JL, Ebling FJG, eds. *Textbook of Dermatology.* 5th ed. Oxford, UK: Blackwell Scientific Publications; 1992:115–125.

3. Habif TB. Principles of diagnosis and anatomy. In: *Clinical Dermatology.* Saint Louis, MO: Mosby; 1990:1–10.

4. Sams UM Jr. Structure and function of the skin. In: Lynch PJ, Sams WM Jr, eds. *Principles and Practice of Dermatology.* New York, NY: Churchill Livingstone Inc; 1990:3–14.

5. LeBlanc K, Baranoski S; Skin Tear Consensus Panel Members. Skin tears: state of the science: consensus statement for the prevention, prediction, assessment, and treatment of skin tears.© *Adv Skin Wound Care.* 2011;24(9 Suppl):2–15.

6. Tagami H, Ohi M, Iwatsuki K, Kanamaru Y, Yamada M, Ichijo B. Evaluation of the skin surface hydration *in vivo* by electrical measurement. *J Invest Dermatol.* 1980;75(6):500–507.

7. Stott NA, Wipke-Tevis DD, Hopf HW. Cofactors in impaired wound healing. In: Krasner DL, Rodeheaver GT, Sibbald RG, eds. *Chronic Wound Care: A Clinical Source Book for Healthcare Professionals.* 4th ed. Malvern, PA: HMP Communications; 2007:215–220.

8. Johnson C, Shuster S. The measurement of transepidermal water loss. *Br J Dermatol.* 1969;81(Suppl S4):40–46.

9. Lynde CW. Moisturizers: what they are and how they work. Available at: http://www.skintherapyletter.com/2001/6.13/2.html. Accessed January 22, 2012.

10. Ryan S, Fowler E, Coutts P, Sibbald RG. Approaches to the wound edge: a toolkit. Presented at the Symposium on Advanced Wound Care and Medical Research Forum on Wound Repair in San Diego, CA, April 21–24, 2005.

11. Saap L, Fahim S, Arsenault E, et al. Contact sensitivity in patients with leg ulcerations: a North American study. *Arch Dermatol.* 2004;140(10):1241–1246.

12. Tavadia S, Bianchi J, Dawe RS, et al. Allergic contact dermatitis in venous leg ulcer patients. *Contact Dermatitis.* 2003;48(5):261–265.

13. Saary J, Qureshi R, Palda V, et al. A systematic review of contact dermatitis treatment and prevention. *J Am Acad Dermatol.* 2005;53(5):845.

14. Kalish RS. Recent developments in the pathogenesis of allergic contact dermatitis. *Arch Dermatol.* 1991;127(10):1558–1563.

15. Rietschel RL, Fowler JF. The pathogenesis of allergic contact hypersensitivity. In: *Fisher's Contact Dermatitis.* 4th

ed. Baltimore, MD: Williams & Wilkins; 1995:1–10.

16. Cameron J. The importance of contact dermatitis in the management of leg ulcers. In: Moffatt C, Harper P, eds. *Access to Clinical Education: Leg Ulcers.* New York, NY: Churchill Livingstone Inc; 1997:182–185.

17. Fräki JE, Peltonen L, Hopsu-Havu VK. Allergy to various components of topical preparations in stasis dermatitis and leg ulcer. *Contact Dermatitis.* 1979;5(2):97–100.

18. Dooms-Goossens A, Degreef H, Parijs M, Kerkhofs L. A retrospective study of Patch test results from 163 patients with stasis dermatitis or leg ulcers. I. Discussion of the Patch test results and the sensitization indices and determination of the relevancy of positive reactions. *Dermatologica.* 1979;159(2):93–100.

19. Malten KE, Kuiper JP, van der Staak WB. Contact allergic investigations in 100 patients with ulcus cruris. *Dermatologica.* 1973;147(4):241–254.

20. Kulozik M, Powell SM, Cherry G, Ryan TJ. Contact sensitivity in community-based leg ulcer patients. *Clin Exp Dermatol.* 1988;13(2):82–84.

21. Wilson CL, Cameron J, Powell SM, Cherry G, Ryan TJ. High incidence of contact dermatitis in leg-ulcer patients—implications for management. *Clin Exp Dermatol.* 1991;16(4):250–253.

22. Gallenkemper G, Rabe E, Bauer R. Contact sensitization in chronic venous insufficiency: modern wound dressings. *Contact Dermatitis.* 1998;38(5):274–278.

23. Renner R, Wollina U. Contact sensitization in patients with leg ulcers and/or leg eczema: comparison between centers. *Int J Low Extrem Wounds.* 2002;1(4):251–255.

24. Barbaud A, Collet E, Le Coz CJ, Meaume S, Gillois P. Contact allergy in chronic leg ulcers: results of a multicentre study carried out in 423 patients and proposal for an updated series of patch tests. *Contact Dermatitis.* 2009;60(5):279–287.

25. James WD, Rosenthal LE, Brancaccio RR, Marks JG Jr. American Academy of Dermatology Patch Testing Survey: use and effectiveness of this procedure. *J Am Acad Dermatol.* 1992;26(6):991–994.

26. Smart V, Alavi A, Coutts P, et al. Contact allergens in persons with leg ulcers: a Canadian study in contact sensitization. *Int J Low Extrem Wounds.* 2008;7(3):120–125.

27. Wetter DA, Davis MD, Yiannias JA, et al. Patch test results from the Mayo Clinic Contact Dermatitis Group, 1998–2000. *J Am Acad Dermatol.* 2005;53(3):416–421.

28. Rietschel RL, Fowler JF. Reactions to selected topical medications-lanolin. In: *Fisher's Contact Dermatitis.* 4th ed. Baltimore, MD: Williams & Wilkins; 1995:162–163.

29. Oleffe JA, Blondeel A, Boschmans S. Patch testing with lanolin. *Contact Dermatitis.* 1978;4(4):223–247.

30. Giorgini S, Melli MC, Sertoli A. Comments on the allergenic activity of lanolin. *Contact Dermatitis.* 1983;9(5):425–426.

31. Kligman AM. Lanolin allergy: crisis or comedy. *Contact Dermatitis.* 1983;9(2):99–107.

32. Breit R, Bandmann HJ. Contact dermatitis XXII. Dermatitis from lanolin. *Br J Dermatol.* 1973;88(4):414–416.

33. Reischel RL, Fowler JF. Fragrance allergy. In: *Fisher's Contact Dermatitis.* 4th ed. Baltimore, MD: Williams & Wilkins; 1995:448–460.

34. Sasseville D, Tennstedt D, Lachapelle JM. Allergic contact dermatitis from hydrocolloid dressings. *Am J Contact Dermat.* 1997;8(4):236–238.

35. Rietschel RL, Fowler JF. Vehicles and preservatives including formaldehyde, cosmetics and personal-care products. In: *Fisher's Contact Dermatitis.* 4th ed. Baltimore, MD: Williams & Wilkins; 1995:257–330.

36. Rietschel RL, Fowler JF. Local anesthetics. In: *Fisher's Contact Dermatitis.* 4th ed. Baltimore, MD: Williams & Wilkins; 1995:236–248.

37. Rietschel RL, Fowler JF. Reactions to topical antimicrobials. In: *Fisher's Contact Dermatitis.* 4th ed. Baltimore, MD: Williams & Wilkins; 1995:205–225.

38. Chung CW, Carson TR. Sensitization potentials and immunologic specificities of neomycins. *J Invest Dermatol.* 1975;64(3):158–164.

39. Schorr WF, Ridgway HB. Tobramycin-neomycin cross-sensitivity. *Contact Dermatitis.* 1997;3(3):133–137.

40. Sibbald RG. Hand eczema. *Ostomy Wound Manage.* 1998;44(8):68–78.

41. Arndt KA. *Manual of Dermatologic Therapeutics.* 5th ed. Boston, MA: Little, Brown, and Company; 1995:299–308.

42. Arndt KA. *Manual of Dermatologic Therapeutics.* 5th ed. Boston, MA: Little, Brown, and Company; 1995:53–54.

43. Hengge UR, Ruzicka T, Schwartz RA, Cork MJ. Adverse effects of topical glucocorticosteroids. *J Am Acad Dermatol.* 2006;54(1):1–15.

44. Ghasri P, Scheinfeld N. Update on the use of alitretinoin in treating chronic hand eczema. *Clin Cosmet Investig Dermatol.* 2010;3:59–65.

45. Tarlo SM. Latex allergy: a problem for both healthcare professionals and patients. *Ostomy Wound Manage.* 1998;44(8):80–88.

46. Slater JE. Rubber anaphylaxis. *N Engl J Med.* 1989;320(17):1126–1130.

47. Tarlo SM, Wong L, Roos J, Booth N. Occupational asthma caused by latex in a surgical glove manufacturing plant. *J Allergy Clin Immunol.* 1990;85(3):626–631.

48. Tarlo SM, Sussman G, Contala A, Swanson MC. Control of airborne latex by use of powder-free latex gloves. *J Allergy Clin Immunol.* 1994;93(6):985–989.

49. Wrangsjö K, Osterman K, van Hage-Hamsten M. Glove-related skin symptoms among operating theatre and dental care unit personnel (II). Clinical examination, tests and laboratory findings indicating latex allergy. *Contact Dermatitis.* 1994;30(3):139–143.

50. Sussman GL, Lem D, Liss G, Beezhold D. Latex allergy in housekeeping personnel. *Ann Allergy Asthma Immunol.* 1995;74(5):415–418.

51. Tarlo SM, Sussman GL, Holness DL. Latex sensitivity in dental students and staff: a cross-sectional study. *J Allergy Clin Immunol.* 1997;99(3):396–401.

52. Nieto A, Estornell F, Mazon A, Reig C, Nieto A, Garcia-Ibarra F. Allergy to latex in spina bifida: a multivariate study of associated factors in 100 consecutive patients. *J Allergy Clin Immunol.* 1996;98(3):501–507.

53. Blanco C, Carrillo T, Castillo R, Quiralte J, Cuevas M. Latex allergy: clinical features and cross-reactivity with fruits. *Ann Allergy.* 1994;73(4):309–311.

54. Beezhold DH, Sussman GL, Liss GM, Chan NS. Latex allergy can induce clinical reactions to specific foods. *Clin Exp Allergy.* 1996;26(4):416–422.

55. Gold M, Swartz JS, Braude BM, Dolovich J, Shandling B, Gilmour RE. Intraoperative anaphylaxis: an association with latex sensitivity. *J Allergy Clin Immunol.* 1991;87(3):662–666.

56. Sibbald RG, Fryer P. Latex allergy. An institutional approach, questionnaire and information for healthcare workers. *Ostomy Wound Manage.* 1998;44(9):88–91.

57. Effendy I, Kolczak H, Ossowski B, Höhler T. Topical therapy of onychomycoses with 8% ciclopirox laquer. An open, non-comparative study. *Fortschr Med.* 1993;111(12):205–208.

58. Gupta AK, Sauder DN, Shear NH. Antifungal agents: an overview. Part I. *J Am Acad Dermatol.* 1994;30(5 Pt 1):677–698.

59. Gupta AK, Sauder DN, Shear NH. Antifungal agents: an overview. Part II. *J Am Acad Dermatol.* 1994;30(6):911–933.

60. Sibbald RG, Woo K, Ayello EA. Increased bacterial burden and infection: the story of NERDS and STONES. *Adv Skin Wound Care.* 2006;19(8):447–461.

61. Rolstad BS, Ermer-Seltun J, Bryant RA. Relating knowledge of anatomy and physiology to peristomal skin care. *Gastrointestinal Nursing.* 2011;9(1 Suppl):3–9.

62. Woo KY, Sibbald RG, Ayello EA, Coutts PM, Garde DE. Peristomal skin complications and management. *Adv Skin Wound Care.* 2009;22(11):522–534.

63. Martins L, Tavernelli K, Serrano JLC. Introducing a peristomal skin assessment tool: the Ostomy Skin Tool. *WCET Journal.* 2008;28(2 Suppl):8–13.

64. Colwell JC, Ratliff CR, Goldberg M, et al. MASD part 3: peristomal moisture-associated dermatitis and peri-wound moisture-associated dermatitis: a consensus. *J Wound Ostomy Continence Nurse.* 2011;38(5):541–553.

65. Cottam J, Richards K, Hasted A, Blackman A. Results of a nationwide prospective audit of stoma complications within 3 weeks of surgery. *Colorectal Dis.* 2007;9(9):834–838.

66. Herlufsen P, Olsen AG, Carlsen B, et al. Study of peristomal skin disorders in patients with permanent stomas. *Br J Nurs.* 2006;15(16):854–862.

67. Claessens I, Serrano JLC, English E, Martins L, Tavernelli K. Peristomal skin disorders and the Ostomy Skin Tool. *WCET Journal.* 2008;28(2):26–27.

68. Martins L. Case study--using the Ostomy Skin Tool to justify the resources needed for your patients. *WCET Journal.* 2008;28(2 Suppl):16–17.

69. Porrett T, Rolstad BS, Ermer-Seltun J, et al. Selecting the appropriate skin barrier in ostomy care. *Gastrointestinal Nursing.* 2011;9(9 Suppl):1–16.

70. Perrin A. Case study--using the Ostomy Skin Tool to assist communication between ostomy care nurses. *WCET Journal.* 2008;28(2 Suppl):14–15.

71. Tavernelli K, Reif S. Case study--how the Ostomy Skin Tool can help people with peristomal skin disorders. *WCET Journal.* 2008;28(2 Suppl):18–19.

72. Nichols T, Menier M, Purnell P. Evaluating the process of skin barrier selection through use of a specific tool. *Gastrointestinal Nursing.* 2011;9(1 Suppl):10–14.

73. Purnell P. Proactive decisions vs reactive responses. *Gastrointestinal Nursing.* 2011;9(1 Suppl):15.

Wound Dressing Product Selection: A Holistic, Interprofessional, Patient-Centered Approach©

Diane L. Krasner, PhD, RN, CWCN, CWS, MAPWCA, FAAN;
R. Gary Sibbald, BSc, MD, FRCPC(Med, Derm), MACP, FAAD, MEd, MAPWCA;
Kevin Y. Woo, PhD, RN, FAPWCA

© 2010 Kestrel Health Information, Inc. Used with permission.

Objectives

The reader will be challenged to:
• Apply a wound dressing product selection framework to clinical practice
• Assess dressing performance parameters for holistic, interprofessional patient-centered care
• Identify web-based resources for up-to-date dressing product information.

Introduction

Many wound care clinicians remember the "good old days" when wound dressing product selection simply involved choosing from a handful of products that were essentially variations on the same theme. There was gauze, impregnated gauze, and filled gauze pads. In the earlier 20th century, clinicians added antimicrobial solutions, creams, and ointments (like Dakin's solution developed during World War I and silver sulfadiazine developed in the 1960s), and the wound care formulary was limited and simplistic.

Fast forward to the 21st century and wound care clinicians are confronted with a totally different situation: hundreds of products, scientific rationale for moist interactive dressings, and an emerging evidence-base for product selection.

Current wound care expertise encompasses numerous dressing-related skills, including:

• *Treating the cause of the wound* and addressing *patient-centered concerns* to set the stage for local wound care
• Properly *assessing the wound* and identifying the dressing requirements
• Selecting *dressings based on their form and function* for an individual wound's needs
• Meeting *setting–specific requirements* for dressing change frequency and maintenance
• Addressing *formulary or healthcare system availability* as well as reimbursement requirements.

Wound care product selection today must be as sophis-

Reprinted from Krasner DL, Sibbald RG, Woo KY. Wound dressing product selection: a holistic, interprofessional patient-centered approach©. *WoundSource: The Kestrel Wound Product Sourcebook.* September 2010. Available at: http://www.woundsource.com/wound-dressing-product-selection-white-paper#. © 2010 Kestrel Health Information, Inc. Used with permission.

Holistic Perspectives
Total Patient Care

Pathway 1: Aggressive/Active
Pathway 2: Maintenance
Pathway 3: Palliative/Nonhealable

Woud Care Local Treatment Pathway:
Wound Assessment

Identification of Wound Dressing
Product Requirements

- Wound bed preparation (DAMP© Krasner, Sibbald, Woo)
  - **D**ebridement
  - **A**ntimicrobial/inflammation control
  - **M**oisture balance/exudate management
  - **P**ain/comfort (eg, temperature control, protection)

Interprofessional Considerations
Frequency of dressing changes
Wound access
Consistent with other treatments
  (local topical, regional, systemic)
Patient not allergic to component
Not a common sensitizer

© 2010 Krasner, Sibbald, Woo

Patient-Centered Concerns
Ease of use
Pain management
Odor control
Compatible with activities of
  daily living (ADLs)
Body image/psychosocial
Reimbursement/costs

Figure 1. Conceptual Framework for Wound Dressing Product Selection©.

ticated and as evidence-based as possible. This chapter presents a conceptual framework for the wound dressing product selection process that is based on 3 principles:

- Holistic perspectives[1]
- Interprofessional considerations[2]
- Patient-centered concerns.[3]

This conceptual framework is illustrated in Figure 1 and is discussed in detail in this chapter.

Wound Dressing Product Selection for the 21st Century

For every complex problem, there is a simple solution, and it is wrong. — *H. L. Mencken*

Selecting appropriate wound dressing products and supportive care to maximize healing and patient outcomes is a complex process. Dressing and local wound care options based on science and best practices must be filtered by clinical experience and must be consistent with patient preferences, caregiver requirements, and setting/access issues.[4] Additionally, effective dressing selection and local wound care planning involve the perspectives of the entire interprofessional team.[2]

Knowing the performance parameters of dressing categories/individual products and matching these attributes to an individual's wound can optimize the healing process.[5] However, dressings are only one piece of the puzzle. Dressings alone will not promote wound healing, unless the underlying causes for the wound are also addressed (eg, treatment of the wound cause, blood supply, nutrition, patient-centered concerns, local wound care). As the wound changes, the plan of care must change and dressing products may have to be changed. ***Appropriate dressing product selection:***

- Optimizes the local wound healing environment
- Reduces local pain and suffering
- Improves activities of daily living and quality of life.

Inappropriate dressing selection can:

- Cause the wound status to deteriorate (eg, wound margin maceration, increased risk of superficial critical colonization or deep infection, skin stripping)
- Increase local pressure or pain, especially at dressing change (dressing removal and cleansing)
- Increase costs with the need for frequent dressing changes or the selection of an inappropriate advanced or active dressing.

National and international wound care guidelines and best practice documents mean that there is no longer a local standard of care. No matter where you practice, you will be held to national/international standards of wound care practice.[6] Some experts have argued that the selection of the wrong dressing is just as problematic as the administration of the wrong drug and the clini-cian would be just as liable in a court of law. If dressings can be shown to delay the healing process (eg, wet-to-dry gauze dressings in a wound that requires moist wound healing, pain from inappropriate adhesives, failure to treat critical colonization that can lead to deep infection), their use might be deemed negligent by a jury in a court case.

Holistic Perspectives

Wound dressing product selection must be consistent and congruent with the total plan of care for the person with a wound. Four questions that the clinician should consider are:

1. What type of wound is it? What is the underlying etiology/cause and can you treat or correct the cause (eg, pressure, venous, neuropathic, neuroischemic, ischemic)?
2. Is it healable, maintenance, or nonhealable/palliative?[7]
3. Is the wound colonized, critically colonized, or infected in the deep tissue or wound margin?[8,9]
4. Is the plan of care aggressive/active, maintenance, or palliative/nonhealable?

If the overall plan of care for the person is aggressive/active, the dressing plan should be aggressive/active. For example, if a person has an exudating, infected diabetic foot ulcer with osteomyelitis that is being treated with hyperbaric oxygen therapy and serial debridements, a dressing, such as a silver alginate or a silver foam dressing, would be the dressing of choice.[10] On the other hand, if a person is dying and on hospice and the goal of care is to palliate an exudating, infected diabetic foot wound with osteomyelitis, then a topical antimicrobial, such as cadexomer iodine, povidone-iodine, or chlorhexidine or its derivatives (polyhexamethylene biguanide or PHMB), might be a congruent choice.

In clinical practice, occasions occur frequently when patients are too sick to choose an aggressive pathway for their wound care. A common scenario is when a patient is in critical condition in an intensive care unit, on a respirator, immobilized, and anticoagulated and his life hangs in the balance. The patient develops a sacral pressure ulcer that quickly goes from a partial-thickness lesion to a full-thickness wound with eschar. A holistic approach to wound care would lead to the maintenance pathway. Aggressive/active care in a critically ill patient would be unreasonable. Debridement of eschar in an anticoagulated patient with little healing potential is not a reasonable or prudent practice. A more reasonable option is to maintain the wound using a dressing that would protect the area and keep the eschar stable until the patient improves (at which point the aggressive/active pathway kicks in) or the patient deteriorates (at which point the palliative/nonhealable pathway is chosen).

Wound Assessment and Identification of Wound Dressing Requirements

Wound care requires a holistic approach, looking at the *whole patient* and not just the *hole in the patient*. The very first step of the assessment should aim to determine the accurate wound diagnosis and the cause of the wound. Despite the importance of dressings, wound healing can only be optimized when the underlying wound cause is corrected. For example, strategies to reduce tissue deformation (pressure, friction, and shear) are crucial to promote healing of pressure ulcers. Patients with venous leg ulcers benefit from venous congestion-improving compression therapies (bandages for healing or support stockings to prevent recurrence). Footwear or devices should be considered to redistribute pressure away from diabetic or other neurotrophic foot ulcers. It is important to remember that wounds are not likely to heal if arterial supply is deficient unless patients undergo bypass or dilation of the affected arteries. Other related factors that may influence wound healing and warrant regular evaluation include nutrition, coexisting medical diseases, and certain medications. When healing is not the realistic objective, moisture is contraindicated; instead, conservative debridement without cutting into living tissue, bacterial reduction, and moisture reduction should be considered.

The first step in wound care is to carefully document the wound characteristics:

- Location
- Size: Longest length and the widest width (at a right angle to the longest length or oriented by a head-to-foot perspective)
- Depth as usually measured by a cotton swab or sterile probe
- Undermining and tunneling: location on the clock and extent as measured by a probe
- Wound margin: normal, macerated, erythema, edema, warmth, or increased temperature
- Wound base: by percentage
  - Black-brown firm eschar
  - Brown-yellow soft slough (harmful)
  - Yellow firm tissue that may serve as a foundation for granulation (healthy)
  - Pink, firm, healthy granulation tissue or unhealthy red, friable tissue
  - Exudate:
    - Serous, sanguinous, or pustular or combinations
    - Large, moderate, scant, absent
  - Epithelial edge
  - Sloped purple of advancing, healing epithelial margin
  - Steep slope of stalled chronic wound
- Exposed tissues (tendon, bone) that may not allow granulation on top
- Foreign bodies (eg, gauze fragments, sutures, hardware).

To prepare a wound bed for healing, devitalized and damaged tissue, such as firm eschar, or sloughy materials that promote bacterial growth should be removed or debrided. Topical dressings are used to promote autolytic debridement through the activities of phagocytic cells and endogenous enzymes. Another key function of wound dressings is to manage localized wound infection. All chronic wounds are colonized by bacteria. If bacteria were allowed to proliferate, crossing a critical threshold, local tissue damage can lead to delayed healing. *Many modern dressings contain active antimicrobial ingredients* that are released into the wound surface compartment in an exchange with wound fluid. Dressings with silver are one of the most popular choices of topical agents. Alternatively, bacteria can be entrapped and sequestered in the micro-architecture of a dressing where they may be inactivated. For nonhealable wounds, topical antiseptics dry the wound surface and provide bacterial reduction.

For wounds that have the potential to heal, moisture balance (not too much or too little) is essential for all phases of wound repair. An ideal dressing should be able to keep the wound bed moist for cellular proliferation and migration but at the same time sequester excess drainage to avoid periwound damage.

The major categories of wound dressings are foams, alginates, hydrofibers, hydrogels, and hydrocolloids. These are discussed briefly below.

Foam dressings are designed to wick up a large volume of exudate. The fluid-handling capacity of various foams can be affected by the polyurethane film backing and its ability to transfer moisture vapor out of the dressing but form a barrier to bacterial contamination. Depending on the level of wound exudate, foams have a wear time of 1 to 7 days.

Foams absorb moisture but also give moisture back to a wound if the gradient on the surface becomes dehydrated. This function can lead to periwound maceration, but advanced foam dressings have variable pore sizes that will facilitate partial moisture retention and partial moisture exchange with the wound surface. These second generation foams are less likely to macerate the wound margin. Foams also have been combined with antiseptics (silver, PHMB) and other agents to serve as a delivery vehicle for active therapies at the wound surface (third generation of foam development). Foams that are associated with excessive periwound maceration can be cut to the wound size, fenestrated on the top to wick to a secondary dressing, or changed more frequently.

Alginate dressings are also capable of handling copious exudate, while the gelling effect of these materials will keep the wound base moist. Unlike foams, calcium alginates are bioresorbable (may disappear) and bind fluid to the outside of the fibers rather than the inner pores. Alginates are derived from brown seaweed or kelp. Depending on the species and origin of the calcium alginate (leaf, stem), they may have more gelling (high manuronic acid concentration) or a higher fiber strength (high galuronic acid concentration). These dressings are manufactured in sheets (lateral fluid wicking) or in ropes (vertical fluid wicking). When the alginate is extracted from kelp, it is a sodium hydrogel that can be combined with calcium to form a fibrous structure. When they are applied to the wound, the calcium as part of the alginate is released into the wound and may also trigger the coagulation cascade to facilitate hemostasis. The sodium is exchanged for calcium at the level of the alginate, recreating a sodium alginate hydrogel. In comparison to foams, calcium alginates are less absorptive, but they have

the ability to act as excellent autolytic debriders. Dressings with alginates are often changed daily or as infrequently as 3 times a week.

Hydrofiber dressings consist of carboxymethylcellulose and have a water-hating (hydrophobic) component (methylcellulose) that gives the dressing its tensile strength and a water-loving (hydrophilic) component (carboxy) that acts as a fluid lock. As the dressing absorbs fluid, the hydrofiber is converted into a gel consistency. Hydrofiber dressings are thin and have moderate absorbency, forming a fluid lock. When the hydrofiber is saturated, wound fluid strike-through will occur. These dressings require a secondary dressing to keep them in place because the addition of an adhesive will interfere with the fluid absorption properties of the dressing.

Hydrogel dressings are usually indicated for dry wounds. The major ingredient of hydrogels is water (70% to 90%), which donates moisture into the wound base. The backbone for a hydrogel may be a hydrocolloid, propylene glycol, saline, or other substance. This backbone gives them their viscosity or tack to stay on the wound bed. They are excellent autolytic debriders and preserve moisture balance, largely through donating moisture to the wound surface. They are often changed daily to 3 times a week.

Hydrocolloid dressings consist of a backing (often a film or polyurethane) with carboxymethylcellulose, water–absorptive components (such as gelatin and pectin), and an adhesive. Hydrocolloids are designed for wear times of 1 to 7 days, and for this reason, their absorbency is lower than foams or calcium alginates but similar to hydrogels. When these dressings are used for autolytic debridement, they may need to be changed more frequently and may require the removal of nonviable slough from the surface of the wound to prevent odor or secondary bacterial proliferation under the dressing. These dressings often lower the wound surface pH that may contribute to their antimicrobial effect. Some hydrocolloids leave more residue on the wound surface than others, and this residue may contribute to wound odor under the hydrocolloid dressing.

Film dressings are often used for local protection. The choice of a nonadherent (no adhesive) versus a film with adhesive backing should be determined by the fragility of the surrounding skin.

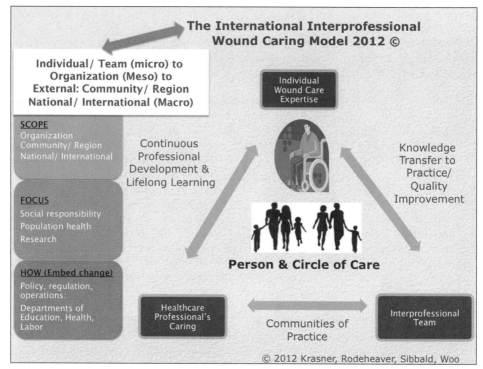

Figure 2. The International Interprofessional Wound Caring Model 2012.
© 2012 Krasner, Rodeheaver, Sibbald, and Woo.

Film materials are semi-occlusive with various degrees of permeability (referred to as the moisture vapor transmission rate or MVTR) that allow a water molecule to pass through the dressing and evaporate into the ambient environment at a variable rate, depending on the MVTR. They are not designed for fluid accumulation below the film. When fluid develops under the dressing, it needs to be evacuated or the dressing changed because the relatively alkaline pH under these dressings with fluid accumulation will promote bacterial proliferation. As an alternative to traditional adhesives (acrylates, hydrocolloids), silicone coatings have been used to reduce local trauma and prevent pain on dressing removal.

Interprofessional Considerations

When different professional groups are involved in a wound patient's care, there may be interprofessional considerations that will have bearing on the dressing selected. Finding a way to accommodate each discipline's unique per- spectives and needs enhances interprofessional wound care (Figure 2).[2] Here are several common examples:

- In an acute care facility, the surgical team wants to examine a dehisced surgical wound on daily rounds, so a dressing that is changed daily and can be lifted off and replaced without compromising the dressing adherence is the best choice (eg, silicone foam versus adhesive foam or gauze dressing).
- In any setting, the physicians need to measure the output from a draining tube site (eg, nephrostomy tube site). Discontinue absorbent gauze pads (eg, abdominal dressings or ABDs) and use cut-to-fit urostomy pouches to allow accurate measurement of the drainage and protect the periwound skin from maceration and erosion.
- In an outpatient wound center, the hyperbaricist needs to assess the wound daily following hyperbaric treatment. A nonadhesive, daily or between-treatment dressing change

CHRONIC WOUND CARE, 5th Edition

is needed (eg, hydrogel, hydrocolloid, or other modern moist interactive dressing).

- In a nursing home, the physical therapy department will begin rehabilitation therapy on a resident with a diabetic foot ulcer. A dressing that minimizes pressure on the wound bed when the resident ambulates is optimal (eg, a piece of alginate rope versus a gauze 2 x 2) with a thin but secure secondary dressing to avoid interfering with the plantar pressure redistribution.

Interprofessional collaboration on dressing selection can prevent complications (such as skin stripping or skin tears) from changing dressings too frequently, having inappropriate adhesive backing or inadequate moisture balance, or lacking required antimicrobial properties. Careful coordination reduces costs and dressing-associated labor.

Another occasion when careful dressing coordination is needed is during wound patient/client transfers from one healthcare setting or service to another, including a discharge home. For example, the optimal dressing for acute care may not be available or reimbursed in long-term care or home care. In the United States, if the person has been a resident in long-term care and is moved to hospice care, the hospice will provide the dressings for the resident while he or she is in the nursing home as part of the per diem hospice benefit. This may necessitate a change of dressing, depending on the hospice dressing formulary.

Finally, is your interprofessional team up to standards? Are you able to provide holistic, patient-centered care? Ask yourself the following 3 questions:

- Does your wound team have the resources (human and otherwise) and knowledge to provide advanced patient-centered wound care?
- Do you have the referral sources in place to meet the needs of selected wound patients (especially their psychosocial and social needs) along with rehabilitation support?
- Does your wound team and dressing formulary enable you to address the needs of special populations (such as bariatric, diabetic, frail elderly, and palliative) in a timely and appropriate manner?

Patient-Centered Concerns

Individualized wound care plans that address specific patient-centered concerns are most likely

European Pressure Ulcer Advisory Panel:
www.epuap.org

European Wound Management Association:
www.ewma.org

World Union of Wound Healing Societies:
www.wuwhs.org

World Wide Wounds:
www.worldwidewounds.org

WoundPedia:
www.woundpedia.com

WoundSource:
www.woundsource.com

Figure 3. Websites with dressing-related information.

to succeed and promote the best outcomes for the patient with a wound. Standardized, "canned" wound care plans often fail because they do not promote patient adherence/coherence. The patient may be labeled "noncompliant" when the real problem is that the care plan has not been properly individualized to the person's specific needs/problems and he or she cannot possibly comply with the routine way. The road to wound care planning success is paved with careful attention to patient-centered concerns, including pain management, odor control, body image and psychosocial concerns, and reimbursement/cost issues.

Common examples of patient-centered concerns that impact dressing product selection include:

- Premedicating patients who experience dressing change pain prior to dressing changes and allowing adequate time for the premedication to take effect
- Selecting, when appropriate, nonadherent dressings to reduce pain and trauma at dressing change
- Addressing odor control issues by utilizing absorbent and/or charcoal dressings and adjusting dressing change frequency
- When possible, selecting secondary dressings that enable patients to shower, bathe, and perform other usual activities of daily living
- Choosing dressings that are easy to apply and that address the needs of the person with a wound and his or her circle of care.

Whenever possible, order dressings that are reimbursed by the person's insurance and that are easily purchased/accessed.

Conclusion

When developing wound dressing product formularies and clinical practice guidelines, be sure to follow a formal process that includes a review of relevant existing clinical practice guidelines and regulatory requirements, such as those in the United States from the Centers for Medicare & Medicaid Services. For guidance on this process, readers are referred to *SELECT: Evaluation and Implementation of Clinical Practice Guidelines: A Guidance Document from the American Professional Wound Care Association*.[11]

Two excellent online wound dressing product resources are available to help build a dressing formulary by generic category: WoundSource (Kestrel Health Information, Inc.), www.woundsource.com/product-category/dressings, and World Wide Wounds (United Kingdom), www.worldwidewounds.com. Websites with dressing-related information are listed in Figure 3.

Practice Pearls

- Incorporating a wound dressing product selection conceptual model into your practice will assure that your product selection is holistic, interprofessional, and patient-centered.
- Individualized wound care plans that address specific patient-centered concerns are more likely to succeed and promote the best outcomes for the patient with a wound.
- Web-based resources for dressing information help you keep updated and evidence-based.

Self-Assessment Questions

1. Which of the following issues is NOT a patient-centered concern?
   A. Pain at dressing change
   B. Odor
   C. Difficult dressing for the staff and caregivers to apply
   D. Color of dressing calls attention to the fact that the person has a wound

2. Common wound dressing performance parameters that can have a significant impact on a dressing's applicability for a particular wound and a specific patient include all of the following EXCEPT:
   A. Ability to handle exudate
   B. Adhesive with low tack
   C. Packaged in boxes of 10
   D. Daily dressing changes are not required

Answers: 1–C, 2–C

References

1. Sibbald RG, Krasner DL, Lutz JB, et al. The SCALE Expert Panel: Skin Changes at Life's End. Final Consensus Document. October 1, 2009. Downloadable at www.gaymar.com.
2. Krasner DL, Rodeheaver GT, Sibbald RG. Interprofessional wound caring. In: Krasner DL, Rodeheaver GT, Sibbald RG, eds. *Chronic Wound Care: A Clinical Source Book for Healthcare Professionals*. 4th ed. Malvern, PA: HMP Communications; 2007:3–9. www.chronicwoundcarebook.com
3. Osterberg L, Blaschke T. Adherence to medication. *N Engl J Med*. 2005;353:487–497.
4. Sackett DL, Straus SE, Richardson WS, Rosenberg W, Haynes RB. *Evidence-based Medicine: How to Practice and Teach EBM*. 2nd ed. Edinburgh, Scotland: Churchhill Livingston; 2000.
5. Cockbill SME, Turner TD. The development of wound management products. In: Krasner DL, Rodeheaver GT, Sibbald RG, eds. *Chronic Wound Care: A Clinical Source Book for Healthcare Professionals*. 4th ed. Malvern, PA: HMP Communications; 2007:233–248. www.chronicwoundcarebook.com
6. Ayello EA, Capitulo KL, Fife CE, et al. Legal issues in the care of pressure ulcer patients: Key concepts for healthcare providers. A consensus paper from the International Expert Wound Care Advisory Panel. June 22, 2009. Downloadable at www.medline.com.
7. Ferris FD, Al Khateib AA, Fromantin I, et al. Palliative wound care: managing chronic wounds across life's continuum: a consensus statement from the International Palliative Wound Care Initiative. *J Palliat Med*. 2007;10:37–39.
8. Sibbald RG, Woo K, Ayello EA. Increased bacterial burden and infection: the story of NERDS and STONES. *Adv Skin Wound Care*. 2006;19:447–461.
9. Woo KY, Sibbald RG. A cross-sectional validation study using NERDS and STONEES to assess bacterial burden. *Ostomy Wound Manage*. 2009;55:40–48.
10. Krasner DL, Sibbald RG. Dressings and local wound care for people with diabetic foot wounds. In: Armstrong DG, Lavery LA, eds. *Clinical Care of the Diabetic Foot*. 2nd ed. Alexandria, VA: American Diabetes Association; 2010:69–78.
11. SELECT: Evaluation and Implementation of Clinical Practice Guidelines. A Guidance Document from the American Professional Wound Care Association (APWCA). 2009. Downloadable at www.apwca.org.

Interprofessional Perspectives on Individualized Wound Device Product Selection©

Diane L. Krasner, PhD, RN, CWCN, CWS, MAPWCA, FAAN;
R. Gary Sibbald, BSc, MD, FRCPC(Med, Derm), MACP, FAAD, MEd, MAPWCA;
Kevin Y. Woo, PhD, RN, FAPWCA; **Linda Norton**, OT Reg(ONT), MScCH

Objectives

The reader will be challenged to:
- Articulate the benefits of interprofessional collaboration to optimize device product selection
- Identify important clinical considerations for compression therapy devices, off-weighting devices, electrical stimulation, ultrasound, hyperbaric oxygen therapy, negative pressure wound therapy, and pressure redistribution surfaces
- Appreciate the complexities of implementing interprofessional individualized selection in clinical practice.

Introduction

Like many aspects of wound care, wound device product selection has become an increasingly complex and sophisticated process over the past several decades. Not only are more products available, but the challenge of matching the appropriate device for a specific patient's profile has become a rising expectation. From pressure redistribution surfaces to negative pressure wound therapy, the process of device selection requires careful interprofessional consideration of the individual's wound as well as his or her holistic, biopsychosocial needs and the setting/environment/ access (Figure 1).[1] By utilizing interprofessional collaboration, healthcare teams can "propose" solution(s) that would have been unattainable through single disciplinary means.[2]

The following general categories of wound care-related devices will be reflected in this chapter. Specific category and/or product information can be found at www.woundsource.com.

- Compression therapy devices
- Off-weighting devices (also known as off-loading devices)
- Adjunctive therapies, such as electrical stimulation, ultrasound, and hyperbaric oxygen therapy (HBOT)
- Negative pressure wound therapy (NPWT)
- Pressure redistribution surfaces (also known as specialty beds and support surfaces).

These devices cover a wide range of products: some are prescription; some are over-the-counter (OTC). Many are regulated or classified by the Food & Drug Administration

Reprinted from Krasner DL, Sibbald RG, Woo KY, Norton L. Interprofessional perspectives on individualized wound device product selection©. *WoundSource: The Kestrel Wound Product Sourcebook*. November 2011. Available at: http://www.woundsource.com/ wound-device-white-paper#. © 2011 Kestrel Health Information, Inc. Used with permission.

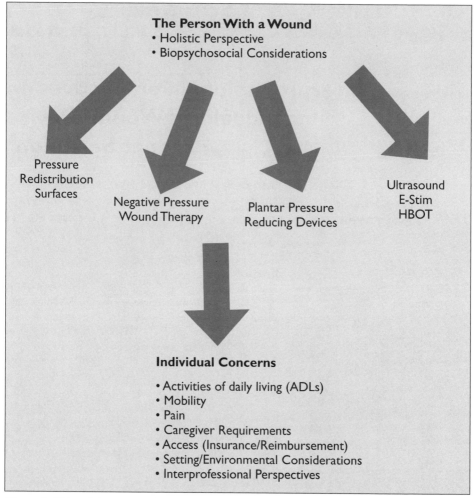

The Person With a Wound
- Holistic Perspective
- Biopsychosocial Considerations

Pressure
Redistribution
Surfaces

Negative Pressure
Wound Therapy

Plantar Pressure
Reducing Devices

Ultrasound
E-Stim
HBOT

Individual Concerns

- Activities of daily living (ADLs)
- Mobility
- Pain
- Caregiver Requirements
- Access (Insurance/Reimbursement)
- Setting/Environmental Considerations
- Interprofessional Perspectives

Figure 1. Wound device considerations for the person with a wound. © 2011 Krasner, Sibbald, Woo, and Norton.

(FDA) in the United States or a comparable agency in other countries. In the United States, the Centers for Medicare & Medicaid Services (CMS) may or may not reimburse for devices based on specific policies and criteria (eg, Group 1, 2, and 3 support surface criteria; hyperbaric oxygen therapy coverage policies). Individual medical necessity, if it can be demonstrated by the prescriber, may enable an individual to obtain a reimbursed device under circumstances that usually would not be covered.

Wound care devices may or may not have indications, contraindications, or precautions — just like medications. These are particularly important for such wound devices as NPWT and HBOT. The prescriber (physician or his or her designee, eg, physician's assistant, nurse practitioner) is responsible for knowing the indications, contraindications, and precautions and ascertaining whether a specific device is appropriate for an individual patient. Failure to do so can result in serious adverse outcomes with legal consequences.

Wound Device Product Usage Issues

In addition to labeled product usage guidelines from the manufacturer, facilities often have their own *policies and procedures* or *protocols* for using

232

National Pressure Ulcer Advisory Panel (NPUAP) Support Surface Standards Initiative: Terms and Definitions Version 01/29/2007 http://www.npuap.org/NPUAP_S3I_TD.pdf	
Cochrane Review on Support Surfaces McInnes E, Bell-Syer SE, Dumville JC, Legood R, Cullum NA Support Surfaces for Pressure Ulcer Prevention. Cochrane Database Sept Rev. 2008; 4:CD001735	
Websites with Device-Related Information	
European Pressure Ulcer Advisory Panel	www.epuap.org
European Wound Management Association	www.ewma.org
World Union of Wound Healing Societies	www.wuwhs.org
World Wide Wounds	www.worldwidewounds.org
WoundPedia	www.woundpedia.org
WoundSource	www.woundsource.com

Figure 2. National and international device-related guidelines, resources, and websites.

devices. It is important that such documents be updated on a regular basis; be updated whenever the manufacturer updates its *guidelines* for product use; and reflect national and international best practices and guidelines (Figure 2).[3] All prescribers must be aware of such documents. Legal advisors suggest the facilities should call such documents guidelines instead of policies and procedures or protocols to reflect the need to individualize them for each patient and to reduce legal exposure.[4] All prescribing healthcare professionals should be trained in the use of the device they are prescribing, and if certification courses are available from the manufacturer, having prescribers certified is highly recommended by legal counsel and risk managers. Other process issues with legal ramifications related to device usage include:

• Appropriate orders by appropriate prescribers
• Timely device initiation and discontinuation
• Documentation of device efficacy
• Patient/caregiver education regarding device use, troubleshooting, and who to contact in case of emergency
• Seamless transitioning across the continuum of care.

Devices are frequently rented through a vendor or other external source. These relationships should be acknowledged by written contracts or agreements that specify vendor and facility responsibilities. Issues to consider include:

• Timely delivery and pickup
• Support for problems/device malfunction
• For devices that are purchased and owned by the facility, the process for annual inspection by the manufacturer or in-house bioengineering.

The "lens" through which wound device product selection is viewed, is — in part — a function of our professional training, considerations, and vantage points. Three international thought leaders in wound care will now present their perspectives from the physician, nurse, and therapist perspectives.

The Physician's Perspective on Individualized Wound Device Product Selection

Compression and venous stasis ulcers. In the *wound bed preparation paradigm*,[5] members of the interprofessional wound care team need to treat the cause and address patient-centered con-

Type of System Pattern of Pressure	Elastic	Non-elastic
	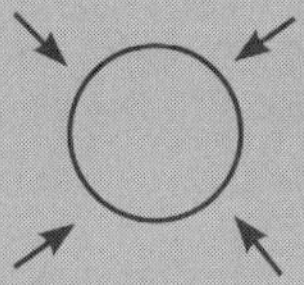 (circle diagram, arrows inward)	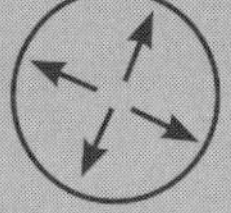 (circle diagram, arrows outward)
Rest	High Pressure	Low Pressure
Muscle Contraction	High Pressure but less	High Pressure
Low	Single Layer Elastic bandages	Unna Boot
High	Long stretch 4 layer	Short stretch Modified Unna Boot (Duke Boot)

Figure 3. Non-elastic systems have low pressure at rest. © 2007 Sibbald.

cerns before considering the components of local wound care. In the case of venous ulcers, clinicians must rule out arterial disease with an ABPI (ankle brachial pressure index). If the ABPI (ankle systolic pressure over brachial systolic pressure expressed as a ratio) is between 0.8 and 1.2, persons with venous leg ulcers should receive compression bandages for healing and stockings to prevent recurrences post-healing. The Cochrane Review on compression therapy[6] evidence base has concluded:

- Compression increases ulcer healing rates compared with no compression
- Multicomponent systems are more effective than single-component systems
- Multicomponent systems containing an elastic bandage appear more effective than those composed mainly of inelastic constituents.

There are several multilayered elastic and inelastic systems available that deliver high compression.[7] Two elastic systems are the 4-layer bandage systems and long-stretch bandages. For high-compression systems that are inelastic, there is the zinc oxide paste boot (Unna boot) that can be made more rigid with an outer layer of a flexible cohesive bandage (Coban™ over zinc oxide paste bandage = Duke boot) or the Coban™ 2-layer bandage. After healing, it is recommended that patients with venous disease are transitioned into the appropriate compression stockings to help prevent recurrence.

That pain is much more common with venous disease has been discussed by Krasner[8] and the World Union of Wound Healing Societies consensus statements on pain.[9,10] A patient with pain due to venous edema prior to the application of compression therapy may tolerate an inelastic support system and move up to an elastic system as the pain and edema are controlled. As illustrated in Figure 3,[7] non-elastic systems have low pressure at rest (less squeezing) and may increase patient adherence until edema and pain control have been optimized. If appropriate, an elastic system can then be introduced. Individuals with mixed venous and arterial disease but who have an ABPI between 0.65 and 0.80 should modify their compression therapy with modified product kits delivering lower compression (eg, Profore lite™, Coban 2 lite™).

Plantar pressure redistribution for diabetic and other neuropathic and neuroischemic foot ulcers. Persons with loss of protective sensation are unaware of trauma or injury to the foot. These individuals often develop plantar calluses (increased pressure) and blisters (friction or shear) with the foot sliding or moving in relation to their footwear. These individuals have 3 important components[11,12] to address before considering sharp surgical debridement of the callus. Using the mnemonic **VIP**, they are:

V — Vascular supply. Must be adequate to heal: Palpable pulse or, when the pulse is not palpable, a biphasic or triphasic Doppler signal, toe pressure over 55, or transcutaneous oxygen saturation over 30 mmHg.

I — Infection. There should be no signs of increased surface bacterial burden (any 3 signs from the **NERDS** mnemonic: Non-healing, ↑Exudate, Red friable granulation, Debris on the wound surface or Smell = use a topical antimicrobial) or deep and surrounding tissue infection (any 3 of the **STONEES** mnemonic: ↑Size, ↑Temperature, Os [Latin for bone exposed or probes], New areas of breakdown, Erythema or Edema = cellulitis, or ↑Exudate, Smell = use a systemic antimicrobial). If increased exudate and smell are present, an additional NERDS criteria is needed for a topical antimicrobial or an additional STONEES criteria for systemic antimicrobials or both.[13,14]

P — Plantar pressure redistribution. The gold standard is the contact cast that the patient cannot remove and will download the forefoot where 80% of neuropathic ulcers are usually located. Removable cast walkers (eg, air cast or CROW walker) can be made non-removable by securing them with a fiberglass, flexible cohesive or zinc oxide bandage to increase adherence to treatment. Less expensive alternatives include the half shoe (absent forefoot for forefoot ulcers and absent heel for heel area ulcers) that comprises 10%–15% of neuropathic ulcers. Many of these devices will have a rocker bottom surface. Other custom orthotics and footwear may be ordered in selected cases.[15]

It is also important after the healing of a foot ulcer to order the correct orthopedic deep-toed shoes and orthotics.

The last two treatments in this section are reserved for individuals with chronic wounds that have the cause corrected or compensated and there is adequate blood supply to heal. In addition, local wound care should be optimized: adequate debridement, infection and persistent abnormal inflammation controlled, and moisture balance optimized and still a healable wound is stalled. There are certain indications where acute wounds may have evidence for hyperbaric oxygen therapy and NPWT at an earlier stage.

Hyperbaric oxygen. HBOT is the administration of 100% oxygen at airtight pressures greater than 1 atmosphere absolute (ATA). Adequate tissue oxygen tension is essential to wound healing. Diminished circulation and hypoxia increase lactate production that is deleterious to wound healing. HBOT sessions usually entail approximately 45 to 120 minutes in the chamber once or twice daily for 20–30 sessions. In-vivo studies have shown that elevated arterial oxygen tensions can increase regulation of growth factors, decrease regulation of inflammatory cytokines, promote angiogenesis, and exert antibacterial effects in wounds.

Hyperbaric oxygen is often beneficial with overwhelming infection as long as there is enough blood supply to heal and maintain the healing response. Pooled data from 6 randomized controlled trials on diabetic foot ulcers suggested a significant reduction in the risk of major amputation with HBOT,[16] but there was no significant change in wound size reduction and number of healed wounds.

High doses of oxygen are toxic, particularly to the brain and lungs. Other potential drawbacks of HBOT include damage to the ears and sinuses, time and direct cost associated with daily travel to and from the treatment center, and the psychological effect of confinement.

Negative pressure wound therapy. NPWT is the delivery of intermittent or continuous sub-atmospheric pressure to the wound bed.[17] There have been many interface surfaces between the wound and the NPWT suction device, including gauze or open-celled foam composed of either polyurethane or polyvinyl alcohol that is cut and placed onto the surface of the wound. The foam is then sealed over with a transparent drape to create a closed airtight system. Contraction of the foam dressing exerts a centripetal effect at the wound edges and a mechanical force at the interface of the foam and wound. The suction effect and mechanical stress are transmitted to cellular and cytoskeletal levels, causing deformation of extracellular matrix (ECM) and cells that is postulated to promote cellular proliferation. Other potential advantages of NPWT are:

- Removal of excess interstitial fluid to reduce the intercellular diffusion distance
- Improvement of local wound blood flow

- Potential reduction of bacterial colonization
- Sequestration of excess matrix metallopro-teinases (MMPs) and pro-inflammatory/ab-normal wound exudate.[18]

Armstrong conducted a multicenter, random-ized, controlled trial (N = 162) to examine the effect of NPWT in complex wounds after partial foot amputation to the trans-metatarsal level in patients with diabetes.[19] Fifty-six percent of the patients healed in the NPWT group compared to 39% of the control group (*P* = .04). Investigations pertaining to the management of acute post-surgical wounds using NPWT also demonstrated positive results.[20,21] Many wound care experts uti-lize NPWT after acute surgical procedures, es-pecially when secondary infection is present (eg, dehiscence of post-sternotomy wounds).

The Ontario Health Technology Advisory Committee performed a systematic review on NPWT[22] in 2010 and concluded:

- NPWT is an effective option in the manage-ment of diabetic foot ulcers
- NPWT is an appropriate option for use following skin grafting of medium-sized (around 30 cm^2) vascular ulcers and burns
- To optimize patient outcomes and safety, ap-propriate guidelines should be adhered to in the application of this technology.

In conclusion, devices are important to facili-tate the treatment of the cause of chronic wounds (compression for venous stasis and plantar pres-sure redistribution for neurotrophic foot ulcers). Other devices (HBOT, NPWT) optimize local wound care for stalled chronic but also healable wounds as well as selected indications in acute wounds.

The Nurse's Perspective on Individualized Wound Device Product Selection

Pressure ulcers are a significant problem across the continuum of healthcare settings. The overall prevalence was 12.3% (N = 92,408) in 2009 ac-cording to a national survey in the United States.[23] The burden of pressure ulcers is significant with the average cost associated with the treatment of deep pressure ulcers and related complica-tions being US $129,248 in acute care. People with pressure ulcers are beset by limited mobil-ity, social isolation, depression, and persistent pain.

In reviews of 53 studies, support surfaces (eg, medical grade sheepskin, high-specification foam mattresses) have been recognized to reduce the incidence of pressure ulcers. Appropriate surfaces or mattresses facilitate pressure redistribution, re-move pressure from injury-prone areas (especially bony prominences), and spread weight evenly to avoid pressure buildup. Foam, gel/water-filled, and low-air-loss mattresses are commonly used. They are considered *reactive* because the effect of pressure redistribution is based on the surface area that the body is in contact with the mattress; the larger the area of the body that is supported by the mattress, the lower the pressure at any given point of contact.

The majority of specialty surfaces are expen-sive, but taking into account the number of ul-cers that can be prevented, the calculated cost of using therapeutic surfaces and other preventative measures is approximately 40 times less than the standard care approach.[24] Amid the wide variety of options, clinicians should understand how to make the selection of the right mattress/surface for the right person (who), the right clinical indication/circumstances (when), the right length of time (how long), and the right health outcomes (what to expect). Remember, there are 5 rights for the use of therapeutic surfaces. The mnemonic *MAT-TRESSES* (Table 1) highlights 10 key factors that should be considered prior to using a support sur-face to ensure cost-effective use of resources to prevent pressure ulcers.

M — Microclimate and moisture. Increasing attention is drawn to the role of microclimate in pressure ulcer care. Microclimate refers to the en-vironment at or near the skin surface that is influ-enced by the combined effect of skin temperature, humidity/moisture, and air movement. An increase of 1°C in skin temperature results in an approxi-mately 13% increase in tissue oxygen demand, making the skin more vulnerable to mechanical damage. Excess moisture from incontinence, sweat-ing, and wound exudation can cause skin macera-tion, weakening the connections between epider-mal cells and collagen fibers. The interruption of normal barrier function increases skin permeability to irritants and pressure damages. Certainly, heat and moisture accumulation is directly related to air movement at the interface between the skin and the supporting surface. Some of the foam mattresses

Table 1. MATTRESSES

	Indication	Rationale
M	Microclimate and moisture	Low air loss for moisture problems (eg, sweating) and heat accumulation
A	Activity levels	Certain surfaces may hinder mobility in bed and patient's ability to get out of bed
T	Tissue tolerance	Tolerance to pressure and other mechanical forces is determined by local perfusion and oxygen delivery
T	Total body weight	People with extreme body mass indices (BMIs, high or low) are more susceptible to pressure damage
R	Repositioning needs	Lack repositioning surface or difficulty with repositioning
E	Edema	Alternating pressure or pulsating surfaces may reduce edema and promote circulation
S	Shear and friction	Surfaces that conform to the body may prevent sliding and associated shear damage to the tissue
S	Symptom management	Pain, shortness of breath, fatigue, and other associated symptoms
E	Existing pressure ulcer(s)	Existing pressure ulcers indicate that the person is at risk for further skin breakdown
S	Sites	Heels are more prone to pressure ulcers; heels should be managed independently of the support surface

have poor heat properties and tend to "hug" the body, limiting airflow. In contrast, low-air-loss or air-fluidized beds (with vapor-permeable covers) promote air circulation that cools the skin through convection and evaporation of moisture from the skin. This type of mattress may be beneficial for patients with severe burns. Other simple measures to control the microclimate include reducing the layers of pads underneath the patient as well as using incontinent briefs, covering, and clothing that is breathable (avoid plastic). It is important to monitor the skin hydration status to avoid excessive dryness that can also cause skin breakdown.

A — Activity level. Accumulating evidence suggests that people with restricted physical activities and mobility are at risk for pressure ulcers. Norton and colleagues have recently proposed[25] that activity levels should be considered when selecting a supporting surface. To optimize activities, clinicians must be aware of the potential of certain therapeutic support surfaces (ie, foam, gel-filled, and air-fluidized mattresses) that tend to mold around body contours (envelopment) and allow the body to sink into the surface (immersion), compromising the patient's ability to get in and out of bed and his or her independence.

T — Tissue tolerance. Skin breakdown is inevitable when metabolic demand outstrips the supply of oxygen and vital nutrients. The extent and severity of tissue injury is, however, dependent on a number of intrinsic factors that predispose individuals to the development of pressure ulcers. Some of these key factors are poor nutritional intake, low BMI (BMI < 18.5), hypoproteinemia, low systolic blood pressure, anemia, contractures and prominent bony prominences, vascular disease, neuropathy, and uncontrolled diabetes. Because many of these factors are not addressed by pressure ulcer risk instruments, selection of support surfaces should be individualized, taking assessment of tissue tolerance to injury into consideration.

T — Total body weight. Pressure and other mechanical forces compress, stretch, and distort the normal alignment of the soft tissue, leading to potential injury. The impact of mechanical distortion of the tissue is more pronounced in patients who are emaciated. In one study, the maximum shear force at the coccyx was higher ($P < .01$) in slender than obese individuals when the head of the bed was raised from the supine position.[26] On the other extreme of the body weight spectrum, bariatric patients are also at high risk for pressure ulcer development due to a substantial stress that is put on the skin. Patients with either high or low BMI should be carefully evaluated for a support surface to prevent skin breakdown.

R — Repositioning challenges. While frequent repositioning is deemed essential to manage pressure, it is not always feasible in critically ill patients, as positioning may precipitate vascular collapse or exacerbate shortness of breath (eg, advanced heart failure). A therapeutic surface is recommended for patients who cannot tolerate frequent repositioning or the head of the bed less than 30 degrees (due to dyspnea or to prevent aspiration during enteral feeding). The turning frequency can be reduced by the use of redistributing support surfaces; however, prolonged exposure to low pressure can be equally damaging to tissue. Clinicians must not forget the need for repositioning despite the type of mattresses or specialty surfaces being utilized.

E — Edema. Edema, which stretches the skin and impairs the delivery of oxygen, is considered a risk factor for skin breakdown. By alternating air pressures in compartments of the mattress under the torso and leg that emulates the body's natural intermittent movements, it is hypothesized that the massage movements may reduce edema by improving capillary blood flow and oxygenation to the wound and skin. Further research evidence is needed to substantiate the physiological impact of alternating mattresses. Despite the potential benefits, alternating air mattresses may not be suitable for individuals with spinal instability, motion sickness, protracted pain, and nausea. Individualized assessment is warranted.

S — Shear and friction. Development of pressure ulcers is a dynamic and complex process that involves the combined effect of mechanical forces including shear and friction in addition to pressure. Pressure is defined as the perpendicular force that is applied to the skin, distorting and compressing underlying soft tissues, especially over bony prominences.[27] Shear or shear stress is produced by displacement or deformation of tissue (usually in a diagonal direction), altering the original alignment of tissue as one layer of tissue slides over the deeper structure in opposite directions (bony skeleton moving in an opposite direction to the surface skin). Deformation disrupts the cell structure, obstructs lymphatic drainage, reduces blood flow, and potentiates ischemia.

In contrast, friction describes the resistance to movement created between 2 surfaces, such as the superficial layers of skin and the adjoining support surface. By simply instituting measures to reduce friction, up to 16% of pressure ulcers can be prevented.[28]

S — Symptom management. A support surface is often considered for palliative patients to promote comfort. The primary purpose may not be focused on pressure ulcer prevention but to ensure comfort at the end of life.

E — Existing pressure ulcer(s). Patients with existing pressure ulcers are usually at risk for developing further skin breakdown. For patients who have multiple ulcers, a support surface should be considered due to the lack of appropriate turning surfaces.

S — Sites. One of the areas that is most vulnerable to pressure-related skin damage is the heel. The heel has a pointed shape with a limited surface area of contact to redistribute pressure, and when this is combined with the low subcutaneous tissue volume, this area is prone to pressure damage. Heel tissue is enveloped within the fibrous septa that allow pressure to build up easily and occlude vascular supply. Boots with the heel area cut out to allow the heel to be completely lifted off the surface are useful to prevent and treat pressure ulcers. Many different heel boots and positioning devices are available;

however, no one device works best in all circumstances. Special attention must be paid to potential damage to the lower leg areas where the pressure is redistributed.

The Therapist's Perspective on Individualized Wound Device Product Selection

Reflecting back to the wound bed preparation paradigm,[5] allied health professionals can be especially helpful to manage the cause of wounds while addressing patient-centered concerns. Regardless of the type of wound, until the cause has been addressed, the wound will not progress to closure. The challenge, though, is to address the cause in a way that can be incorporated into the individual's lifestyle. Evidence-based practice is the integration of the best research evidence with clinical expertise and patient values.[29] This approach is helpful when considering the prescription of devices to prevent or manage wounds, as the best device is not helpful if the patient does not use it or the care providers do not know how to use or maintain the device.

When interpreting the evidence, clinical expertise is required, as many of the studies have small sample sizes, are completed by the manufacturer, and, in the case of support surfaces, compare therapeutic support surfaces to standard hospital mattresses (ie, foam and coil).[30] These studies also usually only consider an indirect measure (such as interface pressure) rather than an outcome measure (eg, wound prevention or wound closure).[30] In addition, they do not address the impact on the individual's lifestyle or his or her safety. For example, when considering support surfaces in bed, healthcare providers must consider the risk of entrapment. Health Canada[31,32] and the FDA have released documents defining the 7 zones of entrapment and guidance measurements:

1. Within the bed rail
2. Under the rail
3. Between the rail and the mattress
4. Under the rail at rail ends
5. Between split bed rails
6. Between the end of the rail and the side edge of the head or footboard
7. Between the head or footboard and the mattress end.

Prescription of a therapeutic support surface,

whether an overlay or mattress replacement, may impact several of these zones (eg, zone 2, 3, and 7). A standard measuring device is available to check to see if the new support surface increases the risk of entrapment by allowing spaces greater than those outlined in the guideline. The risk of entrapment also may be greater with support surfaces with large air bladders (these are usually found on low-air-loss, alternating, or rotating surfaces). These surfaces tend to collapse the further the individual moves to the edge[33] of the surface, even when a perimeter border is present within the mattress.

When an entrapment risk has been identified, bed rails should only be used with extreme caution and be based on the needs of the individual patient. Some patients find the half bed rail at the head section helpful for repositioning. Another approach for people at high risk is to use an adjustable bed with a very low deck height and a floor mat. This approach allows the bed to be raised to a comfortable height for care providers during care but allows the bed to be low enough to help prevent injury if the person falls out of bed. Foam wedges and other devices are also available to help reduce the risk of entrapment.

In terms of pressure ulcer prevention and management, there is evidence that the use of a pressure management cushion reduces the risk of pressure ulcers and extends the number of pressure ulcer-free days for those who do eventually develop pressure ulcers.[34] It has been demonstrated that higher peak pressures under the ischial tuberosities have been associated with increased pressure ulcer development.[35] One way to evaluate pressure is through use of a pressure-mapping device. This device helps the clinician visualize the interface pressure between the individual and the surface upon which he or she sits. Pressure maps must be interpreted with caution, however, as this technology does not measure shear or consider other factors relevant to the prescription of a seat cushion. Other factors to consider include comfort, postural stability, balance, cost, weight capacity, and maintenance.

When considering an evidence-based approach, the individual's perspectives and values play a pivotal role. The literature suggests that anywhere ***between 30% and 70% of devices pre-***

scribed are abandoned by the user.[36] The main reasons for abandonment include:[36]

- Device did not provide the type or extent of assistance required
- Draws unwanted attention to the user
- Individual does not perceive he or she needs the device
- Fit between the individual's environment and the device
- User does not feel his or her opinions were considered
- Training not provided.

In addition, the impact of the device on the person's independence also influences its use. For example, compression stockings are usually prescribed for people with venous insufficiency. Once a venous leg ulcer has closed, however, these stockings can be difficult for people to don and duff independently. Many devices have been designed to assist with this process, however, for people with arthritis or issues with mobility, even when these devices do not foster independence. Many individuals do not want to be dependent on others, as this may increase caregiver burden.

To summarize, an evidence-based approach should be taken in the selection and prescription of equipment to prevent and manage wounds. As the specific devices are often changing, the studies are often conducted by the manufacturers, and the sample sizes are small, studies need to be interpreted with caution. Reviews, such as the **Cochrane Review** on Support Surfaces,[37] and clinical practice guidelines, such as the **Registered Nurses' Association of Ontario** Best Practice Guideline for the Prevention of Pressure Ulcers[38] or the **European Pressure Ulcer Advisory Panel** and **National Pressure Ulcer Advisory Panel** guidelines,[39] may be more helpful for clinicians. Clinical judgment enables the healthcare provider to evaluate new products in relationship to the known evidence and the needs of their individual patients. Patients need education regarding the impact of the device and its use. The patient's perspective needs to be identified and integrated into the plan of care, as the best device is the one the individual will use.

Conclusion

This chapter illustrates how by blending the vantage points from different disciplines, a stronger plan of care can be developed for the person with a wound or at risk for developing one. An interprofessional team approach to wound care enhances patient outcomes. When wound device product selection is viewed through multiple professional lenses, patient-centered care is optimized.

Practice Pearls

- The challenge of matching the appropriate device for a specific patient's profile has become a rising expectation.
- Wound care devices may or may not have indications, contraindications, or precautions — just like medications.
- Evidence-based practice is the integration of the best research evidence with clinical expertise and patient values.[29] This approach is helpful when considering the prescription of devices to prevent or manage wounds, as the best device is not helpful if the patient does not use it or the care providers do not know how to use or maintain it.

Self-Assessment Questions

1. Effective use of devices involves all of the following EXCEPT:
   A. Appropriate orders by appropriate prescribers
   B. Discontinuing all devices prior to transitioning a person from one care setting to another
   C. Documentation of device efficacy
   D. Patient/caregiver education regarding device use, troubleshooting, and who to contact in case of emergency

2. Factors that negatively influence adherence to wound device use include:
   A. The device draws unwanted attention to the user
   B. Training was not provided
   C. The individual does not perceive that he or she needs the device
   D. All of the above

Answers: 1–B, 2–D

References

1. Krasner DL, Rodeheaver GT, Sibbald RG. Interprofessional wound caring. In: Krasner DL, Rodeheaver GT, Sibbald RG, eds. *Chronic Wound Care: A Clinical Source Book for Healthcare Professionals.* 4th ed. Malvern, PA: HMP Communications; 2007:3–9. www.chronicwoundcarebook.com

2. Miller M, Boix-Mansilla V. Thinking across perspectives and disciplines. Harvard Graduate School of Education, Interdisciplinary Studies Project; Project Zero, 2004.

3. Norton L, Coutts P, Sibbald RG. Beds: practical pressure management for surfaces/mattresses. *Adv Skin Wound Care.* 2011;24(7):324–332.

4. Fife CE, Yankowsky KW, Ayello EA, et al. Legal issues in the care of pressure ulcer patients: key concepts for healthcare providers — a consensus paper from the International Expert Wound Care Advisory Panel. *Adv Skin Wound Care.* 2010;23(11):493–507.

5. Sibbald RG, Goodman L, Woo KY, et al. Special considerations in wound bed preparation 2011: an update©. *Adv Skin Wound Care.* 2011;24(9):415–436.

6. O'Meara S, Cullum NA, Nelson EA. Compression for venous leg ulcers. *Cochrane Database Syst Rev.* 2009;(1):CD000265.

7. Sibbald RG, Alavi A, Norton L, Browne AC, Coutts P. Compression therapies. In: Krasner DL, Rodeheaver GT, Sibbald RG, eds. *Chronic Wound Care: A Clinical Source Book for Healthcare Professionals.* 4th ed. Malvern, PA: HMP Communications; 2007:481–488. www.chronicwoundcarebook.com

8. Krasner DL, Papen J, Sibbald RG. Helping patients out of the SWAMP: Skin and Wound Assessment and Management of Pain. In: Krasner DL, Rodeheaver GT, Sibbald RG, eds. *Chronic Wound Care: A Clinical Source Book for Healthcare Professionals.* 4th ed. Malvern, PA: HMP Communications; 2007:85–97. www.chronicwoundcarebook.com

9. Woo KY, Sibbald RG, Fogh K, et al. Assessment and management of persistent (chronic) and total wound pain. *Int Wound J.* 2008;5(2):205–215.

10. Principles of best practice: Minimising pain at wound dressing-related procedures. A consensus document. Toronto, Ontario, Canada: © WoundPedia Inc 2007.

11. Orsted HL, Searles G, Trowell H, Shapera L, Miller P, Rahman J. Best practice recommendations for the prevention, diagnosis and treatment of diabetic foot ulcers: update 2006. *Wound Care Canada* Reprinted. 2006;4(1):R39–R51.

12. Botros M, Goettl K, Parsons P, et al. Best practice recommendations for the prevention, diagnosis and treatment of diabetic foot ulcers: update 2010. *Wound Care Canada.* 4(1):R39–R51.

13. Sibbald RG, Woo K, Ayello EA. Increased bacterial burden and infection: the story of the NERDS and STONE. *Adv Skin Wound Care.* 2006;19:447–461.

14. Woo K, Sibbald RG. A cross-sectional validation study of using NERDS and STONEES to assess bacterial burden. *Ostomy Wound Manage.* 2009;55(8):40–61.

15. Woo KY, Ayello EA, Sibbald RG. The edge effect: current therapeutic options to advance the wound edge. *Adv Skin Wound Care.* 2007;20(2):99–117.

16. Kranke P, Bennett MH, Debus SE, Roeckl-Wiedmann I, Schnabel A. Hyperbaric oxygen therapy for chronic wounds. *Cochrane Database Syst Rev.* 2004;(2):CD004123.

17. World Union of Wound Healing Societies (WUWHS). *Principles of Best Practice: Vacuum Assisted Closure: Recommendations for Use.* A consensus document. London: MEP Ltd, 2008.

18. Buttenschoen K, Fleischmann W, Haupt U, Kinzl L, Buttenschoen DC. The influence of vacuum assisted closure on inflammatory tissue reactions in the postoperative curse of ankle fractures. *Foot Ankle Surg.* 2001;7:165–173.

19. Armstrong DG, Lavery LA, pour le Diabetic Foot Consortium. Negative pressure wound therapy after partial diabetic foot amputation: a multicentre, a randomised controlled trial. *Lancet.* 2005;366(9498):1704–1710.

20. Luckraz H, Murphy F, Bryant S, Charman SC, Ritchie AJ. Vacuum-assisted closure as a treatment modality for infections after cardiac surgery. *J Thorac Cardiovasc Surg.* 2003;125(2):301–305.

21. Song DH, Wu LC, Lohman RF, Gottlieb LJ, Franczyk M. Vacuum assisted closure for the treatment of sternal wounds: the bridge between debridement and definitive closure. *Plast Reconstr Surg.* 2003;111(1):92–97.

22. Ontario Health Technology Advisory Committee (OHTAC) Recommendations: Negative Pressure Wound Therapy, Dec 2010.

23. VanGilder C, Amlung S, Harrison P, Meyer S. Results of the 2008–2009 International Pressure Ulcer Prevalence Survey and a 3-year, acute care, unit-specific analysis. *Ostomy Wound Manage.* 2009;55(11):39–45.

24. Padula WV, Mishra MK, Makic MB, Sullivan PW. Improving the quality of pressure ulcer care with prevention: a cost-effectiveness analysis. *Med Care.* 2011;49(4):385–392.

25. Norton L, Coutts P, Sibbald RG. Beds: practical pressure management for surfaces/mattresses. *Adv Skin Wound Care.* 2011;24(7):324–332.

26. Mimura M, Ohura T, Takahashi M, Kajiwara R, Ohura N Jr. Mechanism leading to the development of pressure ulcers based on shear force and pressures during a bed operation: influence of body types, body positions, and knee positions. *Wound Repair Regen.* 2009;17(6):789–796.

27. Black JM, Edsberg LE, Baharestani MM, et al; National Pressure Ulcer Advisory Panel. Pressure ulcers: avoidable or unavoidable? Results of the National Pressure Ulcer Advisory Panel Consensus Conference. *Ostomy Wound Manage.* 2011;57(2):24–37.

28. Smith G, Ingram A. Clinical and cost effectiveness evaluation of low friction and shear garments. *J Wound Care.* 2010;19(12):535–542.

29. Kitson A, Harvery G, McCormack B. Enabling the implementation of evidence based practice: a conceptual framework. *Qual Health Care.* 1998;7(3):149–158.

30. McInnes E, Bell-Syer SEM, Dumville JC, Legood R, Cullum NA. Support surfaces for pressure ulcer prevention. *Cochrane Database Syst Rev.* 2008;(4):CD001735.

31. Adult Hospital Beds: Patient Entrapment Hazards, Side Rail Latching Reliability, and Other Hazards, © Minister of Public Works and Government Services Canada 2006, Revised Date: 2008/02/29; Effective Date: 2008/03/17.

32. US FDA Guidance entitled *Hospital Bed System Dimensional and Assessment Guidance to Reduce Entrapment,*

published March 10, 2006. http://www.fda.gov/medi-caldevices/deviceregulationandguidance/guidancedocu-ments/ucm072662.htm.

33. Adult Hospital Beds: Patient Entrapment Hazards, Side Rail Latching Reliability, and Other Hazards, © Minister of Public Works and Government Services Canada 2006, Revised Date: 2008/02/29; Effective Date: 2008/03/17.

34. Brienza D, Kelsey S, Karg P, et al. Randomized clinical trial on preventing pressure ulcers with wheelchair seat cushions. *J Am Geriatr Soc.* 2010;58:2308–2314.

35. Brienza D, Karg PE, Geyer MJ, Kelsey S, Trefler E. The relationship between pressure ulcer incidence and buttock-seat cushion interface pressure in at-risk elderly wheelchair users. *Arch Phys Med Rehabil.* 2001;82:529–533.

36. CAOT Position Statement Assistive Technology and Occupational Therapy (2006), http://www.caot.ca/default.asp?pageid=598.

37. McInnes E, Bell-Syer SEM, Dumville JC, Legood R, Cullum NA. Support surfaces for pressure ulcer prevention. *Cochrane Database Syst Rev.* 2008;(4):CD001735.

38. Registered Nurses Association of Ontario Risk Assessment & Prevention of Pressure Ulcers Guideline Supplement. Registered Nurses Association, Toronto 2011.

39. European Pressure Ulcer Advisory Panel and National Pressure Ulcer Advisory Panel. Prevention and treatment of pressure ulcers: quick reference guide. Washington DC: National Pressure Ulcer Advisory Panel; 2009.

Alternative and Complementary Therapies for Wound Care

Karen Laforet, MClSc-WH, BA, RN, IIWCC;

Ruth Anne Baron, BSc ND;

M. Gail Woodbury, PhD, BScPT, MAPWCA;

R. Gary Sibbald, BSc, MD, FRCPC(Med, Derm), MACP, FAAD, MEd, MAPWCA

Objectives

The reader will be challenged to:
- Define alternative and complementary therapies
- Distinguish the benefits and potential side effects of commonly used topical and oral herbal therapies
- Analyze and integrate knowledge to counsel patients regarding wound care therapy options.

Introduction

Many people seek alternative therapies to complement their healthcare treatments because they want to have more autonomy in their care. They may feel frustrated that their treatment is not working, and they may perceive natural treatments as safer. It is important that all healthcare providers be informed of the full range of treatments an individual may be using; therefore, therapeutic relationships based on trust will provide a forum for open communication regarding a patient's usage. Alternative therapies are relatively new within North America. A number of cultures use traditional medicines specific to their location or belief system, and the healthcare professional needs to take the time to gain an understanding of these beliefs and practices in order to provide safe and efficacious treatment.

Current practice for both conventional and ***complementary and alternative medicine (CAM)*** includes knowledge acquired over many centuries as well as modern evidence through scientific proof.[1] As healthcare continues moving in the direction of evidence-based practice, clinicians and governments are demanding studies to prove clinical efficacy of treatment modalities. The amount of evidence that is available to support the use of CAM is limited. Difficulties in evaluating the effectiveness of CAM mirror those for the evaluation of wound care practice in many ways — that is, persons with wounds are unique, wounds are complex, the array of ever-changing products from which to choose is extensive (many have limited supporting evidence), and appli-

Laforet K, Baron RA, Woodbury MG, Sibbald RG. Alternative and complementary therapies for wound care. In: Krasner DL, Rodeheaver GT, Sibbald RG, Woo KY, eds. *Chronic Wound Care: A Clinical Source Book for Healthcare Professionals.* Vol 1. 5th ed. Malvern, PA: HMP Communications; 2012:243–252.

cation and quality manufacturing impact results. At this stage in the development of the science of CAM, it is important to know what evidence of effectiveness does exist, whether in the form of case studies, testimonials, proof-of-concept studies, or clinical trials, and to start to build an understanding of how CAM works in wound care.

The approach of *evidence-based medicine (EBM)* strives to synthesize "best evidence" for a particular clinical problem. One of the challenges when seeking to validate CAM therapies within the EBM model is the perception that the "medicalized" version of therapy required for research denies CAM's core components. Any understanding of these modalities demonstrates that the treatment is individualized to each patient's signs and symptoms with a multifaceted approach. For example, when a practitioner of *traditional Chinese medicine (TCM)* diagnoses a patient with pneumonia as having "wind heat in the lungs," that philosophy will determine diagnosis and treatment. While this patient may be diagnosed with deficient lung qi (positive energy) and deficient lung yin (negative energy), another patient may present with a completely different set of signs and symptoms and yet have the same diagnosis of deficient lung qi and deficient lung yin.[2] *Ayurveda medicine* stresses a balance of 3 elemental energies or humors: *vāyu vāta* (air and space — "wind"), *pitta* (fire and water — "bile"), and *kapha* (water and earth — "phlegm"). According to the Ayurvedic theory, these 3 substances exist in equal parts when the body is healthy. A person with pneumonia will present with an imbalance of these 3 elements. One Ayurvedic theory asserts that each human possesses a unique combination of *dosas* (constitution) that defines that person's temperament and characteristics. These examples demonstrate that building a clinical study to determine a particular remedy's therapeutic efficacy for pneumonia will be difficult to interpret if outcomes are measured for one aspect only — as is the current EBM model.

Healthcare professionals are encouraged to critically analyze existing evidence within the context of established evidence-based models for all forms of therapy being considered — conventional and complementary or alternative.

Persons with chronic wounds are seeking information on alternative therapy options. The authors encourage the reader to investigate credible online resources (Table 1) as well as current literature before initiating a new therapy. To encompass traditional therapies across the globe is beyond the scope of this chapter; therefore, recommendations for the more commonly used CAM therapies for wound care will be provided and linked with the conjured patient case of Mrs. Jones.

Defining Complementary and Alternative Medicine

With the wide range of therapies, practices, and products classified under the CAM umbrella, it is difficult to find consistency in definition and scope. For the purposes of this chapter, CAM therapies are classified as healthcare-related therapies, practices, and products that are not considered part of conventional medicine. *Integrative* (formerly referred to as complementary) medicine is used in addition to or incorporated into a patient's plan of care, whereas alternative medicine is used in place of conventional treatment.[3]

Complementary and Alternative Therapies and Wound Care Management

Before deciding if any alternative therapy is appropriate for wound care, evidence-based principles need to guide whatever therapy is considered. These principles provide an organized, holistic approach to care for the whole person before addressing local wound care. Specifically, this approach aims to control and eliminate the causative factors, provide systemic support to reduce existing and potential cofactors, address patient-centered concerns, and maintain a physiological local wound environment. Other issues to remember when caring for wounds are systemic factors (eg, age, anemia, nutrition) and local factors (eg, blood supply, local infection, previous acute or chronic radiation injury) that affect wound healing.[4] These principles compromise the *wound bed preparation (WBP)* paradigm.[5] CAM therapies have been integrated into WBP, providing recommendations for CAM use within an evidence-based model (Figure 1).[3]

Case Study: Mrs. Jones

Mrs. Jones, who is 71 years old, had a knee replacement 3 years ago. Post-operatively she developed a surgical site infection and the incision dehisced leaving her with a nonhealing wound on the lower tibia. Mrs. Jones is obese, has type II diabetes, and is a recent widow. Since her knee replacement, her mobility is limited in part due to the infection but mainly due to poor pain control. The pain affects her sleep and mobility, essentially isolating her at home. The consequence of her isolation is that her diet consists mainly of refined carbohydrate foods — no fresh fruit or vegetables and limited protein sources.

Mrs. Jones has a community nurse visiting once a week for local wound management. Between nursing visits, she is managing her own wound care. Her daughter, a physiotherapist, noted that the wound care team (comprised of the nurse, family doctor, and case manager) had not made any changes to her dressing routine in 6 months. She recommended that Mrs. Jones see her naturopath.

Controlling and Eliminating Causative Factors

One of the most challenging aspects for healthcare professionals is the need to diagnose and treat the wound cause. Within a CAM framework, the whole person is considered, not just the disease symptoms. Therefore, in this aspect of care, the foundational practice works in synergy with the WBP paradigm, directing the clinician to focus on the cause. Although the path of treatment may be different depending on the constitutional therapy chosen (eg, Ayurvedic, Chinese medicine, homeopathy, kampo, naturopathy, or other traditional medicines), all focus on restoring a person's innate natural balance. A major tenet for all these practices is the understanding of how disease is caused by imbalance. Within a CAM model, the restoration process includes a variety of herbal remedies, exercises, food and fluid intake, energy work, orthomolecular therapy, and other treatments aimed at supporting the body's innate ability to heal and to reduce/eliminate factors impacting health. Evidence comparing the effectiveness of one treatment modality over another has yet to be studied.

The naturopathic perspective on any case is to treat the whole person, assessing any causative factors that must be addressed in order for healing to occur. In Mrs. Jones's situation, the naturopath

identified poor nutrition, inadequate sleep, decreased circulation secondary to her primary disease state, catabolic stress response, and depression — all factors negatively impacting her system's ability to heal. The naturopath prescribed essential fatty acids, zinc, vitamin A, and amino acids. Oral supplements and fish oil, along with a series of intravenous nutrient treatments, were initiated.

After 8 weeks of treatment, the inflammation in her knee decreased, the wound surface area had decreased by 25%, and her pain was well managed, resulting in improved sleep. Her mobility increased so that she was able to go for walks in her neighborhood.

Orthomolecular Therapy

The use of vitamins, minerals, amino acids, and trace elements to correct deficiencies is the main focus of *orthomolecular therapy*.[6] Wound healing is closely linked to malnutrition and deficiencies in vitamins, minerals, fats, and proteins. Inadequate nutrient stores negatively impact the inflammatory and proliferative phases of wound healing: collagen synthesis, fibroblast activity, and compromised host response to microorganisms. Vitamins and minerals that are particularly important in wound healing are vitamins A, C, and D and zinc. See Chapter 3.10.

Vitamin A (retinoids, beta carotene) influences the inflammatory phase of wound healing. Vitamin A is responsible for the release of macrophages and monocytes.[7] During the proliferative phase, it stimulates fibroblasts to increase collagen deposition.[8] Retinoids have an effect on bacteria and inflammation and may have a cancer chemotherapy protection effect. They are known to stimulate both humeral- and cell-mediated immune mechanisms, and some studies have shown that they can reverse the wound healing inhibitory effect of oral corticosteroids.[7,8] Stress, such as surgery, loss of a spouse, and nonhealing wounds, as well as comorbidities, such as diabetes, obesity, and old age (as in Mrs. Jones's current state of health), can rapidly deplete vitamin A stores. Supplementation may be recommended; however, practitioners need to proceed with caution, as high doses may inhibit healing. A qualified practitioner should determine the dosage.

Vitamin C (ascorbic acid, L-ascorbic acid) is involved in collagen synthesis — specifically in the hydroxylation of lysine and proline, the enzymes responsible for tensile strength. Vitamin C influences resistance to infection, is essential for neutrophil and fibroblast function, and strengthens and promotes new blood vessel formation.[9] Smoking and alcohol intake will increase excretion of vitamin C. Scurvy (vitamin C deficiency) results in joint pain, poor wound healing, fatigue, depression, and bleeding disorders. Elderly patients, like Mrs. Jones, may be suffering from subclinical vitamin C deficiency, masking the cause of key patient-specific concerns, such as pain, fatigue, and depression.

While multiple micronutrients are involved in homeostasis, *zinc* is important in wound healing for its role in collagen synthesis. Zinc is involved in the catalytic activities of more than 100 enzymes, protein synthesis, collagen cross-bonding, and promotion of re-epithelization.[10]

Zinc is seldom the limiting factor in wound healing. Individuals with zinc deficiency may display a characteristic dermatitis called *acrodermatitis enteropathica* (dermatitis in a distinct circumoral and distal extremity distribution). Any client with a wound needs to be assessed for nutrient deficiencies with therapeutic dosages and monitored by a qualified practitioner.

Addressing Patient-Centered Concerns

Patient-centered concerns, including pain, psychosocial issues (anxiety, fear, depression, and isolation), nutrition, and financial concerns, need to be acknowledged and controlled while attending to local wound care. Pain sets up a chronic stress response resulting in the patient being "sympathetic dominant." The parasympathetic nervous system reduces heart rate and the negative inotropic effects of sympathetic nervous system response (flight or fight): adrenalin, noradrenalin, vasoconstriction, decreased immune system functioning, etc, providing the body with time to concentrate more on resting, digesting, and healing. A number of modalities have proven efficacy in stimulating a parasympathetic response in the body.

Energy Medicine

Energy work is an umbrella term for a number of modalities that use practitioner intent and energy to reduce stress and stimulate a person's healing abilities. Examples include therapeutic touch, reiki, Qi Qong, and color, light, or vibrational therapy. Body work therapies, such as massage and reflexology, are additional forms of energy medicine. Acupuncture has been found to reduce pain through the gate control theory of Melzak and Wall (one sensation from the insertion of the needle displacing a second competing sensation, such as pain).[11] This therapy has been used and evaluated within traditional healthcare; therefore, it will not be discussed in this chapter.

Nurses started therapeutic touch in the late 1980s. It has been used in all care settings with reported benefits, such as decreased anxiety and pain, increased relaxation, and an overall sense of well-being. Systematic reviews have evaluated the current data to explore its role as an adjunctive therapy.[12,13] While the results overall are mixed, the body of evidence does support its use. The healthcare professional needs to examine the evidence in light of the individual patient's needs.

Aromatherapy

Aromatherapy incorporates a variety of botanical extracts that are commonly used throughout the world to manage pain. Extracts from plants, known as essential oils, have been used for over 3 centuries for managing pain, controlling odor, healing wounds, reducing inflammation, and easing anxiety and stress. While few well designed studies exist, the clinical results demonstrate equal or better control for managing agitation.[14] Potential adverse reactions to essential oils include dermal irritation, mucous membrane irritation, phototoxicity, and contact sensitization. Persons with seasonal allergies must use aromatherapy with caution. If this therapy is being used as a complementary modality for wound care, topical localized essential oil massage should only be completed by a registered aromatherapist with wound care training or in consultation with a wound care expert.

Herbal Medicine

Most frequently, patients will turn to the use of *herbal medicine* when seeking an alternative form of therapy. The estimated use for herbal products in one survey[15] was approximately 57%. While a number of products are taken orally, some topical botanical products have been rec-

Table 1. CAM resources
National Center for Complementary and Alternative Medicine (NCCAM): http://nccam.nih.gov
American Botanical Council: http://abc.herbalgram.org
Journal of Alternative & Complementary Medicine: http://liebertpub.com
Alternative Medicine Review: http://altmedrev.com
World Health Organization: http://www.who.int
PubMed: http://www.ncbi.nlm.nih.gov
Medscape: www.medscape.com

ommended for treatment of wound-associated pain (see Figure 1 under Patient-Centered Concerns). Plant extracts are not to be used in open wounds unless specifically identified as safe to do so.

The interactions between herbal products and conventional drugs are significant. Numerous articles have documented real and potential risks. While the significance of many interactions is uncertain, several interactions, particularly those with St John's wort, may have serious consequences.[16] These reactions include an increase in blood pressure especially with asthma inhalants, nasal decongestants, beer, coffee, wine, and chocolate.

Our knowledge of herb-drug interactions is rapidly filling the gaps, and healthcare professionals need to stay informed about such interactions. The scope of this chapter does not permit a detailed review of the current research, and the authors encourage the reader to stay informed using the resources provided[16] (Table 1).

Studies of the use of *arnica* (**A montana***)* in wound healing are few in number, and the results are contradictory. In one older study, Ernst and Pittler conducted a systematic review to determine the efficacy of homeopathic arnica in subjects with various circumstances including healthy volunteers, tooth extractions, and orthopedic conditions and found no more evidence than could be attributed to placebo to support the use of arnica.[17]

In a more recent double-blind, randomized,

controlled trial conducted by Karow et al,[18] *Arnica montana* D4 was compared with diclofenac for healing of wounds after hallux valgus surgery. The results in terms of mobility, healing, and pain were not significantly different between the groups.

Tinctures of diluted arnica in alcohol can be applied externally to intact skin for the treatment of inflammation, bruising, and other injuries. Anecdotally, the use of arnica tincture, ointment, or cream is effective for pain relief in closed acute injuries.

Capsaicin (cayenne) is an extract from pepper used across the globe as a topical analgesic. Capsaicin acts as a counter-irritant, depleting local sensory terminals of substance P (present in inflammatory disorders, such as inflammatory bowel disease and arthritis).[19] In a meta-analysis of 4 trials comparing capsaicin to placebo for neuropathic pain, results favored capsaicin cream ($P < .01$).[20] Capsaicin products should be used only on intact skin, and the sites should be rotated frequently due to the high risk of hyperemia and local nerve damage.[20] Initial burning is common.

Oral horse chestnut seed extract (HCSE, **Aesculus hippocastanum L***)* has been used to treat a wide variety of rheumatic and inflammatory ailments. The active ingredient is aescin, which has been demonstrated to have anti-inflammatory, anti-edema, and venotonic properties.[21] The mechanism of action is through the inhibition of elastase and hyaluronidase, result-

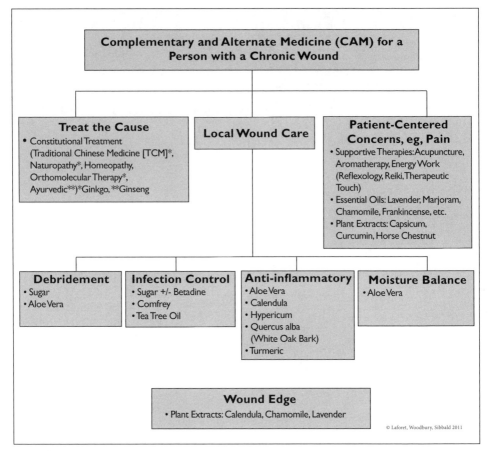

Figure 1. Complementary and alternative medicine (CAM) for a person with a chronic wound

ing in decreased capillary permeability.[22] Ernst and Pittler's systematic review concluded that HCSE is effective in reducing swelling and pain in persons with chronic venous insufficiency.[22] The caveat is that the aescin (active ingredient) dosage is not standardized. Healthcare professionals need to be aware that there is no approved, standardized, oral dose on the market. Topical preparations, while not as effective as the oral preparation, are available with the percentage of aescin generally at 2%.

Turmeric **(Curcuma longa,** *curcumin)* is a standard botanical used in Ayurvedic medicine to treat inflammatory conditions.[23] Turmeric's efficacy as an anti-inflammatory is due to 3 main curcuminoids that inhibit leukotrienes and a number of other molecules associ-

ated with inflammation.[24] Clinical studies have demonstrated consistent anti-inflammatory results. One study compared a nonsteroidal anti-inflammatory analgesic to turmeric with comparable results.[25] Another study focusing on postoperative inflammation demonstrated that turmeric produced a better anti-inflammatory response than placebo.[26] Ayurvedic practitioners blend the powder into a paste or lotion for treatment of a variety of conditions, including partial-thickness wounds. Paste or lotion should be applied only to intact skin.

Local Wound Management

Local wound management consists of 4 key components for assessment and treatment: *de-bridement, infection/inflammation, moisture*

CHRONIC WOUND CARE, 5th Edition

balance, and *wound edge*. Appropriate topical treatment choices need to be matched to the wound characteristics. Numerous botanical extracts are used for wound healing throughout the world. Herbs can be applied as oil, paste, ointment, tincture, or extract or the plant part may be applied fresh to the wound.

The most commonly used herbs are aloe, calendula, hypericum, oak bark, sugar, and tea tree oil (Figure 1). A number of botanicals are used topically within local traditional medicines. The authors discourage the use of the following botanicals for skin and wound care due to their toxicity and potential to cause sensitization: borage, oil of clove, comfrey, Echinacea, goldenseal, horsebaum, willow bark, and marshmallow.

Accounts of using the *aloe plant* (**Aloe vera**) for wounds have been found in the Bible, in the writings of Alexander the Great and Hippocrates, and in Egyptian writings before 150 BC. Its use orally and topically also has been recorded in ancient Polynesian, Indian, and Greek literature.[27]

The *Aloe vera* plant is a green succulent belonging to the lily family. The substance, aloe, is derived from thin-walled mucilaginous cells of the inner central zone of the leaf. The leaf gel is for topical use only and is believed to have emollient and moisturizing effects and therapeutic properties. Pure aloe contains 99% water and more than 75 components, including glucose, uric acid, salicylic acid, creatinine, alkaline phosphate, cholesterol, triglycerides, magnesium lactate, calcium, zinc, sodium, potassium, and chloride.[27]

In addition, aloe is considered anti-inflammatory due to its ability to block prostaglandin release (salicylic acid), to control conversion of histamine through the release of magnesium lactate, and to inactivate bradykinin with the presence of carboxypeptidase.[28] Polysaccharides in the gel activate macrophages, providing an antimicrobial effect.[29]

In-vivo and *in-vitro* studies in acute and chronic wounds have yielded positive and questionable results.[28,30,31] Continued research is needed regarding aloe and how its components specifically affect wound healing. Due to its high moisture content, aloe is an alternative for hydrogels to donate moisture and provide autolytic debridement. An occasional patient may develop an allergy to aloe. Otherwise, adverse reactions

and localized irritation are decreased with pure aloe. Avoid any product containing alcohol.

*Calendula (***C officinalis** *or English [pot] marigold)* has been used on wounds for centuries. It is approved in Germany as an antiseptic and cicatrizant. Calendula is prepared in a variety of ways with a beeswax carrier (being the preferred method for skin and wound care treatment). Generally, beeswax forms are pure; however, beware of the carrier containing propolis (bee glue associated with beeswax), as this may be an allergen. Active components include terpenoids, which were demonstrated by Day 10 in animal studies to stimulate granulation and increase glycoprotein and collagen at wound sites, stimulating epithelization.[32] An *in-vitro* study demonstrated anti-inflammatory effects on par with analgesic medications.[33] In a single-blind, randomized, phase III trial, McQuestion[34] compared calendula cream versus trolamine for radiated breast tissue in 254 women. Calendula reduced occurrence of grade 2 or higher skin reactions ($P < .001$), and associated pain was significantly decreased compared to standard ($P < .03$).

Hypericum (St John's wort), well known for its efficacy in treating depression, also has been used historically to treat local injuries. Hypericum contains a number of active ingredients — two, in particular, make it effective for wound care management. One active component, hypericin, has anti-inflammatory effects, whereas hyperforin has been demonstrated to be effective against gram-positive bacteria.[35] A randomized, double-blind, clinical study was conducted post-cesarean delivery (N = 144). Decreased scar formation was noted on Day 40 versus control; however, the results did not reach statistical significance.[35]

*Oak bark (***Quercus alba***)*, or white oak bark, is an historical anti-inflammatory remedy. The active compound, quercitol, produces a hyperosmolar astringent action on application. In addition, high levels of terpenoids and salicylates elicit anti-inflammatory effects. It has been useful in treating inflammatory skin disorders and partial-thickness wounds. Due to the salicylate level, it is not recommended for large wounds, as it may cause irritant dermatitis. *Individuals allergic to salicylates or related non-steroidal anti-inflammatory agents should avoid oak bark.*[36]

Sugar has a long and steady history dating

back to the 1600s. It is derived from the juice of various plants, such as sugar cane, sugar beet, the date palm, and the maple tree — all produced in a variety of forms. Sugar is thought to enhance wound healing through autolytic debridement as well as via an antimicrobial effect. The mechanism of action is osmosis. The hypertonicity of sugar is part of the antimicrobial effect along with the organic iodine component. The hypertonicity of the sugar reduces periwound edema. This combination as a primary wound dressing is a market leader in Japan.

There is speculation that sugar releases hydrogen peroxide particles in a similar fashion to honey; however, this has not been proven. Honey has been used and clinically studied within traditional healthcare and, therefore, will not be discussed in this chapter.

Murandu et al[37] tested 3 different sugars to determine minimum inhibitory concentration and found that Demerara sugar was not as effective against the 16 bacterial strains tested. Following this *in-vitro* test, a pilot was completed on 22 wounds. Debridement was visible in all wounds by Day 3. Patients stated that there was less localized pain compared to previous dressings, and they found the dressings simple to use.[37] Blood glucose was monitored for persons with diabetes, and no increase in blood glucose was noted during the course of treatment. Murandu's study used sterilized granulated sugar.

The mixture of sugar and povidone iodine is thought to have an antimicrobial effect. Sugar reduces edema in the wound, and at the same time, povidone-iodine is carried to the wound bed, producing the antimicrobial effect. Various commercial preparations have been evaluated with demonstrated efficacy. One animal study showed an increase in fibroblast and keratinocyte activity with the combination of sugar and povidone-iodine.[38]

It is important to remember that table sugar may contain additives (such as cornstarch, coloring, and tricalcium), and it is unknown how these additives may affect the wound. Commercially prepared sugar or sugar and povidone-iodine solutions are recommended for use whenever feasible.

Tea tree oil (TTO, **Melaleuca alternifolia***)* is mostly native to Australia with approximately 230 varieties of species. The chemical composition of the oils is quite complex with more than 15 different terpene hydrocarbons and their associated alcohol present in the standard chemotype.[39] TTO has demonstrated antibacterial, antiviral, antifungal, and anti-inflammatory properties. TTO impacts prostaglandins E2 and interleukin 1B and 10.[40] Edmondson et al[40] did not identify a change in methicillin-resistant *Staphylococcus aureus* status in colonized wounds; however, they noted wound healing was not inhibited. Halcon and Milkus[41] found that TTO was effective as an adjunctive therapy in infected wounds, reducing signs of infection and inflammation. However, clinical efficacy for wound healing remains sparse. One of the authors has patch-tested a number of individuals to TTO with a high percentage of positive patch tests; therefore, the authors recommend that healthcare professionals use only pure tea tree essential oil.

Discussion

Regardless of the CAM therapy considered, it behooves the healthcare professional to gather as much data as possible regarding the intended substance before use. Developing a therapeutic relationship with one's patient is imperative to gain trust and provide an open forum for disclosure of "other" oral or topical therapies the patient is using. Healthcare providers should ask themselves the following questions before considering a CAM therapy: Why am I prescribing this substance? What do I want to accomplish with the wound? What is the expected outcome? How does this therapy work? What evidence do I have that this therapy actually performs as stated? Do I have other more rational choices? The decision to use an alternative therapy can be based upon patient preference as well. In the absence of therapeutic double-blind comparisons, a clinician can perform the following comparative study: Try the alternative therapy, and if a wounded area is not improved (improvement equals $\geq 30\%$ smaller) within 4 weeks or completely healed within 12 weeks, utilize a standard treatment that a wound care professional would recommend.[3]

Conclusion

It is estimated that approximately 80% of patients and 50% of healthcare providers use some form of CAM.[2,42] Given these statistics, it is important that healthcare professionals educate themselves regarding the use, side effects, and contraindications of the various CAM therapies. The information presented in this chapter is a guide only. The authors encourage readers to seek out the articles listed and investigate each therapy thoroughly before recommending or initiating use.

Practice Pearls

- Proactively seek out information from your patients regarding CAM usage.
- CAM therapies, such as energy work, acupuncture, and aromatherapy, have been shown to be effective in managing pain and reducing stress and anxiety.
- Each topical herbal therapy carries with it a known action, an unknown action, and a possible adverse reaction; therefore, it is imperative to research current data before making recommendations.
- The following botanicals are toxic and highly sensitizing: borage, oil of clove, comfrey, Echinacea, goldenseal, horsebaum, willow bark, and marshmallow. They are not recommended for skin and wound care.

Self-Assessment Questions

1. What herbal product would be recommended as an antimicrobial and antifungal?

   A. Aloe

   B. Hypericum

   C. Arnica

   D. Tea tree oil

2. Herbs not recommended for topical wound therapy include:

   A. Aloe

   B. Calendula

   C. Echinacea

   D. Sugar

Answers: 1–D, 2–C

References

1. Knight S. Does complementary therapy have a place in wound care? *Br J Community Nursing.* 2011;16(3):S14–S22.
2. Gardiner P, Legedza A, Woods C, Phillips RS, Kemper KJ. Herb use among health care professionals enrolled in an online curriculum on herbs and dietary supplements. *J Herb Pharmacother.* 2006;6(2):51–64.
3. Laforet K, Woodbury GM, Sibbald RG. Wound bed preparation and complementary and alternative medicine. *Adv Skin Wound Care.* 2011;24(5):226–236.
4. Enoch S, Harding K. Wound bed preparation: the science behind the removal of barriers to healing. *WOUNDS.* 2003;15(7):213–229.
5. Sibbald RG, Orsted HL, Coutts PM, Keast DH. Best practice recommendations for preparing the wound bed: update 2006. *Adv Skin Wound Care.* 2007;20(7):390–405.
6. Kunin RA. Principles that identify orthomolecular medicine: a unique medical speciality. Orthomolecular Medicine Online. Available at: http://www.orthomed.org/home/kunin.html. Accessed June 25, 2011.
7. Arnold M, Barbul A. Nutrition and wound healing. *Plast Reconstr Surg.* 2006;117(7 Suppl):42S–58S.
8. Stechmiller JK. Understanding the role of nutrition and wound healing. *Nutr Clin Pract.* 2010;25(1):61–68.
9. Posthauer ME. The role of nutrition in wound care. *Adv Skin Wound Care.* 2006;19(1):43–52.
10. Langemo D, Anderson J, Hanson D, Hunter S, Thompson P, Posthauer ME. Nutritional considerations in wound care. *Adv Skin Wound Care.* 2006;19(6):297,298,300,303.
11. Melzack R, Wall PD. *The Challenge of Pain.* 2nd ed. London: Penguin Books; 1996.
12. Winstead-Fry P, Kijek J. An integrative review and meta-analysis of therapeutic touch research. *Altern Ther Health Med.* 1999;5(6):58–67.
13. Anderson JG, Taylor AG. Effects of healing touch in clinical practice: a systematic review of randomized clinical trials. *J Holist Nurs.* 2011;29(3):221–228.
14. Lin PW, Chan WC, Ng BF, Lam LC. Efficacy of aromatherapy (Lavandula angustifolia) as an intervention for agitated behaviours in Chinese older persons with dementia: a cross-over randomized trial. *Int J Geriatr Psychiatry.* 2007;22(5):405–410.
15. Adusumilli PS, Ben-Porat L, Pereira M, Roesler D, Leitman IM. The prevalence and predictors of herbal medicine use in surgical patients. *J Am Coll Surg.* 2004;198(4):583–590.
16. Izzo AA, Ernst E. Interactions between herbal medicines and prescribed drugs: an updated systematic review. *Drugs.* 2009;69(13):1777–1798.
17. Ernst E, Pittler MH. Efficacy of homeopathic arnica: a systematic review of placebo-controlled clinical trials. *Arch Surg.* 1998;133(11):1187–1190.
18. Karow JH, Abt HP, Frohling M, Ackermann H. Efficacy of Arnica montana D4 for healing of wounds after Hallux valgus surgery compared to diclofenac. *J Altern Complement Med.* 2008;14(1):17–25.
19. Blumenthal M, Goldberg A, Brinckmann J, eds. *Herbal Medicine: Expanded Commission E Monographs.* Austin, TX: American Botanical Council; 2000.
20. Zhang WY, Li Wan Po A. The effectiveness of topically applied capsaicin. A meta-analysis. *Eur J Clin Pharmacol.* 1994;46(6):517–522.
21. Koch R. Comparative study of Venostasin and Pycnogenol in chronic venous insufficiency. *Phytother Res.* 2002;16 Suppl:S1–S5.
22. Pittler MH, Ernst E. Horse chestnut seed extract for chronic venous insufficiency. *Cochrane Database Syst Rev.* 2006;(1):CD003230.
23. Gernot Katzer's Spice Pages. Turmeric (Curcuma longa

L.). Available at: http://www.uni-graz.at/~katzer/engl/Curc_lon.html. Accessed August 2, 2011.

24. Tyler V. *The Honest Herbal*. 3rd ed. New York, NY: Pharmaceutical Products Press; 1993.

25. Deodhar SD, Sethi R, Srimal RC. Preliminary study on antirheumatic activity of curcumin (diferuloyl methane) [abstract]. *Indian J Med Res*. 1980;71:632–634.

26. Satoskar RR, Shah SJ, Shenoy SG. Evaluation of antiinflammatory property of curcumin (diferuloyl methane) in patients with postoperative inflammation. *Int J Clin Pharmacol Ther Toxicol*. 1986;24(12):651–654.

27. Davis RH, Donato JJ, Hartman GM, Haas RC. Anti-inflammatory and wound healing activity of a growth substance in *Aloe vera*. *J Am Podiatr Med Assoc*. 1994;84(2):77–81.

28. Maenthaisong R, Chaiyakunapruk N, Niruntraporn S, Kongkaew C. The efficacy of aloe vera used for burn wound healing: a systematic review. *Burns*. 2007;33(6):713–718.

29. Leung MY, Liu C, Zhu LF, Hui YZ, Yu B, Fung KP. Chemical and biological characterization of a polysaccharide biological response modifier from *Aloe vera L. var. chinensis* (Haw.) Berg. *Glycobiology*. 2004;14(6):501–510.

30. Khorasani G, Hosseinimehr SJ, Azadbakht M, Zamani A, Mahdavi MR. Aloe versus silver sulfadiazine creams for second-degree burns: a randomized controlled study. *Surg Today*. 2009;39(7):587–591.

31. Bedi MK, Shenefelt PD. Herbal therapy in dermatology. *Arch Dermatol*. 2002;138(2):232–242.

32. Klouchek-Popova E, Popov A, Pavlova N, Krusteva S. Influence of the physiological regeneration and epithelialization using fractions isolated from *Calendula officinalis*. *Acta Physiol Pharmacol Bulg*. 1982;8(4):63–67.

33. Zitteri-Eglseer K, Sosa A, Jurenitsch J, et al. Anti-oedematous activities of the main triterpendiol esters of marigold *(Calendula officinalis L.)*. *J Ethnopharmacol*.

1997;57(2):139–144.

34. McQuestion M. Evidence-based skin care management in radiation therapy: clinical update. *Semin Oncol Nurs*. 2011;27(2):e1–17.

35. Samadi S, Khadivzadeh T, Emami A, Moosavi NS, Tafghodi M, Behnam HR. The effect of *Hypericum perforatum* on the wound healing and scar of cesarean. *J Altern Complement Med*. 2010;16(1):113–117.

36. Molochko VA, Lastochkina TM, Krylov IA, Brangulis KA. The antistaphylococcal properties of plant extracts in relation to their prospective use as therapeutic and prophylactic formulations for the skin [Article in Russian]. *Vestn Dermatol Venerol*. 1990;(8):54–56.

37. Murandu M, Webber MA, Simms MH, Dealey C. Use of granulated sugar therapy in the management of sloughy or necrotic wounds: a pilot study. *J Wound Care*. 2011;20(5):206–216.

38. Nakao H, Yamazaki M, Tsuboi R, Ogawa H. Mixture of sugar and povidone-iodine stimulates wound healing by activating keratinocytes and fibroblast functions. *Arch Dermatol Res*. 2006;298(4):175–182.

39. Carson CF, Hammer KA, Riley TV. Melaleuca alternifolia (Tea Tree) oil: a review of antimicrobial and other medicinal properties. *Clin Microbiol Rev*. 2006;19(1):50–62.

40. Edmondson M, Newall N, Carville K, Smith J, Riley TV, Carson CF. Uncontrolled, open-label, pilot study of tea tree (*Melaleuca alternifolia*) oil solution in the decolonisation of methicillin-resistant *Staphylococcus aureus* positive wounds and its influence on wound healing. *Int Wound J*. 2011;8(4):375–384.

41. Halcon L, Milkus K. Staphylococcus and wounds: a review of tea tree oil as a promising antimicrobial. *Am J Infect Control*. 2004;32(7):402–408.

42. Griffith R, Tengnah C. Regulation of herbal medicines. *Br J Community Nurs*. 2010;15(9):445–448.

Therapeutic Modalities in the Treatment of Chronic Recalcitrant Wounds

Pamela E. Houghton, PT, PhD, MAPWCA;
Karen E. Campbell, RN, MScN, NP/CNS, PhD(Can)

Objectives

The reader will be challenged to:

- Discuss the role of therapeutic modalities (physical agents that promote wound closure)
- Provide an overview of the experimental research that is available for several therapeutic modalities and use this research to describe how each modality affects the wound healing process
- Utilize current clinical research evidence that is available to support the use of these modalities in the treatment of chronic wounds
- Analyze the most common clinical applications and contraindications currently in use for each modality.

Introduction

Therapeutic modalities that are used to stimulate healing of chronic wounds include many physical agents commonly employed by physical therapists and other healthcare professionals. This chapter provides a brief overview of certain electrophysical agents, including electrical stimulation, electromagnetic fields, ultrasound, ultraviolet light, low-level light therapy, hydrotherapy, and pneumatic compression therapy. Several experimental and clinical studies have been published on these topics; therefore, key review articles will be referenced so that readers can obtain a more comprehensive overview of these therapies. These therapies involve applying specialized medical devices to safely and effectively deliver mechanical, light, sound, and electrical energies to healing tissue in selected individuals who will most likely benefit from the therapy.

Identifying the Best Candidates for Therapeutic Modalities

Candidates for therapeutic modalities include people who have chronic wounds that have failed to respond to optimal standard wound care, patients who have any pre-existing medical conditions that are associated with impaired wound healing (eg, diabetes mellitus), and/or patients who prefer a conservative non-surgical option to accelerate wound closure. *Acceleration of wound closure* is particularly important in individuals whose wounds significantly interfere with their ability to perform activities of daily living or result in immobilization for a prolonged period of time. People often

Houghton PE, Campbell KE. Therapeutic modalities in the treatment of chronic recalcitrant wounds. In: Krasner DL, Rodeheaver GT, Sibbald RG, Woo KY, eds. *Chronic Wound Care: A Clinical Source Book for Healthcare Professionals.* Vol 1. 5th ed. Malvern, PA: HMP Communications; 2012:253–270.

prefer a more conservative, non-surgical wound management program, since many individuals who develop chronic wounds are elderly and frequently have several coexisting medical conditions that would contraindicate surgical intervention. The primary care provider is a key person who must be able to identify if the patient is a good candidate for advanced wound therapy using a therapeutic modality. However, all members of the wound care team have an ethical and legal obligation to review available adjunctive therapies with the patient who has a chronic wound. Included in this decision should be consideration of factors affecting healing and a determination of whether the patient has a physical, mental, or medical condition that permits healing. Identification of underlying cause(s) of the wound and any medical conditions that are known to interfere with wound healing (eg, poor glucose control, protein malnutrition, dehydration, anemia, excessive pressure, persistent edema) is critical if the individual is to benefit from a therapeutic modality.

Certain medical conditions have an increased likelihood of producing adverse reactions and therefore prevent or contraindicate the use of some or all therapeutic modalities. *Before applying a therapeutic modality, one must confirm that the patient does not have any of the contraindications for that treatment modality.* Recently, several physical therapists across North America compiled literature and built a consensus regarding relevant contraindications and precautions for several therapeutic modalities.[1] For example, *most therapeutic modalities should not be applied to individuals or wound locations where malignant cells are present* since there is a high likelihood that these forms of external energies will stimulate tumor growth and potentially spread malignant cells. It is also recommended to treat individuals with nonhealing ulcers only after identifying common underlying causes (venous or arterial insufficiency, pressure, and/or neuropathy). Remember that certain inflammatory wounds and dermatological conditions may manifest as unhealed open skin ulcers. Houghton and colleagues also provided an outline of good clinical practices that promote the safe application of these external energies. Paramount in this process is *obtaining informed consent* from the potential recipient or from his or her substitute decision-maker.

This should include an explanation of 1) why the treatment is offered; 2) what patient positioning and clothing are required during the treatment; 3) how the energy should feel; and 4) how long each treatment will take. A clear description of all the risks associated with the treatment, such as skin irritations, electrical surge, and increased pain, must be provided and linked to strategies the clinician will use to reduce the likelihood of these adverse reactions occurring. Regular service and checking of electrotherapeutic devices by qualified biomedical technicians is required to reduce the likelihood of equipment malfunction. An emphasis on open communication between the therapist and the patient while setting stimulus intensity is critical so that the desired sensation is produced without discomfort (to promote treatment adherence). When it is determined that a therapeutic modality is indicated, the next questions to ask are:

1. Who will fund the treatment?
2. Who will deliver the treatment to the patient?
3. Where will the treatment be offered?

Often, the answers to these important practical questions lie within state or provincial restrictions or local agency policies and procedures. For example, ultrasound and diathermy must be administered by a qualified physical therapist in certain sites in the United States and Canada. Ultimately, *the best person to administer the treatment is one who has both knowledge and skill with the therapeutic modality.* The authors have had success in training patients and/or their caregivers to administer daily treatments in under-serviced areas. It can be difficult to identify a single individual who has expertise in both wound care and the application of therapeutic modalities. In the authors' experience, a collaborative approach between a nurse who has extensive training in wound care and a physical therapist with background in the use of therapeutic modalities is ideal.[2] The optimal management of chronic wounds involves the employment of an interprofessional team that includes physicians, nurses, physical therapists, dietitians, and other allied health professionals. It is through this collaborative, interprofessional team approach that individuals with chronic wounds, who often prefer a more conservative, non-surgical approach, can be given the choice of the most effective and safest wound care therapy.

Electrical Stimulation

Endogenous bioelectrical potentials have been measured across the skin of many animals, including humans, and research evidence for the important role of electrical signals in tissue regeneration and repair is compelling. Cheng et al demonstrated that this low level of *electrical current could be measured in wounds that were covered with an occlusive, moisture-retentive dressing* and was absent when wounds were not covered and were allowed to dry out.[3] The presence of these naturally occurring electrical currents prompted early researchers to investigate the benefits of externally applied electrical current. Electrical current has been shown to induce cellular actions in virtually all phases of the wound-healing cascade. Recently, Kloth and Zhao[4] collated and described in detail advances in this area of research. Employment of advanced recombinant DNA technology and epithelial and vascular endothelial cell cultures has led to a better understanding of intracellular mechanisms underlying the effects of electrical fields on wound healing.

Electrical signals applied at physiological levels known to occur at the edge of human wounds have been associated with epithelial cell movement and growth factor and growth factor receptor localization and activation.[5,6] Electrical fields guide epidermal cell migration (electrotaxis or galvanotaxis) mediated by multiple cell pathways including phosphoinositide 3 kinase/phosphatase and tensin homolog, membrane growth factor receptors, and integrins.[7,8] Research performed using cultured fibroblasts suggests that electrical stimulation of these key reparative cells opens voltage-sensitive calcium channels located in the plasma membrane. The resultant influx of intracellular calcium upregulates growth factor receptors, which in turn trigger DNA synthesis and fibroblast proliferation and increase synthesis and secretion of collagen and other extracellular matrix proteins.[8,9] The breaking strength of incisional wounds placed in laboratory animals has been shown to be enhanced by local application of a negative charged electrode.[10]

In summary, this experimental research supports a role for *electrical fields in directing cell migration, regulating the frequency and direction of cell division, and promoting re-epithelization and angiogenic phases of wound healing*. Further,

externally applied electrical currents also stimulate fibroblast activity, resulting in enhanced protein synthesis and collagen reorganization and strength. Two key genes and molecules have been identified that mediate cellular responses to electrical fields produced by externally applied current.

A principle action of electrical stimulation on wound healing is its ability to improve local blood flow and enhance perfusion of injured tissues. Indeed, blood flow enhancement is the main indication recognized by the US Food and Drug Administration (FDA) for electrical stimulation devices used to treat wounds. Experimental evidence suggests that electrical stimulation improves oxygenation of treated tissues in 2 ways. Initially, sensory nerve stimulation using many different forms of electrical stimulation induces vasodilation of local arterioles. Cosmo et al[11] applied electrical stimulation to chronic leg ulcers and detected significant increases in blood flow to the wound and peri-ulcer skin during and up to 60 minutes after electrical stimulation treatment. Improved flap and skin graft survival via electrically induced changes to skin perfusion has been documented by several groups.[12,13]

Electrical stimulation facilitates sustained improvements in blood perfusion of wounds through promotion of many processes involved in angiogenesis. Patterson and Runge have shown that electrical stimulation directly activates vascular endothelial cell function and also stimulates release of VEGF production by muscle cells.[14] Tissue biopsies extracted from venous ulcers in humans after treatment with electrical stimulation have been shown to have greater density of new blood vessels compared to control wounds that did not receive electrical stimulation.[15] These circulatory changes will indirectly stimulate the healing process by facilitating oxygen delivery. *Transcutaneous partial pressure of oxygen (TcPO2) levels have been significantly increased after electrical stimulation* treatment of patient populations with impaired circulation, including individuals with spinal cord injuries[16] and people with diabetes.[17]

An active area of research includes work in both *in-vivo* and cell culture studies examining the effects of electrical current on the growth of many types of bacteria that commonly colonize wounds. Chu et al found that *wounds had fewer bacteria and closed faster when electrical stimulation was applied to silver nylon dressings compared to burn wounds treated with only silver dressings.*[18] This result has stimulated many researchers to investigate a potential synergy between antibacterial effects of positively charged (anodal) electrical current and silver cations (Ag+). Researchers have postulated that the positive charge produced under the anode may promote delivery of silver ions to deeper tissues via iontophoresis.[4] It also has been speculated that concurrent treatment with electrical stimulation may enhance the ability of antibiotics to kill biofilm-associated bacteria.[19]

Because many of the beneficial effects of electrical stimulation are believed to be due to direct cellular actions of the electrical current, most treatment protocols involve techniques to deliver the electrical energy directly to the wound bed.[20] This application technique for electrical stimulation involves using a monopolar setup with specialized electrodes composed of sterile conductive material. *The active electrode is placed directly into the wound, and a larger dispersive electrode is placed on intact skin near the wound.* This direct application technique involves careful removal of wound dressings and judicious use of universal precautions and equipment decontamination procedures to avoid excessive wound manipulation or spread of infection. Newer technologies have incorporated small battery-operated electrical stimulation devices that deliver microamperage current within specialized dressings.[4]

Accelerated wound closure also has been demonstrated following electrical stimulation of distant acupuncture points, paraspinal nerves, and extremities.[21] Protocols with bipolar placement of electrodes on the peri-ulcer skin on either side of the wound have demonstrated significant improvements in wound healing rates.[22] Peters et al have reported improved healing of diabetic foot ulcers when an electroconductive sock was used to apply electrical stimulation to the affected limb.[23] While these *treatments applied outside the wounds offer practical benefits, they typically require longer exposure times and produce less consistent results.*

The optimal stimulus parameters and treatment schedules for the use of electrical stimulation on chronic wounds have not yet been established. Rather, various combinations of stimulus parameters that generate a relatively narrow range of electrical charge (300–500 μC/sec) have been shown to accelerate wound closure.[4] In the literature, treatment schedules vary from as little as 1-hour treatments given 3 times weekly for 4 weeks to as much as 30-minute treatments given twice daily, 7 days a week until closure (approximately 7 weeks).[24] Ahmad found that wound size reduction was greater in subjects receiving 60 minutes versus 45 minutes of high-voltage pulsed current but that further improvements in healing rates were not achieved when electrical stimulation treatment was applied for 120 minutes.[25] This result suggests that longer treatment times may not necessarily produce better outcomes. Thus, *it may be best to optimize the wound environment by coordinating electrotherapy treatments with the timing of wound dressing changes.*

Low-intensity direct current (LIDC) was the electrical waveform utilized predominantly in early clinical studies and has more recently been associated with blood flow changes and antibacterial effects of electrical stimulation. However, this form of current must be used with caution in order to avoid electrochemical burns occurring in tissues underlying the electrodes. High-voltage pulsed current (HVPC) is a form of pulsed current that is commonly used in the treatment of chronic wounds. This form of monophasic pulsed current is known to stimulate several wound healing processes without causing changes in the pH of underlying tissues.[26] While other types of current, including asymmetrical biphasic pulsed current, also have been shown to promote wound closure,[21,22] preliminary data presented from *a recent systematic review suggested that the forms of electrical stimulation that produce bidirectional current flow may not be as effective as unidirectional currents (ie, LIDC, HVPC).*[27]

Stimulus intensity and frequency are adjusted to produce a comfortable tingling sensation, or in insensate skin, the stimulus intensity is adjusted to a sub-motor level (just below the level required to produce visible muscle twitches). Most protocols recommend that the polarity of the electrode in the wound be kept the same throughout a single treatment session; however, in order to avoid a plateau in response to electrical stimulation, the charge of the active electrode should be alternated every 3 to 7 days. It should be noted that *in order to achieve optimal results with this modality, wound desiccation and petrolatum–based products in the wound bed should be avoided*.

Adverse effects associated with electrical stimulation of chronic wounds include only minor discomfort associated with tingling sensations that are produced and/or skin reactions when using self-adhesive electrodes.[28] Frequent checks for reactions (redness) in the skin and tissues under the electrodes are recommended, especially when using devices that emit direct current.

Clinicians require specialized training to learn the proper use of novel equipment and competence with the techniques necessary to apply electrical stimulation safely and effectively to the wound bed.

Electromagnetic Fields

Non-thermal forms of electromagnetic fields (EMFs) do not produce perceptible changes in skin temperature and include pulsed radiofrequency stimulation (PRFS), pulsed short-wave diathermy (PSWD), and pulsed electromagnetic fields (PEMF). The athermal nature of these devices relates to the relatively low power output of high-frequency radio waves, which are modulated through a timing device that produces bursts of millions of low-intensity electrical pulses at preset intervals.[28] *PEMFs commonly used in wound care are typically very low magnetic fields that do not produce heat and are alternated in the range of 1–100 Hz.* Unlike electrical devices that use 2 surface electrodes to emit electrical current (see above), this form of electrical energy is delivered by single coil electrodes at frequencies too high to produce a perceptible sensation in the recipient.

EMFs interact with electrolytes and other charged molecules present in tissue. Movement of these electrically charged molecules induces a small electrical current in tissues. EMFs were first developed for their benefits in bone repair and more recently were found to also accelerate wound closure in soft tissue.[29] Subsequent studies performed in diabetic mice and other animal models showed that EMFs could improve tissue strength,[30] stimulate angiogenesis,[31] and increase the rate of re-epithelization.[32] The main mecha-

nism believed to stimulate tissue repair processes involves acceleration of the binding of di-ionic calcium cations (Ca2+) to calmodulin.[29] The calcium calmodulin molecule activates nitric oxide synthase in endothelial cells, and this results in increased production of nitric oxide.[33] Nitric oxide is a potent anti-inflammatory agent and is known to stimulate the production and release of many different growth factors, including VEGF, tumor necrosis factor-alpha (TNF-α), and transforming growth factor-beta (TGF-β).[1] In *in-vivo* studies, EMFs have been shown to improve tendon strength and result in altered local tissue perfusion, elevated local tissue oxygen levels, and reduced tissue edema.[34]

Some individuals have suggested that it does not matter whether the electrical fields are produced by electrical stimulation devices using 2 electrodes applied in contact with the skin or by inducing an electrical signal by applying EMFs. The net result is accelerated production of granulation tissue during the proliferative phase of the wound healing cascade. However, more research is needed to compare the effects of electrical stimulation and EMFs before this association can be confirmed.

The application of EMFs to wounds is relatively simple since it involves the application of a single electrode that does not need to be placed in direct contact with the wound bed. Smaller, more portable devices that use flexible and disposable coils can easily be placed over wound dressings.[35] This method of producing electrical currents has a distinct advantage, since it does not require placing specialized electrodes in direct contact with the wound or peri-ulcer skin. This is particularly beneficial for painful wounds in which further manipulation of the wound bed is not desirable. This practical benefit is augmented by recent research documenting the analgesic properties of EMFs when post-operatively treating surgical sites.[36] Clinicians should be aware that there is up to a 50-fold difference in the power output used in commercially available EMF devices.[4] This difference in intensity may or may not affect clinical outcomes. Moist wound dressings may need to be removed prior to the treatment, as high water content will tend to produce more superficial heating. Some EMF devices can produce tissue heating that may or may not be desirable depending on the local circulation of the individual patient.

All EMF forms should not be used over metal implants or on patients with cardiac pacemakers or other implanted electronic devices.[37] EMFs travel through air and do not require direct contact to be absorbed by tissues. Therefore, clinicians standing in close proximity to the device may inadvertently receive a small amount of EMF energy. It is recommended that therapists remain at least 1 meter away from functioning EMF machines. The use of relatively short treatment times, appropriate equipment monitoring and maintenance, and careful attention to relevant safety measures should prevent excessive exposure to EMFs.

Ultrasound

Therapeutic ultrasound delivers mechanical energy through conducting media in the form of *high-frequency sound waves that are above the frequency of detection by the human ear.* This traditional form of megahertz (1–3 MHz) ultrasound energy is one of the most commonly used therapeutic modalities by physical therapists across the world. It has been used to treat numerous musculoskeletal and integumentary disorders, including chronic ulcers.

More recently, *low-frequency (kHz) ultrasound devices have been introduced to wound care primarily as a debridement tool* that can rapidly debride wound surfaces. These lower frequency devices produce longer wavelength sound waves and therefore deliver much more acoustic energy per unit time. These kilohertz ultrasound devices are an emerging and popular alternative to sharp or surgical debridement using scalpels and other surgical tools. Because of the enhanced ability to cause tissue damage, the use of low-frequency ultrasound devices requires advanced clinical skills and use of appropriate local anesthesia. Therefore, only clinicians who have the advanced knowledge and sufficient practical experience should employ these devices.

A recent review[38] provides a great overview of the cellular effects of therapeutic ultrasound. Briefly, cell culture studies have demonstrated that therapeutic (MHz) ultrasound stimulates release of chemoattractant and mitogenic factors from inflammatory cells, such as platelets, macrophages, and mast cells; enhances cell proliferation; and upregulates the synthesis and secretion of collagen by wound fibroblasts. Analysis of the histological appearance of tissue exposed to pulsed ultrasound during healing revealed that ultrasound stimulates more rapid progression through the inflammatory phase of wound healing; produces stronger and more elastic scar tissue; enhances angiogenesis and increases capillary density; and causes faster, more pronounced wound contraction to occur. It has been demonstrated that similar improvements in scar tissue strength can be achieved when ultrasound is applied during the inflammatory phase of repair as when sonication is continued throughout all phases of repair.[39] Thus, it has been postulated that the actions of ultrasound produced during the inflammation may underlie changes in the strength or integrity of the scar tissue.

Sound waves have been administered to chronic wounds using different application techniques. More commonly, beneficial effects of ultrasound have been produced by application of relatively low levels of pulsed ultrasound (SATA = 0.5 W/cm^2; duty cycle = 20%; 3 MHz) to the peri-ulcer skin.[40] Specialized dressings have been used as conducting media to deliver mechanical energy produced by ultrasound directly to the base of the wound bed.[41] Accelerated wound closure also has been achieved by delivering low-frequency sound waves from a large stationary sound head immersed in a water bath.[42]

The indirect method of applying ultrasound to the peri-ulcer skin[20] *has tremendous practical advantages*, since it prevents the risk of wound contamination and the tissue dehydration and cooling that can occur when wound dressings are removed. Similar equipment and application techniques commonly used to treat other musculoskeletal conditions can be employed.

Although high doses of ultrasound have the potential to cause tissue cavitation,[43] use of relatively low doses of ultrasound in wound treatment protocols has not yielded any reports of ultrasound-induced adverse effects. The risks of burns produced by this modality are minimal, since ultrasound is used in an interrupted mode that minimizes tissue temperature elevations. Therefore, ultrasound used in the treatment of chronic wounds is a relatively safe and easy-to-use modality that produces minimal disruption to the wound environment.

Lower frequency (kHz) sound waves also have been delivered through a fine mist spray. This form of ultrasound, called non-contact, non-thermal, acoustic therapy, seems to have some unique characteristics. Experimental studies have shown that this form of acoustic therapy can stimulate collagen deposition and increase capillary density of newly formed granulation tissue.[44] Clinical studies have reported that non-contact, non-thermal, acoustic therapy accelerated wound closure of diabetic foot wounds.[45]

Studies conducted in both animal models (pigs) and human wounds showed that non-contact, non-thermal, acoustic therapy could penetrate wounded skin and tissues and lyze bacteria.[46] This form of ultrasound therapy received FDA 510K clearance in June 2005 to "promote wound healing through wound cleansing and maintenance debridement by removal of yellow slough, fibrin tissue exudate, and bacteria."[47]

Ultraviolet Light

Ultraviolet light has long been used by physical therapists for the treatment of various skin conditions. Effects of ultraviolet light that would be beneficial to the wound healing cascade include stimulation of epithelial migration and proliferation and release of chemical mediators, such as prostaglandins and histamine, that stimulate local cutaneous blood flow, erythema,[48,49] and bactericidal effects.[50,51] The type of ultraviolet light is important in determining the tissue response. Ultraviolet light A (UVA) and ultraviolet light B (UVB), which are found in natural sunlight and cause more pronounced cutaneous inflammatory reactions and changes in local skin blood flow,[48,49] have been used to treat dermatological conditions, such as psoriasis. Light of shorter wavelength (180–254 nm) named *ultraviolet light C (UVC) is the type of ultraviolet light most commonly used in the treatment of chronic wounds*. Bactericidal effects are greatest for shorter wavelengths of light (UVC) due to direct effects of UVC on DNA of most prokaryotic bacterium.[52] UVC at a wavelength of 254 nm has been shown to inhibit the *in-vitro* growth of antibiotic-resistant bacteria (methicillin-resistant *Staphylococcus aureus* [MRSA] and vancomycin-resistant

Enterococcus faecalis [VRE]).[51] Subsequent work by the same researchers demonstrated the bactericidal effects of UVC in acute surgical wounds placed in rats.[53] UVC applied directly to the wound base of chronic wounds critically colonized with MRSA produced a significant reduction in bacteria, including MRSA.[54,55] These results remain to be confirmed by other researchers when treating various types of chronic wounds.

Small, portable, relatively cost-effective lamps that deliver UVC at 254 nm are available commercially. Animal studies have shown that ultraviolet lamps that emitted all 3 ultraviolet light bands (UVA, UVB, and UVC) were not as effective as a lamp that only emitted UVC (250–270 nm).[53] Thus, *light sources with specific filters to emit a narrow range of UVC wavelength may be more effective at reducing wound bacteria*. Since even thin transparent dressings have been shown to block the transmission of UVC waves, wound dressings must be removed, and the wound must be properly cleansed prior to UVC treatment. The amount of light energy delivered is known to be dependent on the duration of the treatment and the distance and angle of the light source. Application methods for UVC in wounds are simplified by maintaining the UVC lamp at a consistent angle (perpendicular to the body surface) and distance (approximately 2.5 cm or 1 inch) from the wound. In this way, the desired response is obtained by altering the treatment time. Clinical reports have shown a significant reduction in MRSA following a single 180-second UVC administration to chronic infected wounds.[55] This same exposure time should be used daily to remove MRSA from the wound bed or until the clinical signs of wound infection are no longer observed.[55] Cotton drapes and/or thick petroleum jelly coverings are often used on the peri-ulcer skin to ensure that UVC is only delivered to the infected wound bed and the peri-ulcer skin is protected.[54] This non-contact application technique is often preferred for infected wounds that can be very painful. Judicious use of universal precautions and equipment decontamination procedures are critical when using this modality to treat infected wounds.

Recently, Nussbaum et al concluded a controlled clinical trial where UVC was delivered to the wound and peri-ulcer skin at varied treatment times depending on the wound bed tissue. These findings suggest UVC is effective in promoting wound appearance and stimulating wound closure of pressure ulcers present in people with spinal cord injury.[56] This research suggests that *UVC can induce changes in cells beneath the peri-ulcer skin surface to activate inflammation, natural debridement, and re-epithelization.* If this method of peri-ulcer skin application is chosen, a standardized skin test must be performed to determine the individual's light sensitivity. Since factors that affect an individual's response to light (skin melanin and epidermal thickness) are located in the outer layer of the skin, a similar skin test is not required when treating only the base of an open, infected, chronic ulcer.

Concerns regarding the carcinogenic effects of ultraviolet rays are often raised. It should be noted that carcinogenic effects of ultraviolet light are dependent on the wavelength, depth of light penetration, and duration of light exposure and are related to the occurrence of sun burns.[49] UVC is known to have potent effects on the DNA material; however, it is believed to have minimal ability to induce skin cancer, since it evokes only minimal erythema or burning and penetrates through only the superficial layers of epithelium that are not undergoing cell division. Given that the incidence of skin cancer development is related to the duration of light exposure, prolonged treatment times should be avoided, and UVC treatment should be discontinued when it is no longer indicated. Although the risks of tumorigenesis and skin burns are minimal, even short exposure of UVC to the eye can cause severe retinal damage. Therefore, both the therapist and the patient should wear appropriate eye protection during UVC treatments.

Low-Level Light Therapy

LLLT (low-level light therapy) includes lasers that are a form of monochromatic, coherent, and columnar light. LLLT used by physical therapists, in the red visible wavelength and infrared light, are often class III lasers, which do not result in any significant elevation in tissue temperature. LLLT also can be delivered from light emitting diodes (LEDs) and superluminescent diodes (SLDs) or cluster probes that are made of a mixture of all of these light sources. LEDs and SLDs emit light over a narrow range of wavelengths and produce noncoherent and divergent beams of light and as a result tend to be more readily available and less expensive than laser diodes.[57] The physiological importance of each of these characteristics of laser energy is not known; therefore, for simplicity's sake, the clinical effects of all these light sources will be considered together and called LLLT.

The effects of LLLT on wound healing are complex and variable. A comprehensive review of this topic is recommended.[58] *In-vitro* experiments have demonstrated that LLLT application consistently produces altered cellular activity by directly altering fundamental intracellular processes, such as DNA synthesis, procollagen mRNA expression, calcium flux, membrane permeability, and ATP synthesis. These direct actions of LLLT are believed to underlie several cell processes known to be important in wound healing, including fibroblast migration, collagen and extracellular matrix synthesis, leukocyte proliferation, mast cell degranulation, and keratinocyte migration and secretion. *In-vivo* studies performed in several species, including dogs, rabbits, rats, and mice, have demonstrated that LLLT application to an experimentally induced wound increases collagen deposition and augments wound tensile strength.[59] LLLT also may exert its effects on the wound healing cascade indirectly by inducing the release of chemical mediators and growth factors into the tissue or local blood supply. Other indirect actions of LLLT, including enhanced local blood flow and oxygenation and augmented immune cell activity, have been suggested. However, *results from these experiments in animals have been inconsistent, and several studies have reported no benefit of LLLT on wound healing.*[60,61] Some suggest that effects of LLLT may be dependent on skin structure with loose-skinned animals tending to have more beneficial outcomes compared to tight-skinned animals, such as the domestic pig.[53]

Monochromatic infrared energy (MIRE) has been proposed to be absorbed by hemoglobin and to release nitric oxide, which in turn stimulates microcirculation. However, no significant improvements in tissue oxygenation nor in pain perception were noted when subjects with diabetic neuropathy were treated with MIRE.[62] Other forms of light (polychromatic visible and near infrared light) were found to produce transient elevations in blood flow and these effects were attributed to nitric oxide interactions with vascular endothelium.[63]

Nussbaum and colleagues performed a number of *in-vitro* experiments where cultures of common bacteria species were exposed to various wavelengths and intensities of LLLT.[63] Changes in the number of bacteria induced by (wavelengths) LLLTs ranged between -35% to +190% of baseline. These results raised **concerns that LLLT might accelerate replication of bacteria in colonized wounds.**[64] Until further research results in better understanding of the interaction between bacteria and LLLT, this therapy should be used with caution, especially with patients who have compromised immune function.

A similar LLLT application technique used for the treatment of other musculoskeletal disorders has been described for the treatment of chronic wounds. A transparent film barrier is often employed in conjunction with a contact point application technique in order to prevent cross contamination of the LLLT equipment. A noncontact sweeping technique also can be used. However, using a barrier and holding the LLLT probe further away from the skin would result in significantly less light energy delivered to the wound tissue.[65] A multitude of different LLLT sources, wavelengths of light, dosimetry, treatment techniques, and treatment schedules has been reported in the literature. As a result, optimal treatment parameters for LLLT use cannot be provided at this time.

Further research is needed to determine how various stimulus parameters influence light-induced effects of LLLT and to understand how other factors changing in the wound environment modulate these responses. This will hopefully lead to the development of optimal treatment protocols for LLLT that then can be tested using well designed controlled clinical trials.

Hydrotherapy

Hydrotherapy involving the **delivery of water or other fluids to the wound bed** is one of the oldest therapeutic modalities used by physical therapists in the treatment of chronic wounds. Hydrotherapy is most commonly applied using whirlpools; however, other irrigation systems, such as **pulsed**

lavage with concurrent suction (PLWCS), have been designed for wound care.

Wound cleansing using hydrotherapy removes necrotic and devitalized tissue; debrides loosely adherent yellow fibrinous or gelatinous exudate; and removes any unwanted dirt, foreign contaminants, or harmful residues of topical agents.[66] The removal of foreign matter and non-viable tissue using this non-specific type of mechanical debridement will aid wound healing indirectly due to reduced bacterial burden within the wound.[67] Based on this mechanism of action of **hydrotherapy**, this therapeutic modality **is indicated for open nonhealing wounds that have substantial amounts of necrotic tissue and should be discontinued when wounds are clean.**[20]

Most published protocols for the use of whirlpool on chronic wounds suggest that the limb should be immersed in water of a neutral temperature (92–96 degrees F) for 10 to 20 minutes. If agitation is added to the whirlpool water, care must be taken to ensure that this does not result in excessive pressures that can cause mechanical damage to fragile new tissue deposited in the wound bed. Antimicrobial agents are often added to the whirlpool water to prevent wound infection from waterborne contaminants during hydrotherapy treatments. The benefits of this practice should be weighed against the known cytotoxic effects of these agents on key cells in the wound healing process. **There are reports in the literature of increased wound infection with Pseudomonas aeruginosa for individuals using whirlpool[68] and cross contamination of several individuals with antibiotic-resistant strains of bacteria.**[69,70] This may occur because prolonged water immersion causes superhydration of the skin and can negate the normal skin defenses to bacteria. However, when appropriate protocols outlined by the Centers for Disease Control and Prevention are employed for cleaning, disinfecting, sterilizing, and culturing of the hydrotherapy units, these waterborne infections can be avoided. Other safety considerations for using this modality include the use of appropriate grounding of turbine units, the use of ground fault circuit breakers, and caution when transferring patients to and from the tank.

Whirlpool tanks are not appropriate for all types of chronic wounds or all patients given individual comorbidities. Previously, it was noted that prolonged hydrotherapy treatment (greater than 5 minutes) of chronic venous leg ulcers when the unbandaged lower extremity is in the dependent position can result in increased venous hypertension and vascular congestion leading to limb edema.[71] However, Ogiwara demonstrated that ankle exercises performed while the lower limb is immersed can offset edema formation due to limb dependency during hydrotherapy.[72]

PLWCS is another form of mechanical debridement that applies a stream or spray under controlled pressure to remove loosely adherent necrotic tissue or foreign material. A return suction feature allows for the irrigant, wound exudate, and debris to be collected into a disposable container. One report suggests that PLWCS produces greater rates of granulation tissue production than hydrotherapy treatments using whirlpool.[73] Svoboda et al demonstrated that PLWCS produced better removal of bacteria than a similar volume of fluid delivered with a lower pressure bulb syringe.[74] However, a subsequent experiment showed that bacteria levels rebound back to 95% of original levels within 48 hours of pulsed lavage treatment.[75] This data implies that *removal of bacteria using hydrotherapy may only be transient*. Portable units with disposable attachments make pulsed lavage with concurrent suction very transportable for patients who are immobile, for individuals in whom water immersion is contraindicated or not practically possible, or for patients with venous ulcers in whom the dependent position is not advisable. Care must be taken to avoid irrigation with excessive pressures.

Pneumatic Compression Therapy

Administration of external pressure to reduce tissue edema is considered essential standard therapy for the treatment of chronic leg wounds due to venous insufficiency. This compression therapy is believed to aid wound healing through reducing venous congestion, improving tissue perfusion, and promoting systemic fibrinolytic activity.[76] Direct cellular changes induced by pneumatic compression therapy (PCT) treatment have been noted and include increased production and release of nitric oxide.[77] Several different pneumatic devices have been developed to apply either intermittent or sequential pressures to the edematous extremity in order to relatively rapidly reduce limb girth (within hours).

Application techniques involve placing a neoprene sleeve over the patient's elevated limb and setting the device to deliver a maximum pressure (40–60 mmHg) using a 90 to 30 second on/off cycle for a period of 1 to 4 hours.[20] *The use of pneumatic compression must be combined with post-treatment application of compression bandages in order to sustain the reduction in limb edema.* PCT should not be applied when the patient has deep vein thrombosis, thrombophlebitis, or severe arterial insufficiency. Patients with bilateral limb edema due to congestive heart failure also should not be treated using PCT. Lymphedema occurs commonly with chronic venous insufficiency, and the high protein content of this form of edema may not respond well to higher pressures delivered using PCT.

Review of Clinical Research Evidence

Strong evidence. The 21 controlled clinical trials that have been reported in the literature consistently demonstrated the ability of electrical current to accelerate the healing rate and promote closure for many types of chronic wounds.[2,21-24,78-83] Kloth summarized these studies in a narrative review.[84] New emerging studies suggest that the stimulatory effects of electrical stimulation also work in diabetic foot ulcers[23,83] and venous leg ulcers.[76-80] Of note, several controlled clinical trials showed that electrical stimulation is effective in treating pressure ulcers in a spinal cord injured population.[2,21,25,78]

The European Pressure Ulcer Advisory Panel and the National Pressure Ulcer Advisory Panel recommended the use of electrical stimulation for the treatment of chronic pressure ulcers that failed to heal by conventional treatment. The strength of evidence for the use of electrical stimulation on chronic wounds received the highest rating (Level of Evidence A).[85]

A systematic review conducted as outlined in a protocol published by the Cochrane Library was recently completed.[86] Preliminary findings of this *meta-analysis confirmed commonly held views that electrical stimulation can significantly increase the number of ulcers healed and the rate of healing of various types of chronic wounds.*[27,87] This meta-analysis identified 22 randomized controlled trials involving 1,124 chronic wounds of various etiologies and examined the difference in healing observed between wounds treated with or without electrical treatment. The majority of these studies (18/22) reported accelerated wound closure after treatments involving electrical stimulation compared to appropriate control groups. Eleven of the 22 studies involved exclusively or primarily pressure ulcers. A significant increase in healing rates was detected for pressure and venous leg ulcers.

Application of EMFs has been shown to significantly accelerate wound closure in randomized, controlled, clinical trials involving both pressure ulcers and chronic venous leg ulcers. In addition, significant changes in local blood flow, skin temperature, subcutaneous tissue oxygenation, and local edema have been demonstrated following administration of EMFs to human subjects.[88] This research was recently summarized in a systematic review by McGaughney and colleagues.[89] Only 3 RCTs evaluated the percentage of participants that healed completely,[90-92] and many studies had baseline characteristics that were significantly different between EMF- and control-treated groups. Despite these limitations, they concluded that there was strong evidence that EMFs are more effective than sham EMFs when treating venous leg ulcers but not pressure ulcers. A *Cochrane review* that was recently updated included 3 clinical studies involving 94 subjects with venous leg ulcers.[93] They concluded that there is *no high quality evidence that EMF therapy increases the rate of healing of venous leg ulcers, and further research is needed*. Similarly, another Cochrane review performed by the same group of researchers also concluded that *there currently is no support for use of EMFs on pressure ulcers*.[94] In both cases, these conclusions were based on very few and small studies that met their strict inclusion criteria.

At least 14 controlled clinical trials have been performed on human subjects to assess the effectiveness of ultrasound in the treatment of chronic pressure ulcers and venous leg ulcers. These well designed clinical studies have produced mixed results. When pooled in 2 recent Cochrane reviews evaluating the ability of ultrasound to stimulate healing of pressure[95] and venous ulcers,[96] *limited evidence was found to support ultrasound treat-*

ment of pressure ulcers, but there was good evidence to suggest that ultrasound can help heal venous ulcers.

Several recently published studies examined the effect of ultrasound in healing venous leg ulcers. Franek evaluated low- and high-intensity pulsed ultrasound administered through a water bath for 5–10 minutes 9 times over a 3-week treatment period.[97] Not surprisingly, this short ultrasound treatment protocol resulted in few wound closures. Significantly greater healing rates were detected in the group of subjects receiving the lower dose of ultrasound (0.5 W/cm²).[97] This suggests that higher ultrasound intensities (1.0 W/cm²) may not be beneficial when delivered directly to the wound bed. Two studies produced by the same research group evaluated the merits of combining ultrasound with venous leg surgery in the treatment of chronic venous ulcers.[98,99] They provided ultrasound through a water bath daily for 7 weeks and concluded that adding ultrasound treatment after surgery did not further enhance healing rates of these ulcers. Of note, similar healing rates (57%–58% wound volume reduction in 7 weeks) were reported in the groups of subjects who received only ultrasound treatment and those who underwent surgical procedures including crossectomy, partial stripping, phlebectomy, and ligation of insufficient perforator veins. *Ultrasound treatment may be a preferable choice over surgery for individuals who are not good surgical candidates and if costs of vascular surgery are considered.* A multicenter clinical trial with more than 300 patients who had chronic venous leg ulcers found no benefit of low-dose pulsed ultrasound administered once a week for 12 weeks.[100] A conclusion from this report was that ultrasound does not promote faster healing of venous ulcers. While this study answers calls for research of better methodological quality, unfortunately, the ultrasound treatment protocol was suboptimal. Perhaps a more appropriate conclusion from this work might be that clinicians should refrain from using ultrasound treatment protocols that provide such low exposure to ultrasound energy (12 minutes over 12 weeks).

There is good research evidence to support the use of electrical stimulation therapy treatment of various types of chronic wounds and the use of ultrasound treatment of chronic venous ulcers.

Inconsistent findings. The ability of PCT to heal venous ulcers was examined in 7 controlled clinical trials that involved more than 350 individuals with chronic venous leg ulcers. A systematic review of these research studies found conflicting results.[101] A Cochrane review updated in 2008 concluded that further research is required before it can be determined if PCT can promote healing of venous leg ulcers.[102] Recent work by Nikolovska and colleagues suggested that faster PCT with shorter inflation times (6 seconds on/12 seconds off) may be more effective than traditional treatment cycles (60 seconds on/30 seconds off).[103] Controlled clinical trials have shown other clinical benefits of PCT, including an increase in transcutaneous oxygen tension, improved arterial flow, and reduced edema.[104]

In summary, several controlled clinical trials have been performed to examine the effectiveness of PCT for venous ulcers. However, the results from these trials have been inconsistent. Compilation of data from these reports using meta-analyses has produced no conclusive support for their clinical use. Further research involving larger numbers of subjects is required.

Limited evidence. Inhibitory *effects of UVC* on bacterial growth are well established.[54] Two small, randomized, clinical trials showed that ultraviolet light treatment accelerates closure of chronic infected ulcers.[105,106] These clinical reports together with recent reports of the inhibitory action of UVC on antibiotic-resistant strains of bacteria[54,55] warrant consideration of the use of this modality for the treatment of chronic infected wounds. Should preliminary findings be confirmed, UVC also may be helpful in stimulating re-epithelization of superficial pressure ulcers.[56]

Physical therapists commonly use *hydrotherapy* to aid healing of chronic wounds. However, only 2 relatively small controlled trials exist to support this practice, and little new research has appeared in the current literature.[73,107] Given the paucity of research evidence and the risk of complications, the use of hydrotherapy in promoting new tissue formation in clean, nonhealing ulcers should be evaluated carefully.

Non-contact, non-thermal acoustic therapy is a relatively new modality available to accelerate healing, and initial reports on diabetic foot wounds suggest that this novel treatment approach warrants future consideration.[46] Whether this modality is also of benefit for healing other common types of wounds will be of interest.

Modalities, such as hydrotherapy, UVC, and acoustic therapy, have very limited clinical research evidence of their benefits on chronic wounds. Preliminary findings of 1 or more clinical trials involving less than 100 subjects suggest these therapies could potentially improve healing of certain types of chronic wounds; however, future research involving a greater number of appropriate subjects with a particular type of wound is required to confirm these initial reports.

No benefit. Several clinical trials have tested the ability of LLLT to accelerate closure of chronic wounds over appropriate controls. These include 5 small but well controlled clinical trials that have been published recently.[108–112] Results were inconsistent (3 of 5 studies found no benefit of LLLT).

While differences in the LLLT treatment protocols might explain inconsistent findings, *until factors that dictate biological responses to LLLT are better understood, this therapy will continue to lack research support.* Rather, there appears to be mounting evidence in well designed clinical trials that LLLT, as we are currently using it, has no added benefit to accelerate healing of chronic wounds. This conclusion is controversial, since other experts in this field suggest that positive findings are available in the majority of better designed clinical trials[58,113] and in studies where higher intensity light therapy is provided.[58]

Indications for Therapeutic Modalities for Wound Treatment

Various modalities speed wound closure of chronic wounds by affecting different cellular processes in the wound healing cascade. Research is emerging to suggest that many therapeutic modalities that deliver external *energy in various forms can activate nitric oxide production and release*. This in turn activates growth factors, including VEGF, a potent stimulator of new vessel growth and re-epithelization. It has been suggested that this may be a common pathway by which several agents influence tissue repair and regeneration.[33] Clearly, this hypothesis relies on the assumption that these energies will reach target tissues at an optimal intensity capable of

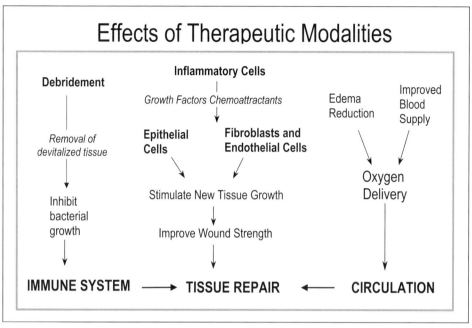

Figure I. Effects of therapeutic modalities.

biostimulation. In light of this recent work, it is possible that clinicians wishing to select the ideal treatment for clients with chronic wounds may have a choice of physical agents that act similarly to stimulate healing. If this is the case, other factors need to be considered, such as clinical research evidence, practical issues associated with accessing the therapy in the local healthcare setting, and patient preference.

Electrical currents applied using 2 electrodes (capacitive coupling) are effective in virtually all phases of wound healing (Figure 1). Electrical stimulation also is known to help reduce bacterial bioburden in wounds, enhance tissue perfusion, and block painful stimuli coming from the wound. Clinical studies suggest that it can speed closure of common types of chronic wounds including pressure ulcers, diabetic foot ulcers, venous leg ulcers, and critically ischemic wounds. Based on both experimental and clinical research evidence, clinicians may find this modality very versatile for a wide range of clinical indications.

Although EMFs are believed to directly stimulate cellular processes of healing similar to electrical fields produced by capacitive cou-

pling, there is compelling research evidence to suggest that this modality can stimulate local circulation and enhance tissue oxygenation. Recent use of EMFs in the discipline of plastic surgery has demonstrated the efficacy of EMF treatment for managing the painful postoperative period for patients undergoing elective cosmetic surgery.[36] *Current research supports the use of EMFs to treat chronic wounds that lack appropriate tissue oxygenation or have impaired local circulation*, such as chronic venous ulcers.

Ultrasound may be best administered early in the healing process to activate the inflammatory process or to stimulate new tissue formation of nonhealing but clean ulcers. There is little evidence to suggest that ultrasound administered during later proliferative or remodeling phases will have any significant effect on the biomechanical properties of the wound tissue. It has been suggested that ultrasound induces circulatory changes that enhance healing via augmentation of local tissue perfusion and oxygenation. However, there is relatively little evidence to show that pulsed ultrasound, which is typically used to treat chronic wounds, can stimulate vasodilation of local arterioles and augment local blood flow in the short term. There is also limited evidence to suggest that pulsed ultrasound delivered at the intensity recommended for wound healing can attenuate pain signals. Perhaps this may occur secondarily to a quicker resolution of the inflammatory phase of repair. However, the ability of ultrasound to alter nerve transmission of pain signals is lacking, and few studies have detected a significant reduction in pain intensity after ultrasound treatment of soft tissue injury. Based on current research involving traditional megahertz ultrasound, it is likely to be most effective when administered to stalled wounds that require stimulation to reactivate the wound healing processes. Acoustic therapy seems to possess some unique bactericidal properties that may help treat locally infected wounds.

Pneumatic compression therapy is a modality that can be used in conjunction with compression bandages for chronic leg ulcers that are not healing due to persistent and extensive leg edema caused by chronic venous insufficiency. Bactericidal effects of UVC suggest that it is indicated for the treatment of chronic infected wounds that are overburdened with surface bacteria or are contaminated with bacteria that have become resistant to antibiotic therapy. Recent clinical research suggests that this modality also may be beneficial in the treatment of non-infected pressure ulcers requiring debridement.[56]

Hydrotherapy is indicated to assist with wound cleansing and non-specific wound debridement. Therefore, short hydrotherapy treatments can be applied to wounds filled with foreign matter, necrotic tissue, or topical treatment residues. Practical considerations have dictated that the majority of wounds treated with hydrotherapy tanks are lower-limb wounds. Because of the risk of acquiring waterborne wound contamination, hydrotherapy treatments should be discontinued once the wound bed is clean and free of devitalized tissues.

Conclusion

The use of therapeutic modalities for the treatment of chronic wounds is an active area of current research. *A growing body of research supports the use of certain therapeutic modalities in the treatment of recalcitrant chronic wounds, in particular the use of electrical stimulation therapy for chronic pressure ulcers and therapeutic ultrasound for the treatment of chronic venous ulcers.* Through the building of interdisciplinary wound care teams and the education of fellow healthcare professionals, these adjunctive therapies can be offered to patients who have chronic wounds and may wish for a more conservative and cost-effective treatment program.

Practice Pearls
- A collaborative approach between a nurse who has extensive training in wound care and a physical therapist with background in the use of therapeutic modalities is ideal.
- Longer treatment times may not necessarily produce better outcomes.
- It may be best to optimize the wound environment by coordinating electrotherapy treatments with the timing of wound dressing changes.
- Clinicians require specialized training to learn the proper use of novel equipment and competence with the techniques necessary to apply electrical stimulation safely and effectively to the wound bed.
- While treatments applied outside the wounds offer practical benefits, they typically require longer exposure times and produce less consistent results.

Self-Assessment Questions

1. The therapeutic modality that currently has the strongest research evidence to support its use in the treatment of chronic pressure ulcers is:
   A. Therapeutic ultrasound
   B. Ultraviolet C therapy
   C. Electrical stimulation
   D. Electromagnetic fields
   E. Hydrotherapy

2. Which of the following therapeutic modalities may increase the possibility of wound infection?
   A. Ultraviolet C therapy
   B. Low-level light therapy including lasers

C. Electrical stimulation

D. Hydrotherapy

E. Both B and D

3. Which of the following therapeutic modalities can be applied to the periwound skin with the wound dressing intact?

A. Electrical stimulation

B. Therapeutic ultrasound

C. Ultraviolet C light

D. Pneumatic compression therapy

E. Both B and D

4. Which of the following therapeutic modalities has/have been shown to improve tissue oxygen perfusion in human subjects with impaired circulation or open wounds?

A. Electrical stimulation

B. Therapeutic ultrasound administered in pulsed mode

C. Hydrotherapy

D. Electromagnetic fields

E. Both A and D

Answers: 1–C, 2–E, 3–E, 4–E

References

1. Houghton PE, Nussbaum E, Hoens A. Safe practice procedures for all electrophysical agents treatments. *Physiotherapy Canada.* 2010;62(5):74–75.
2. Houghton PE, Campbell KE, Fraser CH, et al. Electrical stimulation therapy increases rate of healing of pressure ulcers in community-dwelling people with spinal cord injury. *Arch Phys Med Rehabil.* 2010;91(5):669–678.
3. Cheng K, Davis SC, Oliveria-Gandia M, et al. Confirmation of the electrical potential induced by occlusive dressings. Presented at the Symposium on Advanced Wound Care. 1995.
4. Kloth LC, Zhao M. Endogenous and exogenous electrical fields for wound healing. In: McCulloch J, Kloth L, eds. *Wound Healing: Evidence-Based Management.* 4th ed. Philadelphia, PA: FA Davis Company; 2010:450–513.
5. Nishimura KY, Isseroff RR, Nuccitelli R. Human keratinocytes migrate to the negative pole in direct current electric fields comparable to those measured in mammalian wounds. *J Cell Sci.* 1996;109(Pt 1):199–207.
6. Zhao M, Song B, Pu J, et al. Electrical signals control wound healing through phosphatidylinositol-3-OH kinase-gamma and PTEN. *Nature.* 2006;442(7101):457–460.
7. Zhao M. Electrical fields in wound healing — an overriding signal that directs cell migration. *Semin Cell Dev Biol.* 2009;20(6):674–682.
8. Pu J, McCaig CD, Cao L, Zhao Z, Segall JE, Zhao M. EGF receptor signalling is essential for electric-field-directed migration of breast cancer cells. *J Cell Sci.*

2007;120(Pt 19):3396–3403.
9. Cheng K, Goldman RJ. Electric fields and proliferation in a dermal wound model: cell cycle kinetics. *Bioelectromagnetics.* 1998;19(2):68–74.
10. Smith J, Romansky N, Vomero J, Davis RH. The effect of electrical stimulation on wound healing in diabetic mice. *J Am Pod Assoc.* 1984;74(2):71–75.
11. Cosmo P, Svensson H, Bornmyr S, Wikström SO. Effects of transcutaneous nerve stimulation on the microcirculation in chronic leg ulcers. *Scand J Plast Reconstr Surg Hand Surg.* 2000;34(1):61–64.
12. Im MJ, Lee WP, Hoopes JE. Effect of electrical stimulation on survival of skin flaps in pigs. *Phys Ther.* 1990;70(1):37–40.
13. Kjartansson J, Lundeberg T, Samuelson UE, Dalsgaard CJ. Transcutaneous electrical nerve stimulation (TENS) increases survival of ischaemic musculocutaneous flaps. *Acta Physiol Scand.* 1988;134(1):95–99.
14. Patterson C, Runge MS. Therapeutic angiogenesis: the new electrophysiology? *Circulation.* 1999;99(20):2614–2616.
15. Junger M, Zuder D, Steins A, Hahn M, Klyscz T. Treatment of venous ulcers with low frequency pulsed current (Dermapulse): effects on cutaneous microcirculation. *Hautarzt.* 1997;48(12):897–903.
16. Mawson AR, Siddiqui FH, Connolly BJ, et al. Effect of high voltage pulsed galvanic stimulation on sacral transcutaneous oxygen tension levels in the spinal cord injured. *Paraplegia.* 1993;31(5):311–319.
17. Gilcreast DM, Stotts NA, Froelicher ES, Baker LL, Moss KM. Effect of electrical stimulation on foot skin perfusion in persons with or at risk for diabetic foot ulcers. *Wound Repair Regen.* 1998;6(5):434–441.
18. Chu CS, McManus AT, Pruitt BA Jr, Mason AD Jr. Therapeutic effects of silver nylon dressings with weak direct current on *Pseudomonas aeruginosa*-infected burn wounds. *J Trauma.* 1988;28(10):1488–1492.
19. Costerton JW, Ellis B, Lam K, Johnson F, Khoury AE. Mechanism of electrical enhancement of efficacy of antibiotics in killing biofilm bacteria. *Antimicrob Agents Chemother.* 1994;38(12):2803–2809.
20. Houghton PE. Therapeutic modalities effects on tissue repair and chronic wounds. In: Prentice W, ed. *Therapeutic Modalities for Physical Therapists.* 4th ed. New York, NY: McGraw Hill Inc; 2010.
21. Kaada B. Promoted healing of chronic ulceration by transcutaneous nerve stimulation (TNS). *Vasa.* 1983;12(3):262–269.
22. Baker LL, Rubayi S, Villar F, Demuth SK. Effect of electrical stimulation waveform on healing of ulcers in human beings with spinal cord injury. *Wound Repair Regen.* 1996;4(1):21–28.
23. Peters EJ, Armstrong DG, Wunderlich RP, Bosma J, Stacpoole-Shea S, Lavery LA. The benefit of electrical stimulation to enhance perfusion in persons with diabetes mellitus. *J Foot Ankle Surg.* 1998;37(5):396–400.
24. Feedar JA, Kloth LC, Gentzkow GD. Chronic dermal ulcer healing enhanced by monophasic pulsed electrical stimulation. *Physical Therapy.* 1991;71:639–649.
25. Ahmad ET. High-voltage pulsed galvanic stimulation: effect of treatment duration on healing of chronic pressure

ulcers. *Ann Burns Fire Disasters*. 2008;21(3):124–128.

26. Newton RA, Karselis TC. Skin pH following high voltage pulsed galvanic stimulation. *Phys Ther.* 1983;63(10):1593–1596.

27. Koel G, Houghton PE. A systematic review: effectiveness of electrical stimulation for wound healing. Presented at the European Pressure Ulcer Advisory Panel (EPUAP) in Birmingham, UK, August, 2010.

28. Houghton PE, Nussbaum E, Hoens A. Electrical stimulation therapy (TENS, NMES, and HVPC). *Physiotherapy Canada*. 2010;62(5):27–38.

29. Callaghan MJ, Chang EI, Seiser N, et al. Pulsed electromagnetic fields accelerate normal and diabetic wound healing by increasing endogenous FGF-2 release. *Plast Reconstr Surg*. 2008;121(1):130–141.

30. Strauch B, Patel MK, Rosen DJ, Mahadevia S, Brindzei N, Pilla AA. Pulsed magnetic field therapy increases tensile strength in a rat Achilles' tendon repair model. *J Hand Surg Am*. 2006;31(7):1131–1135.

31. Weber RV, Navarro A, Wu JK, Yu HL, Strauch B. Pulsed magnetic fields applied to a transferred arterial loop support the rat groin composite flap. *Plast Reconstr Surg*. 2004;114(5):1185–1189.

32. Strauch B, Patel MK, Navarro JA, Berdichevsky M, Yu HL, Pilla AA. Pulsed magnetic fields accelerate cutaneous wound healing in rats. *Plast Reconstr Surg*. 2007;120(2):425–430.

33. Ennis WJ, Lee C, Meneses P. A biochemical approach to wound healing through the use of modalities. *Clin Dermatol*. 2007;25(1):63–72.

34. Mayrovitz H, Larsen P. A preliminary study to evaluate the effect of pulsed radio frequency field treatment on lower extremity periulcer skin microcirculation of diabetic patients. *WOUNDS*. 1995;7:90–93.

35. Sussman C. Pulsed short wave diathermy and pulsed radio frequency stimulation. In: Sussman C, Bates-Jensen B, eds. *Wound Care: A Collaborative Practice Manual for Physical Therapists and Nurses*. 2nd ed. Gaithersburg, MD: Aspen Publications Inc.; 2001:405–426.

36. Hedén P, Pilla AA. Effects of pulsed electromagnetic fields on post operative pain: a double-blind randomized pilot study in breast augmentation patients. *Aesthetic Plast Surg*. 2008;32(4):660–666.

37. Houghton PE, Nussbaum E, Hoens A. Short wave therapy: thermal and non thermal. *Physiotherapy Canada*. 2010;62(5):63–73.

38. Watson T. Ultrasound in contemporary physiotherapy practice. *Ultrasonics*. 2008;48(4):321–329.

39. Gan BS, Huys S, Sherebrin MH, Scilley CG. The effects of ultrasound treatment on flexor tendon healing in the chicken limb. *J Hand Surg*. 1995;20B(6):809–814.

40. Callam MJ, Dale JJ, Harper DR, Ruckley CV, Prescott RJ. A controlled trial of weekly ultrasound therapy of chronic leg ulceration. *Lancet*. 1987;July 25:204–205.

41. Brueton RN, Campbell B. The use of Geliperm as a sterile coupling agent for therapeutic ultrasound. *Physiotherapy*. 1987;73(12):653–654.

42. Eriksson SV, Lundeberg T, Malm M. A placebo controlled trial of ultrasound therapy in chronic leg ulceration. *Scand J Rehabil Med*. 1991;23(4):211–213.

43. Houghton PE, Nussbaum E, Hoens A. Continuous and pulsed ultrasound. *Physiotherapy Canada*. 2010;62(5):13–25.

44. Thawer HA, Houghton PE. Effects of ultrasound delivered through a mist of saline to wounds in mice with diabetes mellitus. *J Wound Care*. 2004;13(5):171–176.

45. Ennis WJ, Foremann P, Mozen N, Massey J, Conner-Kerr T, Meneses P. Ultrasound therapy for recalcitrant diabetic foot ulcers: results of a randomized, double-blind, controlled, multicenter study. *Ostomy Wound Manage*. 2005;51(8):24–39.

46. Serena T, Lee SK, Lam K, Attar P, Meneses P, Ennis W. The impact of noncontact, nonthermal, low-frequency ultrasound on bacterial counts in experimental and chronic wounds. *Ostomy Wound Manage*. 2009;55(1):22–30.

47. Unger PG. Low-frequency, noncontact, nonthermal ultrasound therapy: a review of the literature. *Ostomy Wound Manage*. 2008;54(1):57–60.

48. Farr PM, Diffey BL. The erythemal response of human skin to ultraviolet radiation. *Br J Dermatol*. 1985;113(1):65–76.

49. Davidson SF, Brantley SK, Johnson SG, Hsu HS, Das SK. The effects of ultraviolet irradiation on wound contraction in the hairless guinea pig. *Br J Plast Surg*. 1992;45(7):508–511.

50. High AS, High JP. Treatment of infected skin wounds using ultra-violet radiation — an *in-vitro* study. *Physiotherapy*. 1983;69(10):359–360.

51. Conner-Kerr TA, Sullivan PK, Gaillard J, Franklin ME, Jones RM. The effects of ultraviolet radiation on antibiotic-resistant bacteria *in vitro*. *Ostomy Wound Manage*. 1998;44(10):50–56.

52. Hall JD, Mount DW. Mechanism of DNA replication and mutagenesis in ultraviolet-irradiated bacteria and mammalian cells. *Prog Nucleic Acid Res Mol Biol*. 1981;25:53–126.

53. Conner-Kerr TA. Light therapy. In: McCulloch JM, Kloth LC, eds. *Wound Healing Evidence Based Management*. 4th ed. Philadelphia, PA: FA Davis Company; 2010:650–613.

54. Thai TP, Keast DH, Campbell KE, Woodbury MG, Houghton PE. Effect of ultraviolet light C on bacterial colonization in chronic wounds. *Ostomy Wound Manage*. 2005;51(10):32–45.

55. Thai TP, Houghton PE, Campbell KE, Woodbury MG. Ultraviolet light C in the treatment of chronic wounds with MRSA: a case study. *Ostomy Wound Manage*. 2002;48(11):52–60.

56. Nussbaum E, Flett H, McGillivray C. Ultraviolet-C (UVC) improves wound healing in persons with spinal cord injury (SCI). Presented at the International Spinal Cord Society meeting in Washington, DC, June 4–8, 2011.

57. Conner-Kerr TA. Wound technology: the future is now. *Extended Care Product News*. 2005;104:34–39.

58. Nussbaum EL, Baxter GD, Lilge L. A review of laser technology and light tissue interactions as a background to therapeutic applications of low intensity lasers and other light sources. *Physical Therapy Reviews*. 2003;8:31–44.

59. Enwemeka CS. Laser biostimulation of healing wounds: specific effects and mechanisms of action. *J*

Orthop Sports Phys Ther. 1988;9(10):333–338.

60. Allendorf JD, Bessler M, Huang J, et al. Helium-neon laser irradiation at fluences of 1, 2, and 4 J/cm² failed to accelerate wound healing as assessed by both wound contracture rate and tensile strength. *Lasers Surg Med*. 1997;20(3):340–345.

61. Yu W, Naim JO, Lanzafame RJ. Effects of photostimulation on wound healing in diabetic mice. *Lasers Surg Med*. 1997;20(1):56–63.

62. Franzen-Korzendorfer H, Blackinton M, Rone-Adams S, McCulloch J. The effect of monochromatic infrared energy on transcutaneous oxygen measurements and protective sensation: results of a controlled, double-blind, randomized clinical study. *Ostomy Wound Manage*. 2008;54(6):16–31.

63. Nussbaum EL, Lilge L, Mazzulli T. Effects of 630-, 660-, 810-, and 905-nm laser irradiation delivering radiant exposure of 1-50 J/cm² on three species of bacteria in vivo. *J Clin Laser Med Surg*. 2002;20(6):325–333.

64. Cambier D, Vanderstaraeten G. Helium neon laser: a contraindication for infected wounds? *In vitro* study on *Pseudomonas aeruginosa*. *Lasers Med Sci*. 1997;12:151–156.

65. Lilge L, Tierney K, Nussbaum EL. Low-level-laser therapy for wound healing: Feasibility of wound dressing translumination. *J Clin Laser Med Surg*. 2000;18(5):235–240.

66. Niederhuber SS, Stribley RF, Koepke GH. Reduction of skin bacterial load with use of the therapeutic whirlpool. *Phys Ther*. 1975;55(5):482–486.

67. Bohannon RW. Whirlpool versus whirlpool rinse for removal of bacteria from a venous stasis ulcer. *Phys Ther*. 1982;62(3):304–308.

68. Solomon SL. Host factors in whirlpool-associated *Pseudomonas aeruginosa* skin disease. *Infect Control*. 1985;6(10):402–406.

69. Embil JM, McLeod JA, Al-Barrak AM, et al. An outbreak of methicillin resistant *Staphylococcus aureus* on a burn unit: potential role of contaminated hydrotherapy equipment. *Burns*. 2001;27(7):681–688.

70. Stanwood W, Pinzur MS. Risk of contamination of the wound in a hydrotherapeutic tank. *Foot Ankle Int*. 1998;19(3):173–176.

71. McCulloch JM, Boyd VB. The effects of whirlpool and the dependent position on lower extremity volume. *J Orthop Sports Phys Ther*. 1992;16(4):169–173.

72. Ogiwara S. Calf muscle pumping and rest positions during and/or after whirlpool therapy. *J Phys Ther Sci*. 2001;13(2):99–105.

73. Haynes LJ, Brown MH, Handley BC, et al. Comparison of pulsavac and sterile whirlpool regarding the promotion of tissue granulation [abstract]. *Physical Ther*. 1994;74(Suppl 5):54.

74. Svoboda SJ, Bice TG, Gooden HA, Brooks DE, Thomas DB, Wenke JC. Comparison of bulb syringe and pulsed lavage irrigation with use of a bioluminescent musculoskeletal wound model. *J Bone Joint Surg Am*. 2006;88(10):2167–2174.

75. Owens BD, White DW, Wenke JC. Comparison of irrigation solutions and devices in a contaminated musculoskeletal wound survival model. *J Bone Joint Surg Am*. 2009;91(1):92–98.

76. Delis KT, Husmann MJ, Nicolaides AN, Wolfe JH,

Cheshire NJ. Enhancing foot skin blood flux in peripheral vascular disease using intermittent pneumatic compression: controlled study on claudicants and grafted arteriopaths. *World J Surg*. 2002;26(7):861–866.

77. Tan X, Qi WN, Gu X, Urbaniak JR, Chen LE. Intermittent pneumatic compression regulates expression of nitric oxide synthases in skeletal muscle. *J Biomech*. 2006;39(13):2430–2437.

78. Adunsky A, Ohry A; DDCT Group. Decubitus direct current treatment (DDCT) of pressure ulcers: results of a randomized double-blinded placebo controlled study. *Arch Gerontol Geriatr*. 2005;41(3):261–269.

79. Franek A, Taradaj J, Polak A, Cierpka L, Basczak E. Efficacy of high voltage stimulation for healing of venous leg ulcers in surgically and conservatively treated patients. *Phlebologie*. 2006;35:127–133.

80. Jankovic A, Binic I. Frequency rhythmic electrical modulation system in the treatment of chronic painful leg ulcers. *Arch Dermatol Res*. 2008;300(7):377–383.

81. Jünger M, Arnold A, Zuder D, Stahl HW, Heising S. Local therapy and treatment costs of chronic, venous leg ulcers with electrical stimulation (Dermapulse): a prospective, placebo controlled, double blind trial. *Wound Repair Regen*. 2008;16(4):480–487.

82. Santos RP, Nascimento CA, De Andrade EN. Use of high voltage electrical stimulation in healing of venous ulcers [Uso da eletroestimulacao de alta voltagem na cicatrizacao de ulceras venosas]. *Fisioterapia Movemento*. 2009;22(4):615–623.

83. Petrofsky JS, Lawson D, Berk L, Suh H. Enhanced healing of diabetic foot ulcers using local heat and electrical stimulation for 30 min three times per week. *J Diabetes*. 2010;2(1):41–46.

84. Kloth LC. Electrical stimulation for wound healing: a review of evidence from *in vitro* studies, animal experiments, and clinical trials. *Int J Low Extrem Wounds*. 2005;4(1):23–44.

85. European Pressure Ulcer Advisory Panel and National Pressure Ulcer Advisory Panel. Treatment of pressure ulcers: Quick Reference Guide. Washington, DC: National Pressure Ulcer Advisory Panel; 2009.

86. Fernandez-Chimeno M, Houghton PE, Holey L. Electrical stimulation for chronic wounds (Protocol). *Cochrane Database of Systemic Reviews*. 2004;(1):CD004550.

87. Houghton PE, Koel G. Electrical stimulation increases number of ulcers healed. Preliminary findings of a Cochrane review. Presented at the World Confederation of Physical Therapy 2011 in Amsterdam, Netherlands, June 2011.

88. McMeeken JM. Magnetic fields: Effects on blood flow in human subjects. *Physiotherapy Theory and Practice*. 1992;8:3–9.96.

89. McGaughney H, Dhamija S, Oliver S, Porter-Armstrong A, McDonough S. Pulsed electromagnetic energy in management of chronic wounds: a systematic review. *Physical Therapy Reviews*. 2009;14(2):132–146.

90. Ieran M, Zaffuto S, Bagnacani M, Annovi M, Moratti A, Cadossi R. Effect of low frequency pulsing electromagnetic fields on skin ulcers of venous origin in humans: a double-blind study. *J Orthop Res*. 1990;8(2):276–282.

91. Salzberg CA, Cooper-Vastola SA, Perez F, Viehbeck

MG, Byrne DW. The effects of non-thermal pulsed electromagnetic energy on wound healing of pressure ulcers in spinal cord-injured patients: a randomized, double-blind study. *Ostomy Wound Manage.* 1995;41(3):42–51.

92. Comorosan S, Vasilco R, Arghiropol M, Paslaru L, Jieanu V, Stelea S. The effect of diapulse therapy on the healing of decubitus ulcer. *Rom J Physiol.* 1993;30(1-2):41–45.

93. Aziz Z, Cullum NA, Flemming K. Electromagnetic therapy for treating venous leg ulcers. *Cochrane Database Syst Rev.* 2011;(3):CD002933.

94. Aziz Z, Flemming K, Cullum NA, Olyaee Manesh A. Electromagnetic therapy for treating pressure ulcers. *Cochrane Database Syst Rev.* 2010;(11):CD002930.

95. Baba-Akbari Sari A, Flemming K, Cullum NA, Wollina U. Therapeutic ultrasound for pressure ulcers. *Cochrane Database Syst Rev.* 2006;(3):CD001275.

96. Cullum NA, Al-Kurdi D, Bell-Syer SE. Therapeutic ultrasound for venous leg ulcers. *Cochrane Database Syst Rev.* 2010;(6):CD001180.

97. Franek A, Chmielewska D, Brzezinska-Wcislo L, Slezak A, Blaszczak E. Application of various power densities of ultrasound in the treatment of leg ulcers. *J Dermatolog Treat.* 2004;15(6):379–386.

98. Dolibog P, Franek A, et al. Application of different power densities of pulsed ultrasound in the treatment of leg ulcers. *J Dermatol Treatment.* 2004;15(6):379–386.

99. Taradaj J, Franek A, Brzezinska-Wcislo L, et al. The use of therapeutic ultrasound in venous leg ulcers: a randomized, controlled clinical trial. *Phlebology.* 2008;23(4):178–183.

100. Watson JM, Kang'ombe AR, Soares MO, et al. Use of weekly, low dose, high frequency ultrasound for hard to heal leg ulcers: the VenUS III randomised controlled trial. *BMJ.* 2011;342:d1092.

101. O'Sullivan-Drombolis DK, Houghton PE. Pneumatic compression in the treatment of chronic ulcers. *Physical Therapy Reviews.* 2009;14(2):81–91.

102. Nelson EA, Mani R, Vowden K. Intermittent pneumatic compression for treating venous leg ulcers. *Cochrane Database Syst Rev.* 2008;(2):CD001899.

103. Nikolovska S, Arsovski A, Damevska K, Gocev G, Pavlova L. Evaluation of two different intermittent pneumatic compression cycle settings in the healing of venous ulcers: a randomized trial. *Med Sci Monit.* 2005;11(7):CR337–CR343.

104. Iwama H, Suzuki M, Hojo M, Kaneda M, Akutsu I. Intermittent pneumatic compression on the calf improves peripheral circulation of the leg. *J Crit Care.* 2000;15(1):18–21.

105. Burger A, Jordaan AJ, Schoombee GE. The bactericidal effect of ultraviolet light on infected pressure sores. *S Afr J Physiother.* 1985;41:55–57.

106. Wills EE, Anderson TW, Beattie BL, Scott A. A randomized placebo-controlled trial of ultraviolet light in the treatment of superficial pressure sores. *J Am Geriatr Soc.* 1983;31(3):131–133.

107. Burke DT, Ho CH, Saucier MA, Stewart G. Effects of hydrotherapy on pressure ulcer healing. *Am J Phys Med Rehabil.* 1998;77(5):394–398.

108. Dehlin O, Esmståhl S, Gottrup F. Monochromatic phototherapy: effective treatment for grade II chronic pressure ulcers in elderly patients. *Aging Clin Exp Res.* 2007;19(6):478–483.

109. Durovic A, Maric D, Brdareski Z, Jevtic M, Durdevic S. The effects of polarized light therapy in pressure ulcer healing. *Vojnosanit Pregl.* 2008;65(12):906–912.

110. Kaviani A, Djavid GE, Ataie-Fashtami L, et al. A randomized clinical trial on the effect of low-level laser therapy on chronic diabetic foot wound healing: a preliminary report. *Photomed Laser Surg.* 2011;29(2):109–114.

111. Leclère FM, Puechguiral IR, Rotteleur G, Thomas P, Mordon SR. A prospective randomized study of 980 nm diode laser-assisted venous ulcer healing on 34 patients. *Wound Repair Regen.* 2010;18(6):580–585.

112. Minatel DG, Frade MA, Franca SC, Enwemeka CS. Phototherapy promotes healing of chronic diabetic leg ulcers that failed to respond to other therapies. *Laser Surg Med.* 2009;41(6):433–441.

113. Belanger AY. Laser. In: *Evidence Based Guide to Therapeutic Physical Agents.* Philidelphia, PA: Lippincott Williams & Wilkins; 2001:191–222.

Negative Pressure Wound Therapy

Adrianne P. S. Smith, MD, FACEP;
Kathy Whittington, RN, MS, CWOCN;
Robert G. Frykberg, DPM, MPH;
Jean DeLeon, MD

Objectives
The reader will be challenged to:
- Describe the use of negative pressure wound therapy (NPWT) as a standard in advanced wound care
- Review the appropriate most up-to-date information on the use of NPWT in chronic wound care
- Summarize the current understanding of proposed mechanisms of action for NPWT
- Recognize potential complications related to NPWT usage and determine interventions to reduce risks.

Introduction

"Creativity…consists largely of rearranging what we know in order to find out what we do not know. Hence, to think creatively, we must be able to look afresh at what we normally take for granted."
— *George Kneller*

Negative pressure wound therapy (NPWT) is the process by which negative pressure is distributed across a wound base via a dressing with the specific intent to promote wound healing. Over the centuries, popularity for using negative (subatmospheric) pressure to treat wounds has waxed and waned. In medical literature, negative pressure-based therapies used for wound healing have been referred to as *cupping, pneumatic occlusive therapy, passive hyperemia therapy, active drainage, suction drainage therapy, active aspiration, vacuum drainage, vacuum sealing technique (VST), topical negative pressure (TNP), subatmospheric pressure dressings (SPD), NPWT, vacuum sealing dressing (VSD), irrigation drainage,* and a patent filed in China in 2010 brought it full circle with *reduced pressure wound cupping treatment.* With each advancing generation, healthcare practitioners have observed the wound healing potential of negative pressure interpreted through the limitations of their existing knowledge of medical sciences. Spurred by innovative equipment, advances in healthcare technology, and the artistic ingenuity and technical competency of the practitioner caring for the wounded patient, NPWT has been constrained by the risk of complications, technical difficulties, inappropriate patient selection, and the need to develop a clear, defensible evidence base to support

Smith APS, Whittington K, Frykberg RG, DeLeon J. Negative pressure wound therapy. In: Krasner DL, Rodeheaver GT, Sibbald RG, Woo KY, eds. *Chronic Wound Care: A Clinical Source Book for Healthcare Professionals.* Vol 1. 5th ed. Malvern, PA: HMP Communications; 2012:271–299.

the safe and efficacious use of the proposed technique. The advent of new, portable, computer-programmable negative pressure generators, novel treatment materials, newer understandings of *"cellular" healing responses*, and modern cause-effect validation coupled with the healthcare community's burgeoning interest in tissue regeneration created the perfect storm for resurgence of a modern-day platform for NPWT. The utility of NPWT for managing complex wounds, ulcers, burns, post-operative wounds, and non-surgical tissue defects has emerged as a readily available, frequently employed, and internationally adopted therapeutic practice with applicability for acute and chronic wounds in a variety of care settings.[1,2]

The current NPWT platform was built with the full anticipation of eventually using modulations in the negative pressure profile to direct specific cellular responses to improve the healing rate, quantity, and quality of tissue generated. As with all wound care practices, the "evidential clarity and defensibility" for NPWT will be bounded by the capability of the scientific wound care community to understand and judge the merits of the process within the existing conceptual and technological constraints of the era in which they live.

Modern Perspectives of NPWT

"No single achievement in science is possible without the painstaking work of the many hundreds who have built the foundation on which all new work is based." — Nobel Laureate Polykarp Kusch

The current NPWT platform witnessed a surge in popularity when Dr. Louis Argenta and Dr. Michael Morykwas at Wake Forest University developed Vacuum Assisted Closure® (V.A.C.®) Therapy (KCI USA, Inc., San Antonio, Texas) to optimize the benefits of subatmospheric (negative) pressure for wound healing[1,2] with special focus on perfusion and granulation tissue development.[3] This integrated system uses a computerized therapy unit to intermittently or continuously deliver negative pressure through a resilient, open-cell foam surface dressing that is sealed with an adhesive drape. The original tubing design had a terminal pad, sealed in contact with the foam, which delivered wound space pressures and redirected wound exudate into a specially designed, disposable canister.

While the basic components of the NPWT systems remain the same, ongoing research has led to the development of added features and associated benefits for many devices. For example, the Therapeutic Regulated Accurate Care (T.R.A.C.™) Pad used with the V.A.C. Therapy system added pressure sensing ports along the collection tubing to improve monitoring and maintenance of the set target pressure at the wound site as an initial design improvement over the process of inserting the cut end of the collection tube directly into the foam. The SensaT.R.A.C.™ Technology design improvement facilitated increased exudate collection. Improved ability to accurately maintain pressure in a variety of environmental conditions and to alert caregivers through various alarms has contributed to acceptance of NPWT for certification as safe-to-fly on some military air transport vehicles.

Additional refinements have included *Smart Alarms*™ that alert caregivers when corrective action is needed and, in some conditions, interrupt therapy if critical programmed parameters are met. The therapy unit alarms in any of the following conditions:
- The canister is full, missing, or improperly placed
- The tubing is blocked
- The tubing or dressing has air leaks
- Therapy is inactive
- The battery is low.

V.A.C. Therapy is intended to create an environment that *promotes wound healing* by secondary or tertiary (delayed primary) intention by preparing the wound bed for closure, removing exudate and infectious material, reducing edema, promoting granulation tissue formation, and promoting perfusion.[2] V.A.C. Therapy is indicated for patients with chronic, acute, traumatic, subacute, and dehisced wounds; partial-thickness burns; ulcers (such as diabetic or pressure); flaps; and grafts.[4]

NPWT Systems

"Without continual growth and progress, such words as improvement, achievement, and success have no meaning." — Benjamin Franklin

V.A.C. Therapy System, marketed in the United States since 1995, serves as a predicate device for a series of products approved for NPWT. Characteristically described, the current NPWT platform has evolved to include several key components: 1) an electric-powered or non-powered *negative pressure generating "pump"* with continuous and/or intermittent negative pressure modality, 2) *connective tubing* to convey pressure changes to the wound space, provide a conduit to remove exudate, and, in some cases, monitor the pressure delivered to the wound space, 3) a water-impermeable, adhesive-sealed occlusive, *oxygen- and water vapor-semipermeable drape* to protect against pressure loss and wound contamination, 4) an *interface dressing* (with or without a nonadherent intervening contact layer) that interacts with the tissue at the wound base, helps wick exudate from the recesses of the wound, and through which the negative pressure is delivered to the wound space, and 5) an *exudate collection process* to contain exudate removed from the wound.

NPWT System Designs and Innovations

At present, 13 manufacturers of NPWT devices are recognized by the US Centers for Medicare & Medicaid Services (CMS) for reimbursement after undergoing 510K, substantial equivalency determination with the V.A.C. Therapy System as the predicate device. US Food and Drug Administration (FDA)-approved negative pressure pumps span from simple vacuum generators to fully computerized feedback systems, non-powered or electrically powered with and without battery backup, variably capable of generating and monitoring continuous and intermittent negative pressure. *Device alarms* strive to improve the therapeutic safety profile, especially related to identifying situations that may be related to serious and potentially fatal blood loss. NPWT has undergone a tremendous expansion attesting to the extensive applicability of subatmospheric (negative) therapy to multiple clinical situations and care settings. The following generalized, non-comprehensive review of key component modifications is designed to provide insight to the product variation available. Comparative impact of specific therapy and device variances on clinical wound healing outcomes has yet to be fully determined.

Pumps. Prior to the development of computer-regulated pumps, wall suction was used for evacuation of exudate from wounds. While effective for wound exudate management, wall suction techniques create an abrupt drawdown and do not allow for pulsed regulated pressure delivery. Initial modifications on the predicate device were focused on proof of concept and assuring delivery of programmed negative pressure through wound site feedback, monitoring for continuous and intermittent pressure, expanding ranges for negative pressure (-40 mmHg to 230 mmHg) to increase number of approved manufacturers, validating antimicrobial gauze dressing as an appropriate alternative "filler material," decreasing noise, and improving portability. Presumably, modulating pressure cycle times, peak pressure, pressure wave patterns, and treatment regimes influences tissue cellular content, collagen and extracellular matrix deposition, and quantity and rate of generation. "Optimal" tissue healing would be achieved through response-adjusted negative pressure treatment profiles. Previously, lower pressure ranges and gauze were the focus of newer devices to distinguish themselves from the predicate device. Current device improvements seek further portability, ease of use, and universal applicability. Some newer devices are designed for use with both gauze and foam, without preferential styling, thereby securing their utilization independent of the physician's choice of therapy. For instance, XLR8® (Genadyne Biotechnologies, Great Neck, New York) was designed for maximal suitability with low weight (600 g), full-range peak pressure profile capacity (50 mmHg–230 mmHg), continuous and intermittent modality, a built-in Li-Ion battery with minimal 8-hour life, and 3-hour charge time with minimal noise levels.[5]

Power source. Previously, newer models remained electrically powered with a focus on extended battery life. Now attention has turned toward achieving non-powered, alternative energy-sourced devices and devices that are solely battery powered with imminent disposability for short-term, out-of-hospital therapy. Powered and non-powered device clinical safety considerations remain similar to those of the predicate device, even though in the United States non-powered NPWT devices are managed under a separate FDA classification guidance document.[6] The SNaP® Wound Care System (Spiracur Inc., Sunnyvale, California) is an exceptionally lightweight, "ultraportable," non-powered, mechanically generated negative pressure unit that showed special utility for ambulatory, out-of-hospital disaster-injured patients in Haiti where community electricity suffered prolonged disruption.[7]

Portability. Device evolution progressed from remarkably heavy, stationary units to exceptionally lightweight, ultraportable devices, applicable in all care settings from inpatient bedridden to outpatient fully ambulatory. The SNaP device spearheaded this body of devices by switching to a mechanically powered device that maintains a preset constant or intermittent pressure (-75, -100, or -150 mmHg) without electricity or batteries.[8] A novel engineering approach to exceptional portability was achieved through innovative design exemplified by the pocket-sized NPD 1000™ Negative Pressure Wound Therapy device (Kalypto Medical, Mendota Heights, Minnesota) that runs on 3 AA batteries coupled with an antimicrobial combination collection system dressing pad.[9] Other devices followed suit to join the roles of improved portability through "miniaturization," improved economy of size for off-the-shelf availability, and improved "disposability" to optimize application for the post-operative, surgically closed, 7-day treatment, acute wound market (V.A.C.Via™ Negative Pressure Wound Therapy System, KCI USA, Inc.; XLR8 and A4-NWPT pump®, Genadyne Biotechnologies; PICO™ Single Use Negative Pressure Wound Therapy System, Smith & Nephew, Inc., St-Laurent, Quebec, Canada). Accessories also aid portability; for example, car chargers (Vario 18, Medela Inc., McHenry, Illinois) and various out-of-hospital bed connectors, hospital trolley carts, and personal carrying cases provide convenient mobility.[5,10-13]

Device-related clinical safety. Safety considerations for potential complications, such as bleeding, foreign body retention, pain, tissue ingrowth, infection, and exsanguination, exist for all NPWT systems, regardless of care setting, portability, and recommended pressure profiles. Caution should be taken to mitigate potential complications with appropriate patient selection and therapy adjustments, as needed. Alarm types are

variable, but most devices have some ability to notify in the event of an air leak and non-delivery of the intended pressure.[4]

Tubing and collection systems (drains). Tube collection systems remove exudate from the wound and deliver negative pressure to the wound space. Across various systems, tubing differs in lumen length and diameter, which affects the rate of exudate removal and the potential for obstruction development. If blockage occurs without clearance, maceration, infection, and wound deterioration may ensue. Some systems use the collection tubing as a simple conduit; others add the benefit of wound space pressure monitoring through the terminal pad (Prevena™ Incision Management System, T.R.A.C. Pad and SensaT.R.A.C., KCI USA, Inc.).[14,15] Another level of advanced negative pressure therapy delivery is achieved through software programming automatic response feedback loops. The Mobility Solutions Miller drains (Miller Digivac Toe and Finger Chambers, Miller Extremity Garments, Miller DermiVex Drain, and Miller Encompass Drain) are body location-specific silicone drains modified for use with gauze interfaces.[16,17] Dressing techniques that assist with digits and unusual contours, even in pediatric populations, have been described.

Canisters. Exudate collection canisters may be open or sealed with gel packs (isolyzers) for solidification of wound exudate. Out-of-hospital disposal of liquid blood-contaminated waste may be limited, depending upon local restrictions imposed by environmental protection regulations. Rules for collection, storage, and disposal of biohazardous materials, both liquid and solid, may apply. The isolyzer assists in converting restricted liquid waste to disposable solid waste to facilitate disposal. One-way valves between canisters and tubing systems prevent backflow of biohazardous materials onto the wound when negative pressure is discontinued. Similarly, some systems may utilize backflow prevention between the pump and the canister connection system to prevent contamination of the pump system and internal filters. Canister sizes vary depending upon the size of the associated pump, desired portability, and wound type being targeted. Canister capacities range from 25 cc to 1500 cc with and without the ability to be emptied and reused. Procedures and policies must be established for reusable products to reduce the likelihood of cross-contamination. Caution must be used with canisters greater than 500 cc as their use may increase the risk of severe fluid loss, dehydration, and exsanguination. Larger canister sizes are not recommended for neonates, infants, children, or adults with low-volume states or problems with coagulation[18] where the removal of a large percent total body fluid volume or coagulation factors may pose a significant risk. Although evidence supports the safe use of NPWT in children, the therapy should be applied to children with caution to ensure safety.[19–21]

Adhesive drape. Most adhesive drapes used with NPWT consist of water vapor-semipermeable polyurethane film coated with a hypoallergenic, pressure-sensitive acrylate adhesive. Drapes seal the environment, maintaining the negative pressure over the wound, create a barrier to outside contaminants, and provide a moist wound healing environment. This allows the underlying wound exudate to condense into a gelatinous coagulum, which supports re-epithelization at the wound margins. There are no distinctions between the drapes used in foam-based systems versus those used in gauze-based systems, and both systems typically require oxygen and water vapor semipermeability to allow for moisture balance and oxygenation of the periwound skin. Many NPWT providers will contract dressing manufacturers to produce a drape with their specific requirements for size, shape, peel tabs, adhesive content, and branding. Since these products are usually essentially equivalent to 3M™ Tegaderm™ Dressings (3M Health Care, St Paul, Minnesota),[22] transparent films are frequently used to repair leaks when the brand-specific drape is not available. Some dressing systems distinguish themselves through attempts to innovate the dressing application process. The NPD 1000 Negative Pressure Wound Therapy device does not require a secondary occlusive drape because the interface dressing and exudate process are integrated within the pad. Additionally, hydrocolloid wafers and stoma paste are often helpful to achieve a seal in difficult-to-dress locations.[23]

Irrigation systems. *NPWT "instillation systems"* also have undergone design changes for programmed wound irrigation treatments with prolonged, intermittent, or continuous profiles. Although these systems have been used predominantly to treat osteomyelitis and soft tissue infections, they can be used to deliver agents other than antibiotics, such as antimicrobial agents, chemical debriders, anti-inflammatory agents, growth factors, oxygen and energy molecules, chemotherapeutics, "liquefied" cellular and tissue components, and tissue nutritional factors. Appropriate testing to prove the safety and clinical efficacy of expanded indications would be required. This is no small feat, since the medical scientific evidential bar has been set high for demonstrating both mechanisms of action and clinical outcomes. Even with a current, fairly robust clinical retrospective evidence base,[20] achieving full reimbursement approval for NPWT for pediatric indications has been difficult to attain in all countries. The V.A.C. Instill® Therapy Unit (KCI USA, Inc.) and the irrigation systems, Svedman® and SVED® (Innovative Therapies Inc., Gaithersburg, Maryland), are the most commonly used devices.[24]

NPWT pressure treatment modalities. Most manufacturers offer devices with both continuous and intermittent pressure modalities for inpatient and outpatient care settings. Two schools of thought surround the "optimal" negative pressure treatment target: low pressure at -80 mmHg or high pressure at -125 mmHg. Some devices are designed to provide only the lower negative pressure treatment range, while others are designed to treat both the lower and higher ranges. As care setting focus shifts toward alternative care settings/ambulatory out-of-hospital, the trend has shifted to develop NPWT devices specifically designed to target wound types amenable to the continuous pressure modality, simplified operation, and lowered out-of-hospital treatment costs.

NPWT Wound Interface Materials

An interface dressing, with or without a nonadherent intervening contact layer, directly influences 1) microstrain delivery to the tissue surface, 2) exudate removal by helping to wick fluid from the recesses of the wound, and 3) negative pressure modulation as it passes into the wound space and then out to the periwound tissues. The most commonly prescribed NPWT interface dressings are foams composed of either open-cell reticulated polyethylene (PU) foam or polyvinyl alcohol (PVA) foam and an absorbent cotton-blend antimicrobial gauze containing 0.2% polyhexamethylene biguanide hydrochloride (PHMB). Some devices have developed device-specific foams: KCI USA, Inc. with GranuFoam™ and GranuFoam Silver®, Medela Inc. with Avance™ (green foam), Smith & Nephew with RENASYS®-F, and Innovative Therapies Inc. with SVED Svamp® Foam. Most gauze-based dressing kits offer antimicrobial gauze, eg, Kendall™ AMD Antimicrobial Dressings containing 0.2% PHMB (Covidien, Mansfield, Massachusetts).[25] Silverlon® (Argentum Medical, LLC, Chicago, Illinois), a silver-impregnated woven nylon, has received special recognition for utility with NPWT.[26–28] Dressings specifically designed for NPWT systems include the Bio-Dome™ dressing and Bio-Dome EasyRelease (ConvaTec, Inc., Skillman, New Jersey)[29] and the Kalypto collection pad. Adapted for use with any NPWT system, Hydrofera Blue® Bacteriostatic Dressing (Hydrofera, LLC, Willimantic, Connecticut) is a PVA sponge with two broad-spectrum bacteriostatic agents, methylene blue and gentian violet.[30] An intervening nonadherent contact dressing layer (eg, Mepitel® or Mepitel One, Mölnlycke Health Care, Norcross, Georgia) may be applied to any of the dressing systems in an effort to reduce potential complications related to dressing adherence and tissue in-growth.

NPWT foam dressings. PU and PVA are the two most common materials used to create open-cell, hydrophilic or hydrophobic, NPWT foams. Pore size and strut measurements determine the density, tensile strength, and porosity of the foam. Pore diameter, strut (cell or walls of the foam) thickness, and applied negative pressure define the microstrain delivered to the tissue surface.

V.A.C. GranuFoam. The black V.A.C. Granu-Foam PU dressing has reticulated or open pores ranging in size from 400 μm to 600 μm and is considered effective at promoting granulation tissue formation while aiding in wound contraction.[31] It is hydrophobic (or moisture repelling), which enhances exudate removal. Several specialized V.A.C. GranuFoam dressings have also been designed to accommodate the needs of specific wound sites (ie, abdominal cavity, heel, and hand).[32] These facilitate the application of negative pressure to anatomical locations with contours that make it difficult to achieve an airtight seal (Plates 13–16, page 319).

V.A.C. GranuFoam Silver. The V.A.C. GranuFoam Silver Dressing combines the properties of V.A.C. GranuFoam with those of silver. The reticulated or open pores of this dressing have microbonded metallic silver uniformly distributed throughout the dressing, providing continuous delivery of silver.[33] The V.A.C. GranuFoam Silver Dressing is an effective barrier to bacterial penetration and may help reduce infection (Plates 17–20, page 319). Topical silver has broad-spectrum antimicrobial activity. The only silver dressing specifically designed for use with V.A.C. Therapy is the V.A.C. GranuFoam Silver Dressing. This dressing provides continuous release of ionic silver for up to 72 hours and has been shown to be effective against 150 microbial species.[33] A subset of 6 organisms considered clinically relevant was selected for quantitative antimicrobial testing. A sample of the V.A.C. GranuFoam Silver Dressing was added to 50 mL of the challenge organism at approximately 10^5 colony-forming units per milliliter (CFU/mL) and incubated over time. The dressing showed significant antimicrobial activity in as little as 30 minutes after exposure to the organisms. The open-celled, reticulated structure of this dressing allowed for microdeformational changes at the foam-tissue interface in the same manner as the V.A.C. GranuFoam Dressing. A study was conducted on porcine full-thickness wounds treated with either the V.A.C. GranuFoam Dressing or the V.A.C. GranuFoam Silver Dressing to determine if granulation rates would be comparable.[33] There were no significant differences ($P > .05$) in wound granulation rates (as measured using wound volume measurements) between these 2 V.A.C. Therapy dressings. Together, these studies indicate that the properties of the V.A.C. GranuFoam dressing are retained by the V.A.C. GranuFoam Silver dressing, which assists with granulation tissue formation and serves as an effective barrier against microorganism invasion.[34]

V.A.C.® WhiteFoam® Dressing. V.A.C. WhiteFoam PVA dressing is a dense foam with a higher tensile strength that requires higher negative pressures (125 mmHg–175 mmHg) in order to provide adequate distribution of negative pressure throughout the wound. V.A.C. White-Foam is hydrophilic (or moisture maintaining), is premoistened with sterile water, and possesses relatively nonadherent properties.[31] It is generally recommended for use in tunnels and tracts and other situations where special attention is necessary to avoid the possibility of tissue in-growth into the foam.

Hydrofera Blue Bacteriostatic Dressing. Hydrofera Blue Bacteriostatic Dressing ("Blue Foam") is a PVA sponge with two broad-spectrum bacteriostatic agents, methylene blue and gentian violet. These agents are effective against the drug-resistant organisms, methicillin/oxacillin-resistant *Staphylococcus aureus* (MRSA) and vancomycin-resistant enterococci (VRE). The foam's open cell structure naturally provides capillary vacuum action to draw excess fluid and exudate from the wound bed. Hydrofera Blue must be moistened with sterile saline or sterile water and squeezed out before application to the wound bed. Color change from blue to white indicates complete release of antimicrobial agents. Case studies support the use of this foam at negative pressure ranges, both low (-80 mmHg) and high (-125 mmHg), to improve chronic wounds without any significant complications.[35,36]

Avance ("Green Foam") Dressings. Avance Foam is open-cell, hydrophobic polyurethane specifically designed for use with the Avance NPWT device at negative pressure (-120 mmHg) to provide the desired 5%–20% microstrain for enhanced cellular proliferation. Preclinical studies conducted by Malmsjö et al compared Avance Foam's biological effects to the predicate V.A.C. GranuFoam (-125 mmHg) and to AMD gauze (-80 mmHg), with and without intervening contact layers, Mepitel and Mepitel One. Specific investigations related to wound bed granulation tissue quantity, tissue in-growth into the filler material, delivery of negative pressure to the wound bed, and blood flow in the wound bed. Malmsjö and colleagues noted a more pronounced granulation tissue formation with foam (green and black) than with gauze. When a wound contact layer was applied, granulation tissue formation was slightly greater under foam than under gauze, with the degree of granulation tissue development being similar for both Avance Foam and V.A.C. GranuFoam. Both foams showed a slightly greater amount of wound contraction as compared with AMD gauze. The two intervening contact layers supported equal degrees of contraction. The wound bed tissue grew into

foam but not into gauze, and the degree of tissue in-growth was similar for both Avance Foam and V.A.C. GranuFoam. The investigators' results confirmed observations that gauze was easier to remove and antimicrobial AMD gauze does not disrupt the wound bed. Moreover, the presence of an intervening contact layer, such as Mepitel and Mepitel One, hinders in-growth and lessens the force needed for removal of foam in NPWT.[37,38]

RENASYS-F foam. The RENASYS-F foam is open-cell, hydrophobic, black, polyurethane foam developed for specific use with the Smith & Nephew RENASYS EZ and RENASYS GO NPWT systems. Smith & Nephew's EZCARE and VISTA systems (formerly BlueSky Medical devices) utilize AMD gauze dressings at negative pressure ranges from 40 mmHg to 80 mmHg, while the RENASYS system platform uses gauze or foam at negative pressure ranges from 40 mmHg to 200 mmHg. Bondojki et al used the RENASYS-F system to treat 18 patients in a prospective, multicenter study with a variety of wound types, including pressure ulcers, diabetic foot ulcers, and traumatic and surgical wounds. Results showed that at the end of the 14.6 day mean treatment duration, 83% of wounds (15/18) had progressed sufficiently to discontinue NPWT. Reductions in wound dimension, exudate level, odor, and nonviable tissue during the therapy with a significant increase in "beefy red" granulation tissue suggested the viability of utilizing the new RENASYS-F foam.[39]

Svamp Foam. Innovative Therapies Inc. (ITI) combines continuous irrigation with negative pressure therapy in its AC electric-powered NPWT systems: the original larger, 5.5 lb, 18-hour battery Svedman device intended for hospital use and the smaller, more portable, 1.9 lb, 14-hour battery SVED device. The proprietary open-celled, hydrophobic black and hydrophilic white PU Svamp Foams may be used with both devices that provide negative pressure therapy prior to, during, or after irrigation. The dry white foam is denser with a higher tensile strength. Irrigation and negative pressure application are achieved by two different pathways within the tubing system, which allows flexibility in the timing of irrigation in relation to the institution of negative pressure. As with other NPWT devices, the ITI systems are intended for use on patients with chronic, acute, traumatic, subacute, and dehisced wounds; diabetic ulcers; pressure ulcers; flaps; and grafts. Antimicrobial and amino acid preparation may be used with the system and all preparations should be used in accordance with the manufacturer's product instructions for use (IFU). Dressings are changed every 48–72 hours and if the irrigation has been discontinued for more than 2 hours, and nonadherent intervening contact layers may be used to reduce patient discomfort with dressing changes. Both continuous (-70 mmHg, -120 mmHg, and -150 mmHg) and intermittent modalities are available with a negative pressure (-25 mmHg) maintained during the off phase of the on-off cycle (5 min/2 min). Visual and audible alarms alert to notify instances of low pressure, air leaks, and full canister as the volume approaches maximum capacity (SVED 300 cc; Svedman 1,200 cc). Teder, Sandén, and Svedman conducted swine model, infected full-thickness wound healing studies to validate their proof of concept to demonstrate that the passage of fluid cleanses both the NPWT pad and the wound. The irrigation systems assisted with avoiding the collection of blood, exudate, or infectious materials, and the negative pressure treatment facilitated granulation tissue development.[40]

Antimicrobial gauze dressings (cotton blends). NPWT systems using moistened gauze typically recommend the Chariker-Jeter Technique where a nonadherent intervening contact layer covers the wound bed; moistened gauze is lightly layered to fill the wound space surrounding a flat, fenestrated drain and enclosed by a transparent polyethylene adhesive drape. The most frequently recommended gauze has a cotton-nylon blend containing 0.2% PHMB, antimicrobial dressing AMD. PHMB is a polymeric, broad-spectrum, cationic antimicrobial agent that impairs the outer membrane of gram-positive and gram-negative bacteria, showing sustained killing activity against MRSA, VRE, *Escherichia coli, Pseudomonas aeruginosa, Bacteroides fragilis, Clostridium perfringens*, and yeasts, such as *Candida albicans*.[25] Studies show antimicrobial gauze dressings with PHMB may expand options for extended occlusive dressing duration without significantly increasing wound bacterial load or human cellular cytotoxicity profiles. If the negative pressure therapy becomes inactive, dressings do not need

to be removed immediately but may be left intact for 24 hours or more depending upon the manufacturer's IFU. Other attributes of PHMB include the reduction of wound pain, odor, and fibrin slough and the prevention of necrotic tissue build-up in chronic wounds.[41,42] Antimicrobial dressings are more commonly used for infection prevention. Dressings may be used clinically to augment treatment of active infections but are not considered stand-alone therapies.

NPWT devices recommending preferential use of AMD Gauze with pressure ranges 60 mmHg–80 mmHg include Prospera® PRO-I™, PRO-II™, and PRO-III™ (Prospera, Fort Worth, Texas), Versatile1™ (BlueSky Medical, Carlsbad, California), EZCARE and V1STA (Smith & Nephew), Exsudex™ (RecoverCare, Louisville, Kentucky), Invia® Liberty™ and Vario (Medela Inc.), Moblvac® (Ohio Medical Corporation, Gurnee, Illinois), A4-NWPT pump (Genadyne Biotechnologies), VENTURI™ AVANTI and VENTURI COMPACT (Tally Medical USA, Lansing, Michigan), and SNaP (Spiracur Inc.).[5,8,13,43–47]

Silverlon Negative Pressure Dressing (nylon). Silverlon NPD (Argentum Medical, LLC), awarded the Frost & Sullivan 2006 Product Innovation Award for the US antimicrobial dressings market, is an absorbent, nonadherent silver nylon product that releases silver for 7 days. The autocatalytic silver-plating process uniformly and permanently coats the entire polymeric substrate surface circumferentially with silver that is readily released in ionic form when contacted by wound exudate. In the presence of moisture, this unique product continuously emits a very high level of ionic silver into the wound bed. The tight nylon weave resists in-growth and adherence while its porous quality permits negative pressure delivery to the tissue without obstructing exudate evacuation. This product serves as the wound contact layer for the Kalypto collection pad. The use of silver as an antimicrobial agent extends back many centuries. Silver has broad antimicrobial activity against both gram-negative and gram-positive bacteria and has demonstrated minimal development of bacterial resistance.

Bio-Dome and Bio-Dome EasyRelease (ConvaTec). This innovative wound dressing, designed for use with the Engenex® NPWT System (licensed from Boehringer Technologies), is comprised of non-woven polyester layers joined by a silicone elastomer, which effectively fills the wound while permitting exudate fluid transport. The Bio-Dome dressing has specifically engineered open pore spaces that resist collapse under negative pressures 30 mmHg–75 mmHg, presenting an unobstructed area for tissue growth influenced by a 5%–20% cellular microstrain tissue-interface pressure. The product's pore structure was designed to lower risks for in-growth and adherence-related pain, bleeding, and foreign body retention with a higher material tensile strength and a lower bioadhesion profile. The silicone elastomer reduces adherence but the Bio-Dome EasyRelease was specifically designed with a flat profile to further reduce tissue adherence and potential in-growth. Studies conducted by Girolami et al demonstrated the ability of the system to reduce aggressive adherence in the wound bed, eliminate risk of foreign body deposits, and reduce pain during removal and re-application while optimizing granulation tissue proliferation.[48] This is the only non-foam-based dressing system purposely designed to further the application of the new NPWT platform focusing on microstrain to specifically direct cellular proliferative responses. The Engenex has unique software programming to provide patient compliance tracking.[49,50]

Kalypto Negative Pressure Device Collection Pad. The Kalypto NPD pad is an innovative combination "all-in-one" styled negative pressure dressing designed for specific use with the Kalypto Medical NPD 1000 lightweight (8 oz) pump. The design allows for maximum portability. The dressing pad has a Silverlon contact nonadherent layer for minimal adherence and antimicrobial activity. The intermediate layer is composed of a two-fiber, non-woven, exudate collection system where absorbent hydrophilic fibers wick fluids into a super absorbent, bonding inner pad. The inner pad is surrounded by a non-woven, semi-occlusive polyurethane film. The indicated negative pressure is delivered to the tissue even though the pad swells as exudate accumulates in the inner core. The periwound margin is protected by a hydrophobic Gore® membrane, which protects against maceration as long as the system fluid limits are not exceeded (25 cc, 50 cc, 75 cc, 140 cc). The hydrogel adhesive

gasket allows for easy application. The pump runs on 3 AA alkaline batteries, provides negative pressures of 40 mmHg–125 mmHg, and offers both continuous and intermittent pressure modes. The Silverlon-generated antimicrobial activity is present with and without active therapy as established by Davis et al[51,52] measuring bacterial clearance in full-thickness wounds inoculated with *Pseudomonas aeruginosa* ATCC 37312 using a porcine model.

The largest reduction in bacterial concentration was seen at 48 hours after inoculation. Case studies in diabetic foot wounds, venous insufficiency, and chronic leg wounds demonstrated the product's ability to support chronic wound healing with minimal complications as long as the fluid handling capacity of the dressing is observed.[52]

Intervening nonadherent contact layers. Early nonadherent contact layers (primary contact dressings) were designed to address the issues of adherence, tissue trauma, and pain. Subsequent evolution added the qualities of avoiding the deposition of fibers, cytotoxic agents, or irritating extractable additives. Both gauze and foam applied directly to the wound surface have been associated with bio-adherence and tissue in-growth. Additives to the materials, such as soft paraffin, oils, or silicone, may alter the adherence of the product. *The application of intervening contact layers reduces negative pressure transduction to the tissue.* The degree of reduction depends upon the product and number of layers applied. Over the years, the development of potential complications and required corrective surgical intervention has prompted a variety of suggested remedies that still influence clinical practice today: careful patient selection, more frequent dressing changes, institution of intervening nonadherent contact dressings, selection of alternative interface materials, lowered treatment pressures, and, in some situations, postponing the use of negative pressure therapy. These remedies should be considered to reduce complications regardless of the interface being applied (gauze, foam, fabricated construct).

Paraffin-coated dressings. Some of the earliest modern-day nonadherent dressings are cotton blends coated with soft paraffin (eg, Vaseline Petrolatum Gauze, Covidien, and Adaptic™ with knotted viscose, Systagenix Wound Management,

Gargrave, United Kingdom). These are manufactured with and without antimicrobials, such as povidone-iodine (eg, Betadine™ gauze, Purdue Frederick, Norwalk, Connecticut) or 3% bismuth tribromophenate (eg, Xeroform™ gauze, Covidien). Available since the 1900s, tulle gras is absorbent cotton coated with balsam of Peru, paraffin, and oils. Plain cotton has been substituted with nylon-blended cotton to improve strength, and balsam of Peru has been replaced with newer, less sensitizing antimicrobials, such as chlorhexidine acetate 0.5% (eg, Bactigras®, Smith & Nephew) and 0.2% PHMB hydrochloride (eg, AMD). The combination of nonadherence and antimicrobial properties increases application duration for some gauze dressings.

Hydrocolloid pectins. Dressings made with hydrocolloid pectins have been used with NPWT (eg, GranuFlux®, ConvaTec) for their increased absorption and ability to "dissolve" into spaces when contacted by exudate yet still be easily removed with rinsing. Generally recommended for open wounds, hydrocolloid wafers used with NPWT-treated wounds help obliterate air spaces between the tissue and the sealing dressing to facilitate the retention of a seal. This is very important for anatomically difficult-to-dress locations. Some products have the added advantage of paraffin and hydrocolloid pectins for increased nonadherence (eg, Urgotul®, Urgo Medical, Chenove, France).

Silicone preparations and other nonadherent materials. Silicone-coated dressings demonstrate improved nonadherent qualities while minimizing irritation or potential allergic reactions. Paraffin has long been an additive to coat materials to decrease adherence. Meshed and woven characteristics of properties of materials may still allow "in-growth," which also affects adherence, ease of removal, and discomfort with extraction. Nonadherent products, such as Mepitel (Mölnlycke Health Care), Jelonet®, Biobrane® (Smith & Nephew), 3M™ Tegapore™, and Adaptic Touch® (Systagenix Wound Management), have become a product staple used under gauze or foam to reduce in-growth and pain during NPWT treatments. While soft silicone is not intrinsically absorbent, it is usually applied to cotton and cotton-blend gauzes to improve the absorptive capacity of the resultant product

while still maintaining the nonadherent quality. **Inappropriate interface materials.** Some products are deemed to be inappropriate for use with NPWT systems. Those materials that impede delivery of negative pressure to the wound surface or obstruct full evacuation of wound exudate should be avoided.

Natural sponges. Initially, sponge-based dressings were considered as potential alternative wound dressings because of their ability to conform to a space, fluid capacitance, tensile strength, and availability. However, natural sponges have limited application as NPWT dressings due to their "semi-open cell" communication pattern where some pores do not communicate with others. In a sponge and some "closed cell foams," the fluid channeling may flow into a space that does not allow for complete fluid extraction. Variable pore size and communication make pressure transmission and fluid extraction unpredictable. Consequently, exudate fluids and small particulate infectious materials could become trapped within the body of the sponge and the distribution of negative pressures across portions of a sponge could be compromised.

Perforated plastic film and bordered products. Perforated plastic film composed of polyethylene terephthalate (PET), a thermoplastic polymer resin that does not contain polyethelene, can be used as an NPWT dressing cover; however, the ability of the dressing to function properly will depend upon size and number of perforations.[53] The dressing must allow full exudate extraction while delivering negative pressure. Fenestrated film dressings with absorption layers (eg, TELFA™, Covidien) are available but may not be well suited for NPWT because of impermeable linings. Similarly, composite dressings made from absorbable cotton and polyester blends and water impermeable outer borders were created for "low-adherent" treatments (eg, Melolin® with borders, Smith & Nephew), but the impermeable borders make these dressings unsuitable for NPWT.

NPWT Application: Indications and Complications

"Healthcare providers will compete to offer the best record of patient safety at the lowest prices. Hospitals and patients will benefit from having accurate informa-

Table 1. Indications and contraindications for NPWT Therapy[54]

Indications

- NPWT is intended to create an environment that promotes wound healing by secondary or tertiary (delayed primary) intention by preparing the wound bed for closure, reducing edema, promoting granulation tissue formation and perfusion, and removing exudate and infectious material.
- It is indicated for patients with chronic, acute, traumatic, subacute, and dehisced wounds; partial-thickness burns; ulcers (such as diabetic or pressure); flaps; and grafts.
- NPWT combined with antimicrobial dressings (silver, PHMB, etc) is an effective barrier to bacterial penetration and may help reduce infection in the above wound types.

Contraindications

- Exposed blood vessels, organs, or nerves
- Malignancy in the wound
- Untreated osteomyelitis
- Non-enteric and unexplored fistulas
- Necrotic tissue with eschar present
- Sensitivity to additive materials (eg, silver or antimicrobial agents)

Table 2. Safety precautions for NPWT (as stated in the V.AC. Therapy IFU Safety Information Sheet[54])

Category	Suggested NPWT Treatment
• Exposed vessels and organs	• Cover with muscle flaps or other natural tissue or fine-meshed, nonadherent porous material prior to NPWT • Administer NPWT only in inpatient setting with skilled nursing and close monitoring, when vessels or organs are not completely covered and protected with a thick layer of natural tissue or fine-meshed, nonadherent porous material • Stop NPWT and seek immediate medical intervention if sudden, increased, or hemorrhagic bleeding is observed for any reason or if frank blood is seen in the tubing or in the canister
Inadequate hemostasis • Anticoagulants • Platelet aggregation inhibitors	• If wound hemostasis is tenuous, administer NPWT in inpatient setting with skilled nursing and close monitoring
Non-sutured hemostatic agents • Bone wax • Absorbable gelatin sponge • Spray wound sealant	• Protect against dislodging of agents • Start with lowest negative pressure setting then monitor closely while progressing to target treatment pressure, as tolerated • Administer therapy only in inpatient setting with skilled nursing and close monitoring
Sharp edges or bone fragments	• Eliminate sharp edges or bone fragments from wound • Smooth or cover residual edges to decrease the risk of serious or fatal injury, should shifting of structures occur • Use caution when removing dressing components from wound
Blood vessel erosion due to infection (Note: the depth of infection and degree of weakening are not always readily apparent through direct visual inspection of the exposed vessel)	• Protect with thick layer of natural tissue, such as muscle flap, or nonadherent porous material • Administer therapy in inpatient setting with skilled nursing and close monitoring because there is increased risk of vascular rupture when blood vessel is infected

Table 2. Safety precautions for NPWT (as stated in the V.A.C. Therapy IFU Safety Information Sheet[54])

Category	Suggested NPWT Treatment
Infected wounds	• Change NPWT dressings at least every 12–24 hours if wound is infected • Monitor patient closely if there are any signs of possible infection or related complications • Contact physician for immediate treatment if there are any signs of the onset of systemic infection or advancing infection at the wound site; discontinue NPWT until the infection or complication has been diagnosed and proper treatment has been initiated
Tendons, ligaments, and nerves	• Protect with natural tissues or moist, fine-meshed, nonadherent material
Osteomyelitis (Note: V.A.C. Therapy should not be initiated on a wound with untreated osteomyelitis)	• Debride necrotic, nonviable tissue and infected bone (if necessary) • Initiate antibiotic therapy • Apply when osteomyelitis has been addressed
Foam placement	• Always use NPWT dressings from sterile packages that have not been opened or damaged • Do not place any foam dressing into blind/unexplored tunnels; the V.A.C. WhiteFoam dressing may be more appropriate for use with explored tunnels • Do not force foam dressings into any area of the wound, as this may damage tissue, alter the delivery of negative pressure, or hinder exudate removal • Always count the total number of pieces of foam used in the dressing and document that number on the drape and in the patient's chart; also document the dressing change date on the drape
Foam removal	• Ensure that all foam pieces have been removed from the wound with each dressing change, because NPWT foam dressings are not bio-absorbable • Follow manufacturer's recommended time schedule for dressing changes; foam left in the wound for greater than the recommended time period may foster in-growth of tissue into the foam, create difficulty in removing foam from the wound, or lead to infection or other adverse events
Reaction to acrylic adhesive	• Be aware that patients who are allergic or hypersensitive to acrylic adhesives may have an adverse reaction to the acrylic adhesive coating on the V.A.C. Drape • If a patient has a known allergy or hypersensitivity to such adhesives, or if any signs of allergic reaction or hypersensitivity develop, such as redness, swelling, rash, urticaria, significant pruritus, or bronchospasm, discontinue use and consult a physician immediately
Defibrillation	• Remove the NPWT dressing if defibrillation is required in the area of dressing placement

Table 2. Safety precautions for NPWT (as stated in the V.A.C. Therapy IFU Safety Information Sheet[54])

Category	Suggested NPWT Treatment
Magnetic resonance imaging (MRI)	• Do not take the V.A.C. Therapy unit into the MR environment because the unit is MR unsafe • Leave V.A.C. GranuFoam dressing in place if therapy will not be interrupted for more than 2 hours • Leave V.A.C. GranuFoam Silver Dressing in place only under certain conditions and if therapy will not be interrupted for more than 2 hours (Note: MR image quality may be compromised if the area of interest is in the same area or relatively close to the position of the V.A.C. GranuFoam Silver dressing)
Hyperbaric oxygen therapy (HBO)	• Remove V.A.C. Therapy unit prior to HBO; the unit is not designed for this environment and should be considered a fire hazard in this environment • Replace dressing with compatible HBO dressing or cover V.A.C. Therapy dressing and tubing with moist cotton, gauze, or towel prior to HBO treatment
Maceration of periwound skin	• Do not allow foam to overlap intact skin • Protect fragile/friable periwound skin with a skin preparation product, additional V.A.C. Drape, hydrocolloid, or other transparent film • Realize that multiple layers of the V.A.C. Drape will decrease the moisture vapor transmission rate, which may increase the risk of maceration

tion about areas of excellence and areas that must be improved." — *Timothy F. Murphy, US Congressman*

All medical devices approved as substantially equivalent to provide NPWT share similar indications and complications as those reported in Table 1 for the V.A.C. Therapy predicate device. As with any medical therapy, potential risks have been reported. The volume of use may skew the number of reports toward the most frequently used device. Understanding the etiology of potential complications assists with mitigating the root cause regardless of the specific product being used. Table 1 lists indications and contraindications for NPWT,[54] and Table 2 presents safety precautions.[54] Although it rarely occurs, bleeding may result from exposed vessels and organs, inadequate hemostasis, inadequate protection of vital structures from sharp edges, or erosion of infected blood vessels. Other reported risks that may or may not be related to NPWT include wound infection, dressing material retention, irritation, and maceration of periwound skin.[54] Pain also has been noted secondary to mechanical stress applied to the wound, chemical contact irritation, and in-growth of tissue into the dressing material. The use of an intervening nonadherent contact layer or natural tissue should lessen the likelihood of adherence or in-growth to the interface dressing. Decreasing treatment pressure, increasing frequency of dressing changes, and careful patient selection may also lessen the risk of complications.

NPWT Guidelines

General guidelines for NPWT. Several articles describe in detail the general wound care steps associated with the application of NPWT.[55-57] The general process involves the following steps:

• Complete general wound assessment and care
• Debride wound if necessary
• Assess and treat infection
• Assess and protect periwound tissue
• Maintain moist wound environment
• Apply NPWT in accordance with the guidelines and IFU specific for that product and indication (eg, V.A.C. Therapy Clinical Guidelines[31] and V.A.C. Therapy IFU[54])
• Continue therapy until a base of granulation

tissue is robust enough to be maintained after discontinuation of the therapy or epithelization of the wound base.

Guidelines for foam-based NPWT. Articles provide consensus guidelines and/or algorithms that demonstrate how best to incorporate NPWT into the treatment of specific wound types. For example, Andros and members of a multidisciplinary expert panel[58] updated guidelines for the application of V.A.C. Therapy to diabetic foot wounds. This report summarizes clinical evidence, provides practical guidance through a treatment algorithm, offers best practices to clinicians treating diabetic foot wounds, and addresses the appropriate use of V.A.C. Therapy in treating these complex wounds. In 2004, Gupta et al[59] provided guidelines for the treatment of pressure ulcers, including the appropriate use of V.A.C. Therapy. Niezgoda and Mendez-Eastman[60] published an update of these guidelines, including an algorithm to assist in clinical management decisions related to patients with Stage III and Stage IV pressure ulcers and guidelines for incorporating V.A.C. Therapy into a complete clinical program that should include targeted patient education, pressure ulcer prevention, nutrition, aggressive incontinence management, offloading, periwound care, and routine skin surveillance. Other guidelines and algorithms for the use of V.A.C. Therapy also have been published for traumatic wounds, such as the open abdomen,[61] chest wounds,[62] and lower leg trauma.[63] In an international global expert panel, Runkel et al developed recommendations for traumatic wounds and reconstructive procedures and completed a formal consultative consensus involving 422 independent healthcare workers in 2011.[64]

Guidelines for gauze-based NPWT. In 2011, Birke-Sorensen et al reported the determinations of an international consensus panel convened to initiate the steps necessary to determine best practices for treatment variables including treatment pressures, contact layers, and interface dressing selection.[65] Additional information is being published by these and other authors to show the relative risks and benefits of gauze and foam-based dressings for NPWT. In most instances, AMD gauze appears to be similarly beneficial as an NPWT dressing.

Treating Chronic Wounds with V.A.C. Therapy

Diabetic foot wounds. V.A.C. Therapy has been used to treat diabetic foot wounds in randomized and nonrandomized studies (Table 3). Results from small RCTs by McCallon et al[66] and Eginton et al[67] demonstrated the ability of V.A.C. Therapy to reduce wound surface area and volume. Armstrong and Lavery[68] validated these findings in a large RCT in patients with diabetes and partial foot amputation wounds. Of the 77 patients who were randomized to V.A.C. Therapy, 43 (56%) achieved complete wound closure in a median time of 56 days. In a retrospective study, Page et al[69] reviewed the charts of 47 patients with open foot wounds with significant soft tissue defects. Of these patients, 22 (47%) were treated with V.A.C. Therapy. The authors found that V.A.C. Therapy was associated with a reduction in risk of one or more surgical procedures, complications, and admissions related to the treatment of the index wound during the first year after treatment. In another study using administrative claims data from both Medicare and commercial payors in patients with diabetic foot ulcers, the incidence of subsequent amputation was lower in V.A.C.-treated wounds than those treated without NPWT. Of note, while traditionally treated wounds of greater severity/depth had increasing rates of amputation, this trend was not evident for those treated with V.A.C. Therapy.[70] Blume et al conducted a multicenter, randomized, controlled trial, enrolling 342 patients assigned to either NPWT or advanced moist wound therapy (AMWT) that consisted predominantly of hydrogels and alginates, with both treatment groups receiving standard offloading interventions and followed either 112 days or until 100% wound closure by any means. In this study, a greater proportion of diabetic foot ulcers achieved complete closure in the NPWT treatment group (73 of 169, 43.2%) than with the AMWT control (48 of 166, 28.9%) ($P = .007$), without any significant difference in safety profile, including those subjects followed at 6 and 9 months for all wounds achieving 100% closure.[71]

Pressure ulcers. V.A.C. Therapy also has been used to treat Stage III and Stage IV pressure ulcers (Table 4). The findings of 3 RCTs[72–74] demonstrate that V.A.C. Therapy successfully reduced

Table 3. V.A.C. Therapy findings from selected diabetic foot wound articles

First Author (Year)	Study Type	# of V.A.C. Therapy Patients/Wounds Analyzed	V.A.C. Therapy Findings
McCallon[66] (2000)	Randomized, controlled trial	5 patients	• Four patients achieved delayed primary healing in an average of 22.8 days • Wound surface area decreased by an average of 28.4%
Eginton[67] (2003)	Randomized, controlled trial	6 patients with 7 wounds	• Treatment lasted 2 weeks in this crossover design trial • Decreased wound volume 59% and depth 49%
Armstrong[68] (2005)	Randomized, controlled trial	77 patients	• 43 (56%) patients achieved complete wound closure • Median time to wound closure was 56 days • Median time to achieve 76%–100% granulation tissue formation was 42 days
Page[69] (2004)	Comparative, retrospective study	22 patients	• Median time for wound filling was 38 days • Associated with a reduction in risk of one or more surgical procedures, complications, and readmissions related to the treatment of the index wound during the first year after treatment

Table 4. V.A.C. Therapy findings from selected pressure ulcer articles

First Author (Year)	Study Type	# of V.A.C. Therapy Patients/Wounds Analyzed	V.A.C. Therapy Findings
Ford[72] (2002)	Randomized, controlled trial	20 wounds	• Two ulcers healed completely during controlled trial the 6-week treatment phase • Six ulcers underwent flap surgery • 51.8% mean reduction in ulcer volume
Joseph[73] (2000)	Randomized, controlled trial	18 wounds	• 66% reduction in wound depth • 78% final percent reduction in wound volume over time
Wanner[74] (2003)	Randomized, controlled trial	11 patients	• 50% reduction in initial wound volume in a mean (SD) of 27 (10) days • Reduced costs and improved comfort cited by authors as advantages of V.A.C. Therapy
Philbeck[75] (1999)	Retrospective study	43 wounds	• Ulcers averaged 22.2 cm² in area • Average rate of wound closure was 0.23 cm² per day

pressure ulcer size and may have positively affected wound histology. Philbeck et al[75] conducted a retrospective study of Medicare Part B home care patients who had chronic, nonhealing wounds treated with V.A.C. Therapy. The analyzed subset of pressure ulcer patients had an average wound area of 22.2 cm². Their finding that V.A.C. Therapy healed these ulcers at a rate of 0.23 cm² per day supports the findings of the 3 RCTs, which show V.A.C. Therapy to be a successful treatment

Table 5. V.A.C. Therapy findings from other chronic wound or mixed chronic and acute wound RCTs

First Author (Year)	Study Type	# of V.A.C. Therapy Patients/Wounds Analyzed	V.A.C. Therapy Findings
Vuerstaek[76] (2006)	Randomized, controlled trial	30 patients with chronic leg ulcers	• Median total healing time was 29 days • Median wound bed preparation time was 7 days • 90% of ulcers healed within 43 days • Demonstrated cost effectiveness
Braakenburg[77] (2006)	Randomized, controlled trial	32 patients with any type of acute or chronic wound	• V.A.C. Therapy group: 23 (74%) chronic (1 missing value), 2 (7%) acute, and 6 (19%) subacute wounds • An endpoint was a completely granulated wound or a wound ready for skin grafting or healing by secondary intention • Overall median time to healing was 16 days • In subset of 18 diabetic or cardiovascular patients, median wound healing time was 14 days
Moues[78] (2004)	Randomized, controlled trial	29 patients with full-thickness wounds that could not be closed immediately because of infection, contamination, or chronic character	• Wounds stratified by duration: early treated wounds (existing < 4 weeks before hospitalization) and late treated wounds (> 4 weeks) • Overall median time needed to reach "ready for surgical therapy" was 6.00 ± 0.52 days (median ± SEM) • Median time was 5.00 ± 0.85 days for wounds existing < 4 weeks and 6.00 ± 0.99 days for wounds > 4 weeks • The mean rate of wound surface area reduction was 3.8 ± 0.5%/day

for these chronic wounds. Wounds healed faster than standard of care with a higher incidence of closure.

Other V.A.C. Therapy chronic wound studies. In addition to the previously discussed diabetic foot wound and pressure ulcer studies, several RCTs evaluated V.A.C. Therapy in chronic leg ulcers or in study populations that combined chronic and acute wounds (Table 5). Vuerstaek et al[76] conducted an RCT in 60 hospitalized patients with chronic leg ulcers. For the 30 V.A.C. Therapy patients, the median total healing time was 29 days and the median wound bed preparation time was 7 days. Two other V.A.C. Therapy RCTs included chronic and acute wounds in each of the randomized groups. In the Braakenburg et al study,[77] 32 of the 65 patients were treated with V.A.C. Therapy. Twenty-three patients in the V.A.C. Therapy group had chronic

wounds, while the remaining 9 patients had acute or subacute wounds. The median time to healing for the overall V.A.C. Therapy group was 16 days. The median time to healing was 14 days for the subset of 18 V.A.C. Therapy patients with cardiovascular disease or diabetes. The Moues et al RCT[78] evaluated 54 patients with full-thickness wounds that "could not be closed immediately because of infection, contamination, or chronic character." For the 29 patients randomized to V.A.C. Therapy, the median time needed to reach "ready for surgical therapy" was 6.00 ± 0.52 days. The mean rate of wound surface area reduction in V.A.C. Therapy wounds was 3.8 ± 0.5%/day. All of these studies demonstrate that V.A.C. Therapy has been successfully used in the treatment of chronic wounds. NPWT improved the ability to facilitate wound closure in segments of these selected difficult-to-heal populations.

Table 6. V.A.C. Therapy findings from selected skin graft articles

First Author (Year)	Study Type	# of V.A.C. Therapy Patients/Wounds Analyzed	V.A.C. Therapy Findings
Moisidis[79] (2004)	Randomized, controlled trial	20 wound halves	• Positive results in both qualitative and con-trolled trial quantitative measures • All wound halves healed without need for further debridement or regrafting • Dressings were well tolerated by the patients
Jeschke[80] (2004)	Randomized, controlled trial	5 patients	• 5 were treated with fibrin glue-anchored Integra and postoperative V.A.C. Therapy • Integra take rate was 98 ± 2% • Mean period from Integra coverage to skin transplantation was 10 ± 1 days
Genecov[81] (1998)	Prospective, controlled trial	10 patients	• 7 of 10 donor sites re-epithelized by Day 7
Carson[82] (2004)	Retrospective study	70 patients	• 86% overall healing rate (60 out of 70 patients) • All 50 skin grafts healed in 11–24 days and remained stable at 6 months

Skin grafts. When skin grafts are used to close wounds, V.A.C. Therapy can assist in preparing the wound bed and bolstering the graft (Table 6). The Moisidis et al RCT[79] studied quantitative graft take and qualitative graft appearance (as determined by an independent evaluator who was blinded to treatment assignment). V.A.C. Therapy grafts achieved positive results quantitatively and qualitatively. In another RCT, Jeschke et al[80] evaluated 12 patients with large defects who underwent Integra™ Bilayer Matrix Wound Dressing (Integra LifeSciences, Plainsboro, New Jersey) grafting for reconstruction. For the 5 patients treated with fibrin glue and V.A.C. Therapy, the Integra take rate was 98 ± 2% and the mean period from Integra coverage to skin transplantation was 10 ± 1 days. The Genecov et al prospective, controlled study[81] reported positive V.A.C. Therapy results in pigs and in humans. For the human subjects, all donor sites demonstrated re-epithelization at 1 week. Finally, in the Carson et al retrospective study,[82] 50 out of 70 patients received skin grafts bolstered by V.A.C. Therapy. All 50 grafts healed and remained stable for at least 6 months. NPWT appears to support improved graft take in selected large defect wounds.

Incision management of acute post-op-erative wounds. The use of NPWT over closed incisional wounds in patients who have a high likelihood of developing infection or mechanical stress-related dehiscence is increasingly being evaluated. Stannard et al studied this application in the prophylactic use of NPWT in high-risk lower extremity fractures.[83] Kilpadi and Cunningham described their experiences with using NPWT to assist with managing closed incisions, noting reduction of hematoma and seroma formation in a porcine model.[84] Clearly, there may be a role for assisting patients in a prophylactic fashion.

Cost effectiveness of V.A.C. Therapy. Various studies have shown that V.A.C. Therapy is cost effective in a variety of care settings. Philbeck et al[75] considered cost in their retrospective study of Medicare home healthcare patients. In a subset analysis of pressure ulcers, the authors used wound closure rates reported by Ferrell et al[85] in 1993 for patients with trochanteric and trunk pressure ulcers averaging 4.3 cm^2 who were treated with a low-air-loss surface and saline-soaked gauze. Ferrell et al[85] reported that the wounds closed at an average of 0.090 cm^2 per day. Philbeck et al[75] analyzed patients who were treated with a low-air-loss surface and V.A.C. Therapy and who had

Table 7. V.A.C. Therapy findings from selected acute wound articles

First Author (Year)	Study Type	# of V.A.C. Therapy Patients/Wounds Analyzed	V.A.C. Therapy Findings
Burns			
Kamolz[93] (2004)	Case series	7 patients with bilateral hand burns	• Enhanced perfusion reported in the V.A.C. Therapy-treated hand • Reduction in edema was observed • 5 hands healed without skin grafts • V.A.C. Therapy hand dressing did not need additional splinting
Surgical wounds — dehisced/open abdominal			
Garner[94] (2001)	Case series	14 trauma patients with open abdomens	• Early definitive fascial closure achieved in 13 patients (92%) in a mean of 9.9 ± 1.9 days • A mean of 2.8 ± 0.6 dressing changes were performed
Surgical wounds — sternal wound infections/mediastinitis			
Agarwal[95] (2005)	Retrospective study	103 patients treated after median sternotomy	• 64% had a diagnosis of mediastinitis, while 36% had either superficial infections or a sterile wound • Patients were treated for an average of 11 days • 70 patients (68%) achieved definitive chest closure with open reduction internal fixation and/or flap closure
Subacute wounds			
Argenta[1] (1997)	Case series	94 subacute wounds (overall study evaluated 300 wounds)	• 94 subacute wounds included dehisced wounds, open wounds with exposed orthopedic hardware and/or bone, and other miscellaneous wounds open < 7 days • 26 healed completely • 68 reduced in size and were closed with split-thickness skin grafts, secondary closure, or minor flaps • 37 patients with exposed orthopedic hardware or bone were treated successfully with closure of adjacent muscle and granulation tissue over the bone and hardware

Stage III and Stage IV trochanteric and trunk wounds that averaged 22.2 cm² in area. These wounds closed at an average of 0.23 cm² per day. The average 22.2 cm² wound in this study, treated as described by Ferrell et al, would take 247 days to heal, whereas the same wound would heal in 97 days with V.A.C. Therapy. While acknowledging the fact that larger pressure ulcers typically heal faster than smaller pressure ulcers, the V.A.C. Therapy healing rate described by Philbeck et al

could potentially provide financial benefit associated with a reduced treatment course and patient benefit related to improved quality of life. In another large retrospective study of patients with chronic Stage III and Stage IV pressure ulcers in the home health environment, Schwien et al[86] found that V.A.C. Therapy reduced the number of visits to hospitals and emergent care facilities secondary to wound complications. These studies demonstrate that V.A.C. Therapy is an economical, useful treatment modality for a variety of chronic wounds, rendered in a variety of care settings.[87] Additional negative pressure therapy options have been offered for developed and underdeveloped countries.[88–92]

Treating Acute Wounds with V.A.C. Therapy

More than 125 articles report clinical and scientific results related to V.A.C. Therapy treatment of acute wounds, including burns, dehisced wounds, and subacute wounds. Table 7 briefly summarizes the findings of selected V.A.C. Therapy RCTs, case series, and retrospective studies in each of the aforementioned acute wound categories. Kamolz et al[93] evaluated 7 patients with bilateral hand burns. One hand of each patient was treated with V.A.C. Therapy. The authors reported that V.A.C. Therapy helped to promote perfusion and reduced edema. Garner et al[94] concluded that V.A.C. Therapy can "safely achieve early fascial closure," based on their experiences using V.A.C. Therapy to treat 14 patients with open abdominal wounds. V.A.C. Therapy also has been used to treat sternal wound infections/mediastinitis. In a retrospective review of 103 patients who were treated with V.A.C. Therapy after median sternotomy, Agarwal et al[95] reported that V.A.C. Therapy was administered for an average period of 11 days per patient. The authors also stated that definitive chest closure with open reduction and internal fixation and/or flap closure was achieved for 70 of 103 patients (68%).

In a large case series of 300 wounds, Argenta and Morykwas[1] reported that 26 of 94 subacute wounds healed completely after treatment with V.A.C. Therapy. The remaining 68 subacute wounds reduced in size and were closed using split-thickness skin grafts, secondary closure, or minor flaps. The authors noted that in 37 patients with exposed orthopedic hardware or bone, V.A.C. Therapy successfully achieved closure of adjacent muscle and the formation of granulation tissue over the bone and hardware. Thus, the mechanisms of action that make V.A.C. Therapy a successful treatment for chronic wounds also enable this integrated wound care system to achieve positive results in the treatment of a variety of acute wounds. Additional trials are necessary to determine the economic benefit of adding

NPWT to a surgical treatment regime. Certainly, high-risk patients or procedures with increased likelihood of failing would be optimal candidates.

Treating Wounds with Gauze-Based NPWT

Campbell et al[96] performed a retrospective review of 30 patients treated with NPWT using the gauze-based Chariker-Jeter technique[97] at negative pressure (-80 mmHg) to demonstrate the safety and efficacy of NPWT in a long-term care setting with V1STA, Versatile1, and EZCARE devices (Smith & Nephew). Chronic wounds (n = 11), surgical dehiscence (n = 11), and surgical incisions (n = 8) showed significant reduction in wound volume and area to be able to support discontinuation of NPWT after a median 41 days, with an overall median 88% reduction in wound volume, 68% reduction in area, and a 15.1% weekly overall rate of volume reduction, comparing comparably with foam-based systems. Hurd et al reported 80% pain-free dressing changes and 96% lack of tissue damage with dressing changes in a long-term care facility.[98] Dunn et al validated factors associated with positive and negative outcomes in patients treated with gauze-based NPWT; these outcomes were similar to those noted with foam dressings.[99] Gauze- and foam-based NPWT products appear to produce similar proportions of closed split-thickness skin graft (STSG) wounds according to Fraccalvieri et al; however, the wounds closed with a foam-based (-125 mmHg) system applied on average at 25.9 days as compared to a gauze-based (-80 mmHg) system applied on average at 24.7 days were less pliable with a thicker scar beneath the graft.[100] Dunn et al noted a 96% overall STSG take, increase in granulation tissue to 90% median wound area, and a decrease in non-viable tissue (20%–0%) for wounds treated with gauze-based NPWT (-80 mmHg) for 12 days pre-treatment and 5 days post-treatment.[101] Landsman et al demonstrated the effectiveness of a mechanically powered gauze-based dressing system used to treat diabetic lower extremity wounds.[102] Non-inferiority clinical studies performed by Dorfshar et al demonstrated that gauze-based dressings show similar changes in wound volume and surface area as those observed with foam-based therapies in a clinical inpatient setting.[103] Availability of dressing materials, familiarity with product use, required dressing change intervals, and cost may influence a given practitioner's selection.

Mechanisms of Action for NPWT

A clear understanding of how a therapy works is crucial for making the best use of that treatment. Ongoing research into the mechanisms of action for NPWT continues to clarify the effects that produce the overall wound healing outcome. The combined effects of direct mechanical stress on the cell and alterations in the cell's environment unite to promote a positive wound healing response.

Granulation tissue formation. For healing to occur, the wound defect must fill with granulation tissue. Granulation tissue is composed of new blood vessels, fibroblasts, inflammatory cells, myofibroblasts, endothelial cells, and extracellular matrix. In experiments where V.A.C. Therapy was used to treat porcine surgical wounds, it appeared that V.A.C. Therapy assisted in the formation of granulation tissue.[2] Armstrong and Lavery[68] conducted a large RCT of 162 patients with complex diabetic foot amputation wounds. Their study assessed the time to achieve 76%–100% granulation in patients initially presenting with 0%–10% granulation at baseline. Results from the study indicated that V.A.C. Therapy patients achieved this level of granulation in a mean of 42 days. It is believed that mechanical forces resulting from V.A.C. Therapy and their effect on biochemical processes promote granulation tissue formation.

Mechanical forces. Virtually all aspects of cell physiology may be affected by mechanical stimulation. The cellular response to strain has long been known to result in increased tissue formation. Classic examples are the use of the Ilizarov or distraction osteogenesis technique in hard tissue and tissue expanders in soft tissue.[104,105] With V.A.C. Therapy, externally applied forces may be subdivided into 1) macrostrain and 2) microstrain and microdeformations.[106,107]

Macrostrain. When V.A.C. Therapy is applied, air is evacuated from the dressing via the vacuum, and the tissue is drawn up against the foam. The foam's mechanical properties initially resist the force of the tissue against it, but as the air continues to be evacuated and the tissue force pulling inward exceeds that of the foam pushing outward, the foam compresses, and the wound becomes smaller.

By applying this bulk tissue deformation, or macrostrain, NPWT draws the wound edges together and supports wound healing by decreasing the size of the defect to be filled with granulation tissue.

Microstrain and microdeformations. Microdeformations are caused by negative pressure-induced microstrain of the tissue. The negative pressure draws the tissue surface into the foam pores, promoting cellular stretch and proliferation, which may lead to a decrease in wound size. When the foam-tissue interface is more closely examined, microdeformations can be clearly seen once the vacuum is applied. These microdeformations occur due to microstrains that result in 1) tissue being compressed below the struts and 2) tissue being stretched into the foam pores between the foam struts.

Micromechanical forces have long been known to be responsible for the *induction of cell proliferation and division*.[106,108–110] Other cellular responses to micromechanical forces include gene expression,[111] extracellular matrix (ECM) deposition,[111,112] migration,[113] and differentiation.[108] In general, it is theorized that the cells sense these changes in their local environment through transmembrane signaling proteins known as integrins. The integrins transmit signals to the intracellular molecules, which then transmit the signals to the nucleus, leading to changes in gene transcription.[114,115] The resulting cellular proliferation and ECM production result in decreased wound size.

Saxena et al[106] reported that V.A.C. Therapy and open-celled polyurethane foam produced tissue strains in the average range of 5%–20%. These values are consistent with those shown to result in increased cellular proliferation in bench studies.[109,116] Furthermore, the theoretical models developed by Saxena et al[106] correlated well to actual deformations seen in clinical wounds that had been treated for 4–7 days with V.A.C. Therapy. Greene et al[107] investigated the effect of V.A.C. Therapy-induced microdeformations on capillary formation in chronic wounds. The authors performed an intra-wound comparison of tissue samples with and without exposure to the V.A.C. Therapy. The level of cellular microstrain is believed to be directly related to pore diameter of the interface of the dressing structure, strut thickness, and applied pressure. Wound tissue samples in contact with the GranuFoam Dressing (causing microdeformations) showed increased microvessel density, suggesting improved cellular proliferation and angiogenesis.[107] These changes were attributed to the properties of foam in these early trials specifically designed to investigate foam as an interface material.

Collagen deposition. Provisional matrix models have been generated to evaluate the impact of NPWT on cellular division and migration, extracellular matrix deposition, apoptosis, and angiogenesis.[117] Parameters, such as pressure profile and interface material, show a marked influence on the development of key tissue components, such as collagen deposition, cellular composition, and vascularity *in vitro*.[100,118] The full clinical impact of these findings has yet to be validated *in vivo*, where many other factors influence clinical outcomes and high pressures, or the influence of interface materials may potentially adversely influence tissue quality.[119,120]

Extracellular matrix deposition (hyaluronic acid). Hyaluronic acid makes up approximately 80% of the extracellular matrix (ECM). Increased levels of hyaluronic acid may be a factor in the increased levels of granulation tissue formation shown in studies using V.A.C. Therapy.[68,73] Hyaluronic acid is an important non-sulfonated glycosaminoglycan in the ECM. It is an extremely hygroscopic molecule that provides the tissue with resilience to compressive forces. Hyaluronic acid also may have a protective effect on tissues due to its ability to scavenge free radicals.[121] In tissues biopsied from human mucosal wounds, Oksala et al[122] demonstrated that hyaluronic acid levels rose early before decreasing at Day 7 post wounding. In a porcine full-thickness wound model, granulation tissue was biopsied at Day 9 post wounding and analyzed for hyaluronic acid.[123] High levels of hyaluronic acid were measured in the tissue biopsied after 9 days of V.A.C. Therapy.

Infection management. Bacteria colonize all wounds. Infection occurs when the presence of replicating organisms increases to a high titer level, which then leads to the production and accumulation of bacterial toxins and proteases that impair wound healing. Chronic wound infection is associated with reduced fibroblast presence and improper collagen deposition.[124] It is therefore important to control wound infection to ensure optimal wound healing.

Exudate management. A goal in proper wound bed preparation is to provide exudate management.[125] Extensive evidence exists in the wound healing literature to indicate that the presence of edema in the wound bed can negatively impact wound healing. Removal of excess interstitial fluid by NPWT results in decreased tissue turgor, decreased intercapillary distance, increased lymphatic flow, and improved inflow of nutrients to and removal of waste by-products and proteases from the tissue. The ability of V.A.C. Therapy to favorably impact edema removal has been reported experimentally and clinically in diverse wound types, such as chronic wounds, burns, and acute traumatic wounds.[1,93,126] Caution should be taken to avoid dehydration, coagulopathies, and protein nutritional deficits with excessive exudate removal.

Enhanced perfusion. Adequate perfusion is extremely important to the healing process. Nutrients (including oxygen) that are essential for wound healing are transported to the wound via the blood. Improved perfusion also allows for the removal of cellular waste products, such as carbon dioxide. Initial preclinical studies by Morykwas et al[2] showed that compared to baseline levels, intermittent application of V.A.C. Therapy with the GranuFoam Dressing resulted in more than a 4-fold increase in perfusion. Subsequent studies have confirmed the increase in perfusion associated with V.A.C. Therapy.[127–129]

While the aforementioned studies show the immediate effect of V.A.C. Therapy on perfusion, Kamolz et al[93] showed that increased perfusion also may continue later into the wound healing continuum. It is commonly known that certain burn injuries can progress from partial-thickness to full-thickness burns within a few days of injury and that compromised microcirculation is a contributing factor.[130] In a study of 7 patients with bilateral hand burns, Kamolz et al[93] used video angiography to measure perfusion in the burns. They found that use of V.A.C. Therapy was associated with hyperperfusion and that this may have been a contributing factor to the prevention of burn progression. Five of the 7 V.A.C. Therapy-treated hand wounds healed without skin grafts.

NPWT "filler material" debate. Wound dressing materials are the topic of considerable debate. Yet, one of the most important scientific questions needs to be better addressed: the relevant physics of negative pressure on filler substance and its affect to either augment or diminish pressure distribution throughout the entire tissue plane. In an interdependent fashion, the negative pressure profile and the interface material alter exudate evacuation and tissue microstrain and thereby influence the rate, quantity, and quality of tissue generated. Interface material is not simply "filler material;" it impacts distribution of negative pressure within the wound space, modulates pressure waveforms, and dampens peak pressures delivered to tissue surfaces and extending into surrounding periwound tissue planes. The amount and viscosity of the fluid being evacuated also affects negative pressure delivery, and for some materials, this "fluid effect" is further amplified by variability introduced by the dressing material. Gauze, as compared to open-cell foam, is thought to be more likely to alter the programmed pressure based upon the amount of material used, packing density, method of packing, and interaction between the applied layers. The unique open-cell PU and PVA foams created for the modern NPWT platform were designed to transduce negative pressure to the wound surface with minimal pressure alteration regardless of the exudate quantity or quality, amount of filler material used, layers applied, or orientation of insertion. Foam facilitates delivery of negative pressure profiles in a very "exacting" fashion. The specially designed foams can be easily sized for most wounds and are readily available at a relatively low cost.

On the other hand, gauze is an abundant, inexpensive, and familiar wound dressing material. It can be easily molded around irregular contours and packed into wounds and tunnels and is now readily available in economical, antimicrobial, low-bioadherent, noninflammatory product lines utilized for some NPWT wound types, especially where lower peak pressure and the use of a nonadherent contact layer is required to reduce adherence, in-growth, bleeding, and pain. Many believe gauze has a tendency to "mat and wad" during application and under negative pressure, which may affect fluid evacuation and pressure transduction, especially in larger wounds. In confirmation, Anesäter et al performed a series of studies to examine the effect of material type (foam or gauze) and size (small or large)

on wound contraction and tissue pressure in a porcine full-thickness peripheral wound model under exposure to negative pressure ranges (-20 mmHg to -160 mmHg).[119] NPWT application caused a decrease in tissue pressure at 0.1 cm from the wound margin and an increase at 0.5 cm from the wound margin. Tissue pressure at 0.5 cm was higher with smaller amounts of foam, and smaller amounts of foam also caused significantly more wound contraction. In contrast, gauze created intermediate contraction unrelated to the amount of "filler" material used.

In summary, foam is more likely to deliver programmed pressure profiles, but not all clinical situations require that level of "exactness." Gauze or large amounts of foam generate less contraction, which could be less painful and less likely to cause strain-related bleeding, while small amounts of foam would be most beneficial when maximal wound contraction and granulation tissue development are needed. Researchers are still trying to ferret out the interplay between mechanical pressure modulations and tissue responses.

High versus low NPWT peak pressure debate. Recent studies highlight the existence of *3 zones of perfusion established by NPWT*: 1) the wound bed, 2) the wound margin, and 3) the periwound tissue.[119,128] The current NPWT platform dictates a specific range of microstrain at the wound base and derived its justification based upon measurements of increased blood flow in the periwound tissue and the resulting amount of granulation tissue developed.[1,2] Higher peak negative pressure (-125 mmHg) optimized flow in the periwound tissue and supported a significant increase in granulation tissue development. Lower peak negative pressures (-80 mmHg) generated lower levels of periwound tissue perfusion. Studies showed marginal tissue perfusion increased with increasing negative pressure to a plateau then decreased as additional negative pressure was instituted. Hypoxia (low oxygen content) and ischemia (low perfusion pressure) develop at different levels of pressure for different types of tissue. High levels of negative pressures can lead to hypoxia at the wound margin, and excessive pressures cause ischemic tissue breakdown, apoptosis, and necrosis. Certainly, prolonged hypoxia and ischemia have been associated with tissue necrosis; however, intermittent hypoxia and "mild ischemia" are both recognized stimuli for hypoxia–inducing factor (HIF) and other biomolecules that signal wound healing cascades. It is interesting to note that the "hypoxia and potential ischemia" may be associated with at lower overall pressure at that 0.1 cm tissue plane because the applied energy source is a negative (suction) pressure. At present, there is insufficient information to fully interpret the relative importance of wound base, marginal, and distal blood flow in tissue under the influence of negative pressure forces.

Negative pressure profiles and tissue quality. Studies show that higher levels of peak pressure (-125 mmHg) and intermittent modality have been associated with more granulation tissue developed at a faster rate in full-thickness wounds with adequate vasculature for perfusion and a source for fibroblast cells needed for fibroplasias.[1–3] Multiple factors influence the choice of negative pressure therapy parameters. These may relate to the health of the patient, quality of the tissue being treated, amount of exudate, tissue oxygen and perfusion, and other treatment modalities being used. A practitioner may prefer to use higher negative pressure in a large, well vascularized, highly exudative, post-operative, dehisced hip wound but choose a lower pressure level (-80 mmHg) for a dehisced, infected, abdominal wound with substantial amounts of poorly perfused fat tissue in an elderly patient with diabetes. Hypoxic, ischemic fat tissue may develop necrosis at higher pressure settings. Optimal negative pressure should be high enough to draw the wound margins toward each other without creating adverse tension, deliver sufficient tissue microstrain (5%–20%) to activate cellular division to create the desired amount and quality of collagen-ECM mix deposited, and effectively evacuate inflammatory exudate from the wound space to "perfect" the wound environment.

In an effort to adopt evidence-influenced practice models, some practitioners have utilized bedside diagnostics for perfusion (hand-held Doppler) and oxygenation (transcutaneous oxygen, TCPO2) along with patient comfort levels to guide treatment pressure profiles. While Doppler and TCPO2 assessments are not practical for commonplace application today, newer technology may assist with bedside perfusion and oxygenation verification to inform treatment choices

in the future. Additional diagnostics are being developed and marketed to test wound environment matrix metalloproteinases and other inflammatory mediators. Nonetheless, up to this point, there has been a well established *medical practice of reducing the peak negative pressure and slowing the rate of draw down to reduce pain, bleeding, and other potential complications*. Those choices are made at the presumed potential loss of comparative granulation tissue generated. More information is needed to establish how those choices impact the actual rate and quality of tissue generated.

More scientific-focused research is required. Clearly, wound surface microstrain directly influences cellular proliferation, apoptosis, extracellular matrix deposition, and inflammatory mediator profiles; however, the relative importance of that influence to impact final clinical outcomes has yet to be fully delineated. Negative pressure profile may be manipulated to deliver different levels of strain by modulating peak pressure, pressure waveforms, pressure modality (continuous or intermittent), duration and frequency of application, and selection of different interfaces for transduction. Additionally, a host of non-pressure-related factors influences final clinical wound healing outcomes[125] (Table 8). Several key areas need further investigation and definition: 1) interplay between mechanical stress and inflammatory mediator reduction alters the cell's biomolecular profile either directly (microstrain) or indirectly through environmental changes (exudate evacuation) and their effects are interdependent; 2) pressure profile alterations related to dressing materials in the wound space; 3) tissue growth response (fibroplasias, angiogenesis, and collagen-ECM deposition) resulting from varied pressure profiles applied at different times throughout the human wound healing cycle; 4) tissue growth response in relation to varied pressure profiles depending upon initial tissue type (fat, muscle, tendon/ligament, bone); and 5) tissue growth response where various soluble additives are provided (ie, antimicrobials, nutrients, oxygen, nitric oxide, growth factors, cytokines, collagen, ECM, and cells). A great amount of additional research is warranted. In lieu of the current insufficient level of "evidential clarity" and minimal number of comparative clinical trials, it would be premature to designate a "best" dressing or "best"

Table 8. Factors impacting wound healing

NPWT Device-Related Factors

- Interface materials to distribute pressure and interact with the underlying tissues
- Presence or absence of an intervening nonadherent layer
- Pressure profile
  - Peak negative pressure (maximum)
  - Pressure modality — continuous versus intermittent
  - Pressure wave forms — rapidity of pressure onset ("draw down")
  - Treatment regimes — application frequency and overall duration

Wound-Specific Factors

- Etiology of tissue injury (eg, incision, contusion, blast, thermal, pressure, moisture)
- Location, size, shape, depth
- Exposed vital structures (eg, bone, blood vessels, tendons)
- Tissue nutritional state
- Local vascular status and perfusion
- Local tissue inflammatory status
- Infectious status (local, systemic, biofilm, abscess, suppuration)
- Existing cells, extracellular matrix (ECM), and structural support tissues
- Local oxygenation and tissue energy
- Tissue fluid — edema, drainage, exudate
- Temperature, moisture, and pH

General Health-Related Factors

- Overall physical health and emotional status
  - Medical diseases and disorders
  - Medications, prescribed, over-the-counter, herbals, homeopathic
  - Psychiatric and emotional health
- Socio-economic status and ability to access appropriate care

Recommended Treatments and Interventions

- Debridement — selective and non-selective
- Antibiotic, antimicrobial, anti-inflammatory agents
- Offloading therapy and the ability to mitigate future recurrent trauma
- Compression and manual massage therapy — continuous and intermittent pneumatic
- Oxygenation and perfusion support
- Nutritional supplementation
- Temperature and moisture management
- Case management
- Physical therapeutics
- Tissue-based therapy components (eg, growth factors, cytokines, collagen, hyaluronic acid, cells)
- Exogenous energy provision — electric, electromagnetic, infrared, ultrasound, or vibratory

pressure. In all likelihood, it will not be one "best" for all clinical situations.

Conclusion

NPWT has widespread clinical acceptance. A substantial body of evidence reports its clinical utility in the treatment of chronic and acute wounds. NPWT is intended to create an environment that promotes wound healing by secondary or tertiary (delayed primary) intention by preparing the wound bed for closure, reducing edema, promoting granulation tissue formation and perfusion, and removing exudate and infectious material. It is indicated for patients with chronic, acute, traumatic, subacute, and dehisced wounds; partial-thickness burns; ulcers (such as diabetic or pressure); flaps; and grafts. NPWT design innovations have accelerated provider adoption and improved patient compliance, care setting appropriateness, and realized healthcare system cost reductions. Ease of use coupled with positive clinical healing outcomes fueled a rapid, widespread adoption and penetration of NPWT across the spectrum of surgical and non-surgical medical specialties. Modification toward improved lightweight portable to ultra-portability compact modeling, visible and audible alarms, wound site pressure monitoring feedback, and flight certification approval facilitated NPWT expansion across inpatient, out-of-hospital, ambulatory care, disaster preparedness, and military transport care settings. Improved healing times, pain reduction, and fewer restrictions to mobility with potentially fewer interruptions in patient work schedules encourage positive patient adherence and adoption. Focused awareness of potential risks and complications with structured mitigation strategies should support continued positive safety standing. Further research into clinical efficacy, health outcomes, cost effectiveness, and mechanisms of action will assist in defining future NPWT utilization.

Practice Pearls

- NPWT is a proven, clinically effective, and safe process that promotes healing for acute and chronic wounds.
- NPWT provides a mechanical strain that alters cellular proliferation, extracellular matrix deposition, and local perfusion; additionally, the removal of exudate facilitates the reduction of inhibitory mediators.
- Mechanical strain and inflammatory exudate removal act interdependently to positively impact wound tissue healing response.
- The type of material at the interface is not as important as the modification of NPWT pressure profiles and tissue growth responses.
- Adding nonadherent intervening contact dressings at the tissue-material interface helps mitigate complications.

Self-Assessment Questions

1. Which of the following is not an indication for use of NPWT?
   A. Chronic wounds and ulcers (such as diabetic or pressure)

B. Acute, traumatic, subacute, and dehisced wounds
   C. Full-thickness burns
   D. Flaps and grafts

2. Peak pressure may alter which of the following?
   A. Cellular proliferation
   B. Collagen deposition
   C. Local arterial blood flow
   D. All of the above

3. Which of the following mechanisms of action relate to NPWT?
   A. Promoting edema
   B. Inhibiting granulation tissue formation and perfusion
   C. Wound space expansion
   D. Decreasing exudate and infectious material

4. What dressing has the best likelihood of reducing NPWT-related pain?
   A. Gauze
   B. Foam
   C. Bio-Dome
   D. Intervening nonadherent contact layer

Answers: 1-C, 2-D, 3-D, 4-D

References

1. Argenta LC, Morykwas MJ. Vacuum-assisted closure: a new method for wound control and treatment: clinical experience. *Ann Plast Surg.* 1997;38(6):563–576.

2. Morykwas MJ, Argenta LC, Shelton-Brown EI, McGuirt W. Vacuum-assisted closure: a new method for wound control and treatment: animal studies and basic foundation. *Ann Plast Surg.* 1997;38(6):553–562.

3. Morykwas MJ, Simpson J, Punger K, Argenta A, Kremers L, Argenta J. Vacuum-assisted closure: state of basic research and physiologic foundation. *Plast Reconstr Surg.* 2006;117(7 Suppl):121S–126S.

4. Sullivan N, Snyder DL, Tipton K, Uhl S, Schoelles KM. Negative Pressure Wound Therapy Devices. Technology Assessment Report. Available at: http://www.ahrq.gov/clinic/ta/negpresswtd/negpresswtd.pdf. Accessed February 1, 2012.

5. Genadyne Biotechnologies. XLR8® Negative Pressure Wound Therapy. Available at: http://www.genadyne.com/productoverview.php?category=wound_therapy. Accessed January 29, 2012.

6. US Department of Health and Human Services, Food and Drug Administration, Center for Devices and Radiological Health. Guidance for Industry and FDA Staff: Class II Special Controls Guidance Document: Non-powered Suction Apparatus Device Intended for

Negative Pressure Wound Therapy (NPWT). Available at: http://www.fda.gov/downloads/MedicalDevices/DeviceRegulationandGuidance/GuidanceDocuments/UCM233279.pdf. Accessed February 1, 2012.

7. Fong KD, Hu D, Eichstadt S, et al. The SNaP system: biomechanical and animal model testing of a novel ultraportable negative-pressure wound therapy system. *Plast Reconstr Surg*. 2010;125(5):1362–1371.

8. Spiracur Inc. SNaP® Brochure. Available at: http://spiracur.com/for-clinicians/trainingifu/. Accessed January 29, 2012.

9. Kalypto Medical. Guidelines for Use of the NPD 1000™ Negative Pressure Wound Therapy System from Kalypto Medical®. Available at: http://www.kalyptomedical.com/clinical.php. Accessed January 29, 2012.

10. V.A.C. Via™ Negative Pressure Wound Therapy System [instructions for use]. San Antonio, TX: KCI USA, Inc; 2010.

11. Genadyne Biotechnologies. A4-NPWT. Available at: http://www.genadyne.com/productoverview.php?category=wound_therapy. Accessed January 29, 2012.

12. PICO™ Single Use Negative Pressure Wound Therapy System [instructions for use]. St-Laurent, Quebec, Canada: Smith & Nephew, Inc; 2011.

13. Vario [instructions for use]. McHenry, IL: Medela Inc; 2011.

14. Prevena™ Incision Management System [instructions for use]. San Antonio, TX: KCI USA, Inc; 2010.

15. SensaT.R.A.C.™ Technology [information sheet]. San Antonio, TX: KCI USA, Inc; 2009.

16. Miller MS, Ortegon M, McDaniel C. Negative pressure wound therapy: treating a venomous insect bite. *Int Wound J*. 2007;4(1):88–92.

17. Kasukurthi R, Borschel GH. Simplified negative pressure wound therapy in pediatric hand wounds. *Hand (N Y)*. 2009 Jun 27. [Epub ahead of print]

18. US Food and Drug Administration. FDA Safety Communication: UPDATE on Serious Complications Associated with Negative Pressure Wound Therapy Systems. Available at: http://www.fda.gov/MedicalDevices/Safety/AlertsandNotices/ucm244211.htm. Accessed August 26, 2011.

19. Schiestl C, Neuhaus K, Biedermann T, Böttcher-Haberzeth S, Reichmann E, Meuli M. Novel treatment for massive lower extremity avulsion injuries in children: slow, but effective with good cosmesis. *Eur J Pediatr Surg*. 2011;21(2):106–110.

20. Baharestani M, Amjad I, Bookout K, et al. V.A.C. Therapy in the management of paediatric wounds: clinical review and experience. *Int Wound J*. 2009;6 Suppl 1:1–26.

21. Halvorson J, Jinnah R, Kulp B, Frino J. Use of vacuum-assisted closure in pediatric open fractures with a focus on the rate of infection. *Orthopedics*. 2011;34(7):e256–e260.

22. 3M Health Care. The expanding family of Tegaderm™ Brand Dressings [brochure]. St Paul, MN: 3M Health Care; 2005.

23. Rock R. Get positive results with negative-pressure wound therapy. *American Nurse Today*. 2011;6(1):49–51.

24. Giovinco NA, Bui TD, Fisher T, Mills JL, Armstrong DG. Wound chemotherapy by the use of negative pressure wound therapy and infusion. *Eplasty*. 2010 Jan 8;10:e9.

25. Shah CB, Swogger E, James G. Efficacy of AMD™ dressings against MRSA and VRE [white paper]. Montana State University, Bozeman, MT. Mansfield, MA: Covidien (formerly Tyco Healthcare Group LP). September 2008.

26. Rodriguez A, To D, Hansen A, Ajifu C, Carson S, Travis E. Silver dressings used with wound vacuum assisted closure: is there an advantage? Available at: http://www.silverlon.com/studies/dressing_vac_closure.pdf. Accessed August 28, 2011.

27. Krieger BR, Davis DM, Sanchez JE, et al. The use of silver nylon in preventing surgical site infections following colon and rectal surgery. *Dis Colon Rectum*. 2011;54(8):1014–1019.

28. Deitch EA, Marino AA, Gillespie TE, Albright JA. Silvernylon: a new antimicrobial agent. *Antimicrob Agents Chemother*. 1983;23(3):356–359.

29. Penny HL, Dyson M, Spinazzola J, Green A, Faretta M, Meloy G. The use of negative-pressure wound therapy with bio-dome dressing technology in the treatment of complex diabetic wounds. *Adv Skin Wound Care*. 2010;23(7):305–312.

30. Hydrofera Blue® [instructions for use]. Willimantic, CT: Hydrofera, LLC.

31. Kinetic Concepts Inc. V.A.C.® Therapy™ Clinical Guidelines: A Reference Source for Clinicians. San Antonio, TX: Kinetic Concepts Inc; 2005.

32. Kinetic Concepts Inc. KCI 2006 Product Source Guide. San Antonio, TX: Kinetic Concepts Inc; 2006.

33. Ambrosio A, Barton K, Ginther D. V.A.C. GranuFoam Silver Dressing. A new antimicrobial silver foam dressing specifically engineered for use with V.A.C. Therapy [white paper]. San Antonio, TX: KCI Licensing, Inc; 2006.

34. Payne JL, Ambrosio AM. Evaluation of an antimicrobial silver foam dressing for use with V.A.C. therapy: morphological, mechanical, and antimicrobial properties. *J Biomed Mater Res B Appl Biomater*. 2009;89(1):217–222.

35. Peterson DJ, Hermann K, Niezgoda JA. Effectively managing infected wounds with Hydrofera Blue™ and negative pressure wound therapy. Available at: http://www.hydrofera.com/documents/product_literature/hydrofera_blue/hydrofera_blue_NPWT.pdf. Accessed February 2, 2012.

36. Niezgoda JA. Combining negative pressure wound therapy with other wound management modalities. *Ostomy Wound Manage*. 2005;51(2A Suppl):36S–38S.

37. Malmsjö M, Ingemansson R. Effects of green foam, black foam and gauze on contraction, blood flow and pressure delivery to the wound bed in negative pressure wound therapy. *J Plast Reconstr Aesthet Surg*. 2011;64(12):e289–e296.

38. Malmsjö M, Ingemansson R. Green foam, black foam or gauze for NWPT: effects on granulation tissue formation. *J Wound Care*. 2011;20(6):294–299.

39. Bondjoki S, Reuter C, Rangaswamy M, et al. Clinical efficacy of an alternative foam-based negative pressure wound therapy system. Presented at the Symposium on Advanced Wound Care in Anaheim, CA, September

23–25, 2010.

40. Teder H, Sandén G, Svedman P. Continuous wound irrigation in the pig. *J Invest Surg*. 1990;3(4):399–407.

41. Gray D, Barrett S, Battacharyya M, et al. PHMB and its potential contribution to wound management. *Wounds UK*. 2010;6(2):40–46.

42. Gilliver S. PHMB: a well-tolerated antiseptic with no reported toxic effects. *J Wound Care/Activa Healthcare Supplement*. 2009:S9–S14.

43. Prospera® Negative Pressure Wound Therapy [brochure]. Fort Worth, TX: Prospera; 2008.

44. V1STA Negative Pressure Wound Therapy [quick reference guide]. Largo, FL: Smith & Nephew; 2007.

45. EZCARE Negative Pressure Wound Therapy [quick reference guide]. Largo, FL: Smith & Nephew; 2007.

46. Talley Medical. VENTURI™ Negative Pressure Wound Therapy Clinical Guidelines Manual. Romsey, Hampshire, England: Talley Group Limited; 2009.

47. Hirsch T, Limoochi-Deli S, Lahmer A, et al. Antimicrobial activity of clinically used antiseptics and wound irrigating agents in combination with wound dressings. *Plast Reconstr Surg*. 2011;127(4):1539–1545.

48. Girolami S, Sadowski-Liest D. Bio-Dome™ technology: the newest approach to negative pressure wound therapy. Presented at the Symposium on Advanced Wound Care & Wound Healing Society Meeting in Tampa, FL, April 28–May 1, 2007.

49. Hill L, McCormick J, Tamburino J, et al. The effectiveness of engenex™: a new NPWT device. Presented at the Symposium on Advanced Wound Care & Wound Healing Society Meeting in Tampa, FL, April 28–May 1, 2007.

50. Mitra A, Weyrauch B, Bentley L. Engenex™ and Foundation Based Healing™ [white paper]. Available at: http://www.boehringerwound.com/Engenex%20and%20Foundation%20based%20Healing.pdf. Accessed February 2, 2012.

51. Davis SC, Perez R, Gil J, Valdes J. A pilot study to determine the effects of a negative pressure device on full thickness wounds inoculated with *Pseudomonas aeruginosa* [white paper]. Available at: http://www.kalyptomedical.com/clinical.php. Accessed February 2, 2012.

52. Page J, Woodruff D. The performance of a negative pressure device on chronic wounds of the lower leg and foot. A pilot study [white paper]. Available at: http://kalyptomedical.com/clinical.php. Accessed June 6, 2011.

53. Timoney MF, Zenilman ME. How we manage abdominal compartment syndrome. Available at: http://www.contemporarysurgery.com/pdf/6410/6410CS_REVIEW.pdf. Accessed March 5, 2012.

54. Kinetic Concepts Inc. Instructions for Use: V.A.C.® Therapy Safety Information (for V.A.C.® GranuFoam®, V.A.C.® GranuFoam® Silver™ and V.A.C.® WhiteFoam™ Dressings). San Antonio, TX: Kinetic Concepts Inc; 2006.

55. Venturi ML, Attinger CE, Mesbahi AN, Hess CL, Graw KS. Mechanisms and clinical applications of the vacuum-assisted closure (VAC) device: a review. *Am J Clin Dermatol*. 2005;6(3):185–194.

56. Kaufman MW, Pahl DW. Vacuum-assisted closure therapy: wound care and nursing implications. *Dermatol Nurs*. 2003;15(4):317–326.

57. Short B, Claxton M, Armstrong DG. How to use VAC therapy on chronic wounds. *Podiatry Today*. 2002;15(7):48–54.

58. Andros G, Armstrong DG, Attinger CE, et al. Consensus statement on negative pressure wound therapy (V.A.C. Therapy) for the management of diabetic foot wounds. *Ostomy Wound Manage*. 2006;52(6 Suppl):1–32.

59. Gupta S, Baharestani M, Baranoski S, et al. Guidelines for managing pressure ulcers with negative pressure wound therapy. *Adv Skin Wound Care*. 2004;17(Suppl 2):1–16.

60. Niezgoda JA, Mendez-Eastman S. The effective management of pressure ulcers. *Adv Skin Wound Care*. 2006;19(Suppl 1):3–15.

61. Kaplan M, Banwell P, Orgill DP, et al. Guidelines for the management of the open abdomen. *WOUNDS*. 2005;17(Suppl 1):S1–S24.

62. Orgill DP, Austen WG, Butler CE, et al. Guidelines for treatment of complex chest wounds with negative pressure wound therapy. *WOUNDS*. 2004;16(Suppl B):1–23.

63. Hardwicke J, Paterson P. A role for vacuum-assisted closure in lower limb trauma: a proposed algorithm. *Int J Low Extrem Wounds*. 2006;5(2):101–104.

64. Runkel N, Krug E, Berg L, et al; International Expert Panel on Negative Pressure Wound Therapy (NPWT-EP). Evidence-based recommendations for the use of Negative Pressure Wound Therapy in traumatic wounds and reconstructive surgery: steps towards an international consensus. *Injury*. 2011;42 Suppl 1:S1–S12.

65. Birke-Sorensen H, Malmsjo M, Rome P, et al; International Expert Panel on Negative Pressure Wound Therapy (NPWT-EP). Evidence-based recommendations for negative pressure wound therapy: treatment variables (pressure levels, wound filler and contact layer) -- steps towards an international consensus. *J Plast Reconstr Aesthet Surg*. 2011;64 Suppl:S1–S16.

66. McCallon SK, Knight CA, Valiulus JP, Cunningham MW, McCulloch JM, Farinas LP. Vacuum-assisted closure versus saline-moistened gauze in the healing of postoperative diabetic foot wounds. *Ostomy Wound Manage*. 2000;46(8):28–34.

67. Eginton MT, Brown KR, Seabrook GR, Towne JB, Cambria RA. A prospective randomized evaluation of negative-pressure wound dressings for diabetic foot wounds. *Ann Vasc Surg*. 2003;17(6):645–649.

68. Armstrong DG, Lavery LA; Diabetic Foot Study Consortium. Negative pressure wound therapy after partial diabetic foot amputation: a multicentre, randomised controlled trial. *Lancet*. 2005;366(9498):1704–1710.

69. Page JC, Newswander B, Schwenke DC, Hansen M, Ferguson J. Retrospective analysis of negative pressure wound therapy in open foot wounds with significant soft tissue defects. *Adv Skin Wound Care*. 2004;17(7):354–364.

70. Frykberg RG, Williams DV. Negative-pressure wound therapy and diabetic foot amputations: a retrospective study of payer claims data. *J Am Podiatr Med Assoc*. 2007;97(5):351–359.

71. Blume PA, Walters J, Payne W, Ayala J, Lantis J. Comparison of negative pressure wound therapy using vacuum-assisted closure with advanced moist wound therapy in the treatment of diabetic foot ulcers: a multicenter randomized controlled trial. *Diabetes Care*. 2008;31(4):631–636.

72. Ford CN, Reinhard ER, Yeh D, et al. Interim analysis of a prospective, randomized trial of vacuum-assisted closure versus the Healthpoint system in the management of pressure ulcers. *Ann Plast Surg.* 2002;49(1):55–61.

73. Joseph E, Hamori CA, Bergman S, Roaf E, Swann NF, Anastasi GW. A prospective, randomized trial of vacuum-assisted closure versus standard therapy of chronic non-healing wounds. *WOUNDS.* 2000;12(3):60–67.

74. Wanner MB, Schwarzl F, Strub B, Zaech GA, Pierer G. Vacuum-assisted wound closure for cheaper and more comfortable healing of pressure sores: a prospective study. *Scand J Plast Reconstr Surg Hand Surg.* 2003;37(1):28–33.

75. Philbeck TE Jr, Whittington KT, Millsap MH, Briones RB, Wight DG, Schroeder WJ. The clinical and cost effectiveness of externally applied negative pressure wound therapy in the treatment of wounds in home healthcare Medicare patients. *Ostomy Wound Manage.* 1999;45(11):41–50.

76. Vuerstaek JD, Vainas T, Wuite J, Nelemans P, Neumann MH, Veraart JC. State-of-the-art treatment of chronic leg ulcers: a randomized controlled trial comparing vacuum-assisted closure (V.A.C.) with modern wound dressings. *J Vasc Surg.* 2006;44(5):1029–1038.

77. Braakenburg A, Obdeijn MC, Feitz R, van Rooij IA, van Griethuysen AJ, Klinkenbijl JH. The clinical efficacy and cost effectiveness of the vacuum-assisted closure technique in the management of acute and chronic wounds: a randomized controlled trial. *Plast Reconstr Surg.* 2006;118(2):390–397.

78. Moues CM, Vos MC, van den Bemd GJ, Stijnen T, Hovius SE. Bacterial load in relation to vacuum-assisted closure wound therapy: a prospective randomized trial. *Wound Repair Regen.* 2004;12(1):11–17.

79. Moisidis E, Heath T, Boorer C, Ho K, Deva AK. A prospective, blinded, randomized, controlled clinical trial of topical negative pressure use in skin grafting. *Plast Reconstr Surg.* 2004;114(4):917–922.

80. Jeschke MG, Rose C, Angele P, Füchtmeier B, Nerlich MN, Bolder U. Development of new reconstructive techniques: use of Integra in combination with fibrin glue and negative-pressure therapy for reconstruction of acute and chronic wounds. *Plast Reconstr Surg.* 2004;113(2):525–530.

81. Genecov DG, Schneider AM, Morykwas MJ, Parker D, White WL, Argenta LC. A controlled subatmospheric pressure dressing increases the rate of skin graft donor site reepithelialization. *Ann Plast Surg.* 1998;40(3):219–225.

82. Carson SN, Overall K, Lee-Jahshan S, Travis E. Vacuum-assisted closure used for healing chronic wounds and skin grafts in the lower extremities. *Ostomy Wound Manage.* 2004;50(3):52–58.

83. Stannard JP, Volgas DA, McGwin G 3rd, et al. Incisional negative pressure wound therapy after high-risk lower extremity fractures. *J Orthop Trauma.* 2012;26(1):37–42.

84. Kilpadi DV, Cunningham MR. Evaluation of closed incision management with negative pressure wound therapy (CIM): hematoma/seroma and involvement of the lymphatic system. *Wound Repair Regen.* 2011;19(5):588–596.

85. Ferrell BA, Osterweil D, Christenson P. A randomized trial of low-air-loss beds for treatment of pressure ulcers. *JAMA.* 1993;269(4):494–497.

86. Schwien T, Gilbert J, Lang C. Pressure ulcer prevalence and the role of negative pressure wound therapy in home health quality outcomes. *Ostomy Wound Manage.* 2005;51(9):47–60.

87. de Leon JM, Barnes S, Nagel M, Fudge M, Lucius A, Garcia B. Cost-effectiveness of negative pressure wound therapy for postsurgical patients in long-term acute care. *Adv Skin Wound Care.* 2009;22(3):122–127.

88. Perez D, Bramkamp M, Exe C, von Ruden C, Ziegler A. Modern wound care for the poor: a randomized clinical trial comparing the vacuum system with conventional saline-soaked gauze dressings. *Am J Surg.* 2010;199(1):14–20.

89. Lerman B, Oldenbrook L, Eichstadt SL, Ryu J, Fong KD, Schubart PJ. Evaluation of chronic wound treatment with the SNaP wound care system versus modern dressing protocols. *Plast Reconstr Surg.* 2010;126(4):1253–1261.

90. Armstrong DG, Marston WA, Reyzelman AM, Kirsner RS. Comparison of negative pressure wound therapy with an ultraportable mechanically powered device vs. traditional electrically powered device for the treatment of chronic lower extremity ulcers: a multicenter randomized-controlled trial. *Wound Repair Regen.* 2011;19(2):173–180.

91. Hutton DW, Sheehan P. Comparative effectiveness of the SNaP™ Wound Care System. *Int Wound J.* 2011;8(2):196–205.

92. Campbell AM, Kuhn WP, Barker P. Vacuum-assisted closure of the open abdomen in a resource-limited setting. *S Afr J Surg.* 2010;48(4):114–115.

93. Kamolz LP, Andel H, Haslik W, Winter W, Meissl G, Frey M. Use of subatmospheric pressure therapy to prevent burn wound progression in human: first experiences. *Burns.* 2004;30(3):253–258.

94. Garner GB, Ware DN, Cocanour CS, et al. Vacuum-assisted wound closure provides early fascial reapproximation in trauma patients with open abdomens. *Am J Surg.* 2001;182(6):630–638.

95. Agarwal JP, Ogilvie M, Wu LC, et al. Vacuum-assisted closure for sternal wounds: a first-line therapeutic management approach. *Plast Reconstr Surg.* 2005;116(4):1035–1043.

96. Campbell PE, Smith GS, Smith JM. Retrospective clinical evaluation of gauze-based negative pressure wound therapy. *Int Wound J.* 2008;5(2):280–286.

97. Chariker ME, Jeter KF, Tintle TE, Bottsford JE. Effective management of incisional and cutaneous fistulae with closed suction wound drainage. *Contemporary Surgery.* 1989;34:59–63.

98. Hurd T, Chadwick P, Cote J, Cockwill J, Mole TR, Smith JM. Impact of gauze-based NPWT on the patient and nursing experience in the treatment of challenging wounds. *Int Wound J.* 2010;7(6):448–455.

99. Dunn R, Hurd T, Chadwick P, et al. Factors associated with positive outcomes in 131 patients treated with gauze-based negative pressure wound therapy. *Int J Surg.* 2011;9(3):258–262.

100. Fraccalvieri M, Zingarelli E, Ruka E, et al. Negative pressure wound therapy using gauze and foam: histological, immunohistochemical and ultrasonography morpho-

logical analysis of the granulation tissue and scar tissue. Preliminary report of a clinical study. *Int Wound J.* 2011;8(4):355–364.

101. Dunn RM, Ignotz R, Mole T, Cockwill J, Smith JM. Assessment of gauze-based negative pressure wound therapy in the split-thickness skin graft clinical pathway-an observational study. *Eplasty.* 2011;11:e14.

102. Landsman A. Analysis of the SNaP Wound Care System, a negative pressure wound device for treatment of diabetic lower extremity wounds. *J Diabetes Sci Technol.* 2010;4(4):831–832.

103. Dorafshar AH, Franczyk M, Gottlieb LJ, Wroblewski KE, Lohman RF. A prospective randomized trial comparing subatmospheric wound therapy with a sealed gauze dressing and the standard vacuum-assisted closure device. *Ann Plast Surg.* 2011 Jun 27. [Epub ahead of print]

104. Ilizarov GA. The tension-stress effect on the genesis and growth of tissues. Part I. The influence of stability of fixation and soft-tissue preservation. *Clin Orthop Relat Res.* 1989;(238):249–281.

105. Ilizarov GA. The tension-stress effect on the genesis and growth of tissues: Part II. The influence of the rate and frequency of distraction. *Clin Orthop Relat Res.* 1989;(239):263–285.

106. Saxena V, Hwang CW, Huang S, Eichbaum Q, Ingber D, Orgill DP. Vacuum-assisted closure: microdeformations of wounds and cell proliferation. *Plast Reconstr Surg.* 2004;114(5):1086–1098.

107. Greene AK, Puder M, Roy R, et al. Microdeformational wound therapy: effects on angiogenesis and matrix metalloproteinases in chronic wounds of 3 debilitated patients. *Ann Plast Surg.* 2006;56(4):418–422.

108. Danciu TE, Gagari E, Adam RM, Damoulis PD, Freeman MR. Mechanical strain delivers anti-apoptotic and proliferative signals to gingival fibroblasts. *J Dent Res.* 2004;83(8):596–601.

109. Huang S, Ingber DE. Shape-dependent control of cell growth, differentiation, and apoptosis: switching between attractors in cell regulatory networks. *Exp Cell Res.* 2000;261(1):91–103.

110. Ikeda M, Takei T, Mills I, Kito H, Sumpio BE. Extracellular signal-regulated kinases 1 and 2 activation in endothelial cells exposed to cyclic strain. *Am J Physiol.* 1999;276(2 Pt 2):H614–H622.

111. Chiquet M, Renedo AS, Huber F, Flück M. How do fibroblasts translate mechanical signals into changes in extracellular matrix production? *Matrix Biol.* 2000;22(1):73–80.

112. MacKenna D, Summerour SR, Villarreal FJ. Role of mechanical factors in modulating cardiac fibroblast function and extracellular matrix synthesis. *Cardiovasc Res.* 2000;46(2):257–263.

113. Katsumi A, Naoe T, Matsushita T, Kaibuchi K, Schwartz MA. Integrin activation and matrix binding mediate cellular responses to mechanical stretch. *J Biol Chem.* 2005;280(17):16546–16549.

114. Shyy JY, Chien S. Role of integrins in cellular responses to mechanical stress and adhesion. *Curr Opin Cell Biol.* 1997;9(5):707–713.

115. Wang N, Naruse K, Stamenovic D, et al. Mechanical behavior in living cells consistent with the tensegrity model. *Proc Natl Acad Sci U S A.* 2001;98(14):7765–7770.

116. Chen CS, Mrksich M, Huang S, Whitesides GM, Ingber DE. Geometric control of cell life and death. *Science.* 1997;276(5317):1425–1428.

117. McNulty AK, Schmidt M, Feeley T, Kieswetter K. Effects of negative pressure wound therapy on fibroblast viability, chemotactic signaling, and proliferation in a provisional wound (fibrin) matrix. *Wound Repair Regen.* 2007;15(6):838–846.

118. Wilkes R, Zhao Y, Kieswetter K, Haridas B. Effects of dressing type on 3D tissue microdeformations during negative pressure wound therapy: a computational study. *J Biomech Eng.* 2009;131(3):031012.

119. Anesäter E, Borgquist O, Hedström E, Waga J, Ingemansson R, Malmsjö M. The influence of different sizes and types of wound fillers on wound contraction and tissue pressure during negative pressure wound therapy. *Int Wound J.* 2011;8(4):336–342.

120. Goutos I, Ghosh SJ. Gauze-based negative pressure wound therapy as an adjunct to collagen-elastin [corrected] dermal template resurfacing. *J Wound Care.* 2011;20(2):55–56,58,60.

121. Chen WY, Abatangelo G. Functions of hyaluronan in wound repair. *Wound Repair Regen.* 1999;7(2):79–89.

122. Oksala O, Salo T, Tammi R, et al. Expression of proteoglycans and hyaluronan during wound healing. *J Histochem Cytochem.* 1995;43(2):125–135.

123. McNulty AK, Feeley T, Schmidt M, Norbury K, Kieswetter K. Glycosaminoglycan composition of granulation tissue from wounds treated with negative pressure wound therapy or moist wound therapy. Presented at the Symposium on Advanced Wound Care in San Antonio, TX, April 30–May 3, 2006.

124. Bucknall TE. The effect of local infection upon wound healing: an experimental study. *Br J Surg.* 1980;67(12):851–855.

125. Schultz GS, Sibbald RG, Falanga V, et al. Wound bed preparation: a systematic approach to wound management. *Wound Repair Regen.* 2003;11(Suppl 1):S1–S28.

126. DeFranzo AJ, Argenta LC, Marks MW, et al. The use of vacuum-assisted closure therapy for the treatment of lower-extremity wounds with exposed bone. *Plast Reconstr Surg.* 2001;108(5):1184–1191.

127. Timmers MS, Le Cessie S, Banwell P, Jukema GN. The effects of varying degrees of pressure delivered by negative-pressure wound therapy on skin perfusion. *Ann Plast Surg.* 2005;55(6):665–671.

128. Wackenfors A, Sjögren J, Gustafsson R, Algotsson L, Ingemansson R, Malmsjö M. Effects of vacuum-assisted closure therapy on inguinal wound edge microvascular blood flow. *Wound Repair Regen.* 2004;12(6):600–606.

129. Wackenfors A, Gustafsson R, Sjögren J, Algotsson L, Ingemansson R, Malmsjö M. Blood flow responses in the peristernal thoracic wall during vacuum-assisted closure therapy. *Ann Thorac Surg.* 2005;79(5):1724–1731.

130. Zawacki BE. The natural history of reversible burn injury. *Surg Gynecol Obstet.* 1974;139(6):867–872.

The Role of Oxygen and Hyperbaric Medicine

Robert A. Warriner, III, MD, FCCP, FACWS, FAPWCA;
James R. Wilcox, RN, BSN, ACHRN;
Richard Barry, CHT

Objectives

The reader will be challenged to:

- Analyze the impact of local tissue hypoxia on wound healing and response to infection
- Distinguish the physiological benefits to wound healing provided by oxygen delivered by different mechanisms
- Assess the physiological and pharmacological benefits of hyperbaric oxygen treatment to wound healing
- Select appropriate patients for adjunctive hyperbaric oxygen treatment provided in an integrated wound care setting
- Implement essential aspects of safe hyperbaric patient management in the practice setting.

Introduction

Hyperbaric oxygen treatment (HBOT) as adjunctive therapy to aggressive surgical debridement and antibiotic therapy for necrotizing soft tissue infection dates back to the 1960s. Clinicians took advantage of the specific benefits of elevating tissue oxygen levels in the presence of these anaerobic, exotoxin-producing wound infections to improve limb and tissue salvage and overall survival. Subsequent experience and research in other wound healing problems, including radiation bone and soft tissue injury, acute traumatic ischemias, various types of ischemic reperfusion injury states, and a wide range of chronically hypoperfused and hypoxic wounds, has led to the development of the current recommendations for the clinical use of HBOT as outlined in the 12th edition of *Hyperbaric Oxygen Therapy Indications*,[1] which was published by the Undersea and Hyperbaric Medical Society in 2009. Over the past 10 years, a new understanding of the pharmacology of hyperbaric oxygenation of tissues and randomized, controlled, clinical trials of HBOT in radiation tissue injury and refractory diabetic ulcer healing and limb salvage have enhanced the acceptance of adjunctive HBOT for the mainstream management of complex problem wounds.

Adequate molecular oxygen is required for a wide range of biosynthetic processes essential to normal wound healing. Molecular oxygen is required for hydroxylation of proline during collagen synthesis and cross linking as well as provision of substrate for the production of reactive oxygen species during the respiratory burst occurring within leukocytes that have

Warriner RA, Wilcox JR, Barry R. The role of oxygen and hyperbaric medicine. In: Krasner DL, Rodeheaver GT, Sibbald RG, Woo KY, eds. *Chronic Wound Care: A Clinical Source Book for Healthcare Professionals.* Vol 1. 5th ed. Malvern, PA: HMP Communications; 2012:301–309.

phagocytized bacteria within the wound. While short-term hypoxia is one stimulus for angiogenesis in wound healing, adequate local oxygen levels are required to sustain an effective angiogenic response and for the reconstruction of an adequate dermal matrix. Recent research has shown that oxygen also plays an important role in the cell signaling events necessary for tissue repair, which further explains the fragile dynamic between oxygen availability and the increased demands for oxygen during recovery from tissue injury.[2]

When oxygen availability to a wound is reduced by hypoperfusion from macrovascular arterial disease, microvascular failure, local edema, or infection, wound healing is invariably impaired. *Periwound hypoxia* can be objectively determined by transcutaneous PO2 measurement.[3] When identified, periwound hypoxia should be addressed with further vascular assessment and interventions to improve large vessel perfusion, reduce tissue edema, and improve microvascular homeostasis by maintaining normovolemia and vasomotor tone and with therapeutic oxygen administration. The method of administration determines the potential beneficial effects of additional oxygen administration in support of wound healing.

Supplemental Oxygen Breathing at One Atmosphere

Additional oxygen can be provided therapeutically by increasing the inspired oxygen concentration above 21% by use of a nasal cannula or a simple facemask. The maximum achievable intra-arterial PO2 breathing 100% oxygen at 1 ATA (atmospheres absolute) is approximately 670 mmHg. In well perfused tissues, supplemental oxygen breathing at 1 ATA may transiently reverse mild local tissue hypoxia secondary to edema or mild hypothermic vasoconstriction but has not been shown to reduce postoperative wound infections[4] or improve collagen deposition.

Topical Oxygen

HBOT is not provided by devices that apply oxygen at 1 ATA over the surface of the wound, by devices that provide a small pressure differential (usually around 1.04 ATA) by enclosing an appendage in an inflatable bag or plastic cylinder, or by devices providing a surface oxygen blowover using a micro-oxygen concentrator device. None of these devices are considered by the US Food and Drug Administration to provide hyperbaric oxygen, and the misused terminology has led to significant confusion in both the literature and in discussion of the potential merits of oxygen applied by some manner to the wound surface. Two recent reviews[5,6] addressed the potential for topical oxygen to benefit wound healing. While *in-vitro* research has suggested some rationale for topical oxygen,[7] critical questions have yet to be answered. Topical oxygen appears to increase wound surface and subsurface PO2 values but only to a relatively shallow depth. Topical oxygen produces a gradient opposite of what is produced during HBOT, and it is unclear how this reverse gradient might drive the direction of angiogenesis and tissue growth. Clinical trials and case series to date have produced positive and negative effects,[8-12] unlike the consistently positive results seen with HBOT for chronic lower-extremity wounds and diabetic limb salvage cases. The Undersea and Hyperbaric Medical Society published a position statement[13] that discussed these concerns. The proposed recommendations for topical oxygen in lower-extremity wounds[6] require further validation before they are widely accepted in clinical practice.

An alternative to oxygen delivered by low-flow blowover or topical oxygen under pressure is a dressing that might deliver oxygen to the wound surface typically through incorporation of hydrogen peroxide into the dressing core structure. There is little evidence to suggest any benefit on wound healing other than potential suppression of wound surface microorganisms.

Hyperbaric Oxygen

HBOT is defined as *breathing 100% oxygen in an environment of elevated atmospheric pressure typically ranging from 2.0 to a maximum of 3.0 ATA or 2 to 3 times normal atmospheric pressure.* This can occur in a *monoplace (single-patient) chamber* typically compressed with 100% oxygen or, less frequently, in a *multiplace (multiple-patient) chamber* typically compressed with air with the patient breathing 100% oxygen through a specially designed hood or mask. Intravascular PO2 values are in excess of 1700 mmHg.[14]

HBOT provides additional oxygen to the

hypoxic wound and supports wound healing through a variety of mechanisms. The immediate effects of HBOT occurring during treatment improve wound "metabolism" in the setting of acute or chronic local hypoxia. These relatively short-lived effects in support of wound healing include the following:

1) Improved local tissue oxygenation, leading to improved cellular energy metabolism
2) Increased collagen and other extracellular matrix protein deposition and epithelization
3) Decreased local tissue edema due to vaso-constriction of vessels in nonischemic tissues
4) Improved leukocyte-bacterial-killing (adequate leukocyte count critical for benefit)
5) Suppressed exotoxin production
6) Increased effectiveness of antibiotics that require oxygen for active transport across microbial cell membranes.

These effects, while important, would not by themselves account for the degree of improvement in wound healing seen in most diabetic foot ulcers treated with HBOT.

Over the past 15 years, research has led to a somewhat different understanding of the role of HBOT, which has focused on the role HBOT plays in altering the balance of reactive oxygen (ROS) and reactive nitrogen (RNS) species within the wound, fundamentally altering the wound environment and its healing response. In this context, HBOT also must be thought of as providing oxygen as a cell-signaling agent.[15,16] Achieving these effects beneficial to wound healing requires that a minimum PO2 of around 200 mmHg be achieved in the periwound tissues. The effects include:

1) Enhanced growth factor and growth factor receptor production (especially platelet-derived growth factor [PDGF] and vascular endothelial growth factor [VEGF], helpful in wound matrix reconstruction and angiogenesis)
2) Altered leukocyte β-integrin receptor sensitivity (helpful in mitigating ischemia-reperfusion injury, which occurs in many chronic and some acute wound settings)
3) Reduced inflammation and apoptosis (at least in some acute ischemic wound models)
4) Activated stem cell metabolism and release into the circulation from bone marrow reservoirs.

These physio-pharmacological changes have been observed both in vitro and in vivo.[17-20] It is interesting to note that the ROS- and RNS-mediated pathways that can be enhanced by HBOT can have both positive and negative effects on wound healing. The biochemical environment of the wound when exposed to HBOT probably determines these effects. Perhaps in the future we will be better able to characterize these conditions within the wound or ulcer bed as a means to better select specific patients who will respond optimally to HBOT for limb salvage.

Clinical Experience with HBOT in Wound Healing

Prior to 2010, the strongest clinical evidence for HBOT in diabetic limb salvage was the randomized, controlled, clinical trial reported by Faglia et al.[21] This study involved 68 patients randomized to HBOT and standard care groups. Revascularization was provided to all patients where indicated by arteriographic findings. A team comprised of members who were blinded to the core intervention made the surgical decisions. The HBOT group required 3 major amputations (3/35 or 8.6%), while the standard care group required 11 major amputations (11.33, 33%) with a $P = .016$.

Following a review of the Faglia et al study and an independent, evidence-based review in 2002, the Centers for Medicare & Medicaid Services approved HBOT for Wagner grade 3 and greater diabetic foot ulcers. A 2004 Cochrane review concluded that HBOT significantly reduced the risk of major amputation in diabetic foot ulcer patients.[22] In cost-effectiveness studies, Guo et al[23] and the Canadian Diabetes Association[24] demonstrated that HBOT reduced anticipated major amputations and was cost-effective on a long-term basis.

In a *meta-analysis of HBOT* in wound healing and limb salvage, Goldman[25] evaluated published randomized, controlled, clinical trials and observational studies of various designs using the **GRADE criteria** for assigning levels of evidence. Thirty-five studies (excluding the 2010 Löndahl et al study[26]) met the inclusion criteria of original human studies with diabetes-related wound healing, tissue salvage, or limb salvage as the clinical endpoint. Thirty-three of the studies reported positive efficacy, 1 was equivocal, and 1 was negative with a low strength of evidence. In all, 4,057 patients with diabetes were included in the studies reviewed. When the endpoint was limb salvage, HBOT provided a 3-fold reduction in the risk of amputation when compared to conventional wound care alone, providing GRADE level 1 evidence.

The most recent clinical trial of hyperbaric oxygen in diabetic ulcers was published by Löndahl et al in Sweden.[26] The randomized, single-center, double-blind, placebo-controlled, clinical trial was completed at the Institution for Clinical Sciences in Lund, Lund University. Ninety-four patients with Wagner grade 2, 3, or 4 ulcers of greater than 3 months' duration with adequate perfusion or with non-reconstructable peripheral arterial disease were randomized into 2 groups. Patients were treated with 2.5 ATA air or 2.5 ATA 100% oxygen for 85 minutes in a multi-place chamber with a coded gas delivery system. Treatments were administered 5 days per week for 8 weeks (40 treatments) with a study duration of 10 weeks and a 1-year follow-up. This was an intention-to-treat analysis with a primary endpoint of ulcer healing. Complete healing was achieved in 37/94 patients at 1 year, 25/48 (52%) in the HBOT group and 12/42 (29%) in the placebo group ($P = .03$). Subgroup analysis of patients completing > 35 HBOT sessions showed healing in 23/38 (61%) in the HBOT group versus 10/37 (27%) in the placebo group ($P = .009$).

Finally, the Wound Healing Society Clinical Practice Guidelines for diabetic foot ulcer care[27] give HBOT a 1A level of evidence recommendation, and the ischemic ulcer guidelines[28] give it a level IIB recommendation.

Indications for HBOT in Wounds

The Undersea and Hyperbaric Medical Society[3] provides recommendations for the use of HBOT based on a selected expert panel's review of relevant published clinical and experimental data. This report and other published reviews define the specific wound etiologies that may be expected to benefit from intermittent HBOT exposure, including:

- Acute thermal burns
- Clostridial myonecrosis
- Other necrotizing soft tissue infections

- Compromised skin grafts and flaps
- Crush injury and compartment syndrome
- Other acute traumatic ischemias
- Osteoradionecrosis
- Soft tissue radionecrosis
- Refractory osteomyelitis
- Other wounds with demonstrated peri-wound hypoxia, particularly in patients with diabetes mellitus and chronic ischemic ulcers.

Selection of Patients for HBOT

HBOT is best justified within a consistently applied patient selection process that takes into consideration those factors suggested to impact response to this therapy.[29,30] The most critical of these factors is sufficient local blood flow to support the local elevation of tissue PO2 that is possible during the HBOT exposure. The following should be considered in the initial treatment decision:

- Is the clinical presentation of the wound consistent with the published experience of wounds in which HBOT has been demonstrated to be beneficial?
- Is hypoxia as measured by PtcO2 present in tissue adjacent to the wound?
- Does the periwound tissue respond to an increase of inspired oxygen concentration, indicating at least minimally sufficient periwound blood flow to allow a therapeutic increase in local oxygen tension during HBOT?

Based on these considerations, the hyperbaric physician follows a process similar to the following to determine which patients with problem wounds are appropriate candidates for adjunctive HBOT delivered as a component of total wound care:

1. An appropriate wound etiology associated with local hypoxia or persistent infection is identified.
2. Periwound hypoxia is demonstrated by PtcO2 measurement whenever possible. The equipment for this testing is readily available, and an excellent review article described in detail the principles for performance of the test and interpretation of the results obtained. Multiple electrode sites should be selected whenever possible, including sites adjacent to and in the normal anatomical distribution

of blood flow to the wound. PtcO2 measurements have been shown to be of value in predicting wound healing success or failure and in the evaluation of peripheral arterial occlusive disease.[3]

3. All patients considered for adjunctive HBOT undergo a complete medical and nursing evaluation to determine the risks of treatment and the medical and care issues that will have to be addressed by the hyperbaric medicine team. Glycemic control and prevention of hypoglycemia associated with HBOT are of particular importance. Absolute contraindications (untreated pneumothorax, some concomitant chemotherapeutic agents) should be identified and the patient excluded from treatment. Relative contraindications (factors that increase CNS or pulmonary oxygen toxicity risk, such as high fever, some drugs, such as bleomycin, cis-platin, and factors that increase the risk of otic or pulmonary barotrauma, such as reactive airway disease) should be identified and the patient's condition optimized prior to treatment whenever possible. The hyperbaric physician should determine the appropriateness of the treatment for each patient with respect to the best likely achievable outcome. Cost-effectiveness studies based on medical economic modeling have demonstrated the cost and clinical value position of HBOT in diabetic limb salvage.[31,32] While the personal economic impact of daily visits to an outpatient healthcare facility for HBOT and wound care have not been assessed by study, one can consider the impact and the potential value of the outcome as similar to that experienced by cancer patients undergoing protracted radiation therapy treatment. Londahl demonstrated that HBOT improved long-term health-related quality of life.[33]

4. HBOT is initiated. Treatments for wound healing are typically 90 minutes of 100% oxygen breathing at 2.0 ATA in monoplace chambers or 2.4 ATA in multiplace chambers. Air breathing breaks are usually provided, particularly when treatment pressures are greater than 2.0 ATA, to reduce the risk of central nervous system oxygen toxicity.

Treatments for chronic hypoxic wounds are usually administered daily but may be administered more frequently depending on wound severity and patient condition.

5. A therapeutic rise in PtcO2 values during treatment must be demonstrated. These values should be routinely measured in all patients as early in the course of adjunctive HBOT as possible. While some controversy exists as to the optimal PtcO2 values that must be achieved during treatment to predict successful wound healing, 200 mmHg is usually considered to be the minimum value necessary. In all cases, the clinical response of the wound to HBOT determines whether HBOT should be continued, with the PtcO2 value serving only as a general guide to exclude non-responders earlier to avoid futile treatment.

6. The response to treatment and/or evidence of continued requirement for treatment is frequently reassessed. This involves examination of the wound for evidence of resolution of infection and accelerated tissue growth or stability of the treated tissue graft or flap. The decision to discontinue HBOT can be as complicated as the one to initiate it. Is the patient intolerant of treatment or have other medical conditions occurred that limit the application of an effective treatment protocol? Is the wound failing to respond to adjunctive HBOT after a reasonable trial of treatment? Is the original indication for which adjunctive HBOT was initiated no longer present? Have PtcO2 values in the skin reasonably adjacent to the wound been raised to a level above the selection criteria for the particular patient? Has the wound healing response reached a plateau? The answers to these questions should help to determine when to discontinue treatment.

Adverse Events Occurring During HBOT

Although HBOT has been safely and successfully provided to thousands of patients representing a wide range of ischemic/hypoxic wound healing problems, complications associated with the hyperbaric environment can occur and require careful ongoing medical assessment and sometimes emergency intervention. **Untreated pneumothorax and pregnancy** (when not associated with carbon monoxide poisoning or life-threatening necrotizing soft tissue infection) are the only absolute contraindications. Relative contraindications should be considered from a risk-benefit perspective and optimized if the decision is made to initiate HBOT. A full discussion of these complications is beyond the scope of this chapter. However, adverse events from a large case series were recently reported.[34] The series included 17,394 patients with 453,749 HBOT sessions in monoplace chambers (average of 26 treatments per patient) provided primarily in outpatient settings. The authors noted the relative safety of HBOT, especially when patients received standardized medical evaluations prior to initiating treatment, standardized pretreatment education, and standardized assessments prior to each treatment. In 2010, 956 adverse events were reported for 252,599 treatments in 9,638 patients for an overall adverse event rate of 0.38%. In order of decreasing rate of occurrence were **ear pain** (of any description), **confinement anxiety, hypoglycemic events, shortness of breath**, and **seizure** (35 events, 0.02%, in 2009 and 53 events, 0.02%, in 2010).

The Team in Hyperbaric Medicine: The Hyperbaric Physician, Nurse, and Technologist

The **physician trained in hyperbaric medicine** plays a valuable role as the leader of the HBOT team. A specific body of knowledge defines the scope of hyperbaric medicine practice in these patients. The Undersea and Hyperbaric Medical Society has defined minimum training requirements for physicians, nurses, and technicians. This organization also has defined facility operational standards to enhance the appropriateness and safety of HBOT administration in the United States. HBOT should never be administered in isolation from other aspects of care of the wound or the patient. Therefore, the most successful applications of HBOT occur when the treatment and the hyperbaric physician are fully integrated into an interprofessional wound care approach.

Once the physician decides that the patient is a candidate for HBOT, the hyperbaric therapy nurse performs much of the preparatory work. The varied clinical applications for hyperbarics

have led to the development of a unique, highly skilled nursing specialty. Hyperbaric nurses are responsible for the practical implementation of patient care during hyperbaric treatments. The Baromedical Nurses Association (BNA) established standards for practice and published a textbook, *Hyperbaric Nursing*,[35] which was revised in 2010. The BNA also made a copy of their Nursing Standards of Care available on their website (www.hyperbaricnurses.org). These standards of care provide hyperbaric nurses with exact criteria against which patient care can be evaluated for effectiveness and appropriateness.

Hyperbaric nurses start with a comprehensive nursing history and physical assessment, which always includes the assistance of potential hyperbaric patients and their significant others, if possible. The data collected is documented and communicated to all health team members involved in the care of the patient. This information is used to develop a nursing diagnosis, which is expressed as the sum of 3 parts: problem, etiology, and signs/symptoms. The nursing diagnosis must be continuously prioritized, reviewed, and revised as appropriate throughout the continuum of care. The nursing care plan is continuously evaluated for its impact on patient response to goal achievement. Nursing action should be designed to accomplish established goals, which are initiated based on the nursing plan of care.

The third member of the HBOT team is the **qualified hyperbaric chamber operator**, often referred to as the hyperbaric technologist. The technologist is trained in hyperbaric medicine, safety, and technical aspects and plays a valuable role as a member of the wound care team. Training in hyperbaric medicine is not entry-level training but rather an added qualification for someone who has previously received formal training in an allied healthcare profession. Common examples are individuals certified or licensed as respiratory therapists, military corpsmen, EMTs/paramedics, registered nurses or LPNs/LVNs, nurse practitioners, certified nurse aides, and certified medical assistants.

Technologists can obtain certification through the National Board of Diving & Hyperbaric Medical Technology (NBDHMT) by demonstrating competency in specific areas; by documenting clinical practice experience; by possessing a qualifying allied healthcare profession; and by passing an examination, leading to designation as a Certified Hyperbaric Technologist (CHT).[35] The NBDHMT has defined minimum training requirements for hyperbaric nurses and technologists.[36]

The Undersea and Hyperbaric Medical Society and the National Fire Protection Association (NFPA) have defined facility operational guidelines to enhance the appropriateness and safety of HBOT administration in the United States.[37,38] Additionally, NFPA code standards call for a hyperbaric safety director to be designated at every hyperbaric facility. It is common practice for the lead hyperbaric technologist to be the designee. Further training in safety is recommended for the hyperbaric safety director.

The technologist focuses on patient orientation to the HBOT experience. Emphasis is placed upon the purpose of the treatment, the treatment schedule, special precautions to be taken for the patient's comfort and safety, and teaching the patient middle ear pressure equalization (ear clearing) techniques. Patients should be able to explain their role in the treatment to the technologist. During a treatment, it is important to note that the technologist's main role is to monitor patients and equipment in order to respond quickly to possible adverse events.

Conclusion

Gaps in our knowledge remain, especially as it relates to optimal HBOT candidates. However, when integrated into a system of interprofessional wound care, HBOT has been shown in multiple clinical trials over an extended period of time and in extensive clinical experience in inpatient and outpatient clinical settings to be an effective adjunct to wound healing and diabetic limb salvage. Careful attention to initial patient selection and careful ongoing monitoring to minimize the risk of adverse events and to optimize the therapeutic benefit enhance the value of HBOT in these patients. The interprofessional wound care hyperbaric medicine team has contributed significantly to the effectiveness of this intervention. HBOT should be available to all centers providing limb salvage and complex diabetic foot ulcer treatment services.

Practice Pearls
- Topical oxygen, while perhaps finding value in the future, has yet to be established on firm clinical grounds for wound healing.
- The optimal application of HBOT requires an understanding of the physiology and pharmacology of elevated tissue PO2 and a systematic approach to evaluation and management of patients with wounds.
- The interprofessional hyperbaric medicine care team plays an essential role in achieving safe, optimal outcomes in these patients.

Self-Assessment Questions

1. Local hypoxia in the tissue surrounding a chronic wound has been shown to cause all of the following EXCEPT:
   A. Impaired local response of leukocytes to bacterial infection
   B. Improved rate and amount of collagen synthesis by fibroblasts
   C. Decreased effectiveness of certain antibiotics
   D. Decreased angiogenesis into the wound margin

2. HBOT has been shown to do all of the following EXCEPT:
   A. Stimulate angiogenesis
   B. Improve leukocyte response to bacterial infection
   C. Ameliorate post-ischemic reperfusion injury
   D. Restore normal tissue oxygen values in the absence of any local blood flow

3. HBOT provides the greatest benefit in the treatment of chronic wounds when all of the following conditions are met EXCEPT:
   A. It is administered in an interprofessional setting
   B. Prospective patients are evaluated by a physician specifically trained in the use of HBOT
   C. It is used to replace peripheral arterial angioplasty or surgical revascularization

D. PtcO2 measurements are used along with frequent examination of the wound to determine the course and duration of treatment

Answers: 1-B, 2-D, 3-C

References

1. Gesell LB. The Hyperbaric Oxygen Therapy Committee Report. *Hyperbaric Oxygen Therapy Indications.* 12th ed. Durham, NC: Undersea and Hyperbaric Medical Society; 2009.

2. Sen CK. Wound healing essentials: let there be oxygen. *Wound Repair Regen.* 2009;17(1):1–18.

3. Fife CE, Smart DR, Sheffield PJ, Hopf HW, Hawkins G, Clarke D. Transcutaneous oximetry in clinical practice: Consensus statements from an expert panel based on evidence. *Undersea Hyperb Med.* 2009;36(1):43–53.

4. Meyhoff CS, Wetterslev J, Jorgensen LN, et al; PROXI Trial Group. Effect of high perioperative oxygen fraction on surgical site infection and pulmonary complications after abdominal surgery: the PROXI randomized clinical trial. *JAMA.* 2009;302(14):1543–1550.

5. Whitney JD. Enhancing wound oxygen levels: effectiveness of hydration and transdermal oxygen therapies. In: Sen CK, ed. *Advances in Wound Care, Volume 2.* New Rochelle, NY: Mary Ann Liebert, Inc., Publishers; 2011:128–133.

6. Gordillo GM, Sen CK. Evidence-based recommendations for the use of topical oxygen therapy in the treatment of lower extremity wounds. *Int J Low Extrem Wounds.* 2009;8(2):105–111.

7. Said HK, Hijjawi J, Roy N, Mogford J, Mustoe T. Transdermal sustained-delivery oxygen improves epithelial healing in a rabbit ear wound model. *Arch Surg.* 2005;140(10):998–1004.

8. Kalliainen LK, Gordillo GM, Schlanger R, Sen CK. Topical oxygen as an adjunct to wound healing: a clinical case series. *Pathophysiology.* 2003;9(2):81–87.

9. Blackman E, Moore C, Hyatt J, Railton R, Frye C. Topical wound oxygen therapy in the treatment of severe diabetic foot ulcers: a prospective controlled study. *Ostomy Wound Manage.* 2010;56(6):24–31.

10. Bakri MH, Nagem H, Sessler DI, et al. Transdermal oxygen does not improve sternal wound oxygenation in patients recovering from cardiac surgery. *Anesth Analg.* 2008;106(6):1619–1626.

11. Mosteller JA, Sembrst MM, McGarveuy ST, Quinn JL, Klausner EG, Sloat GB. A comparison of transcutaneous oxygen pressures between hyperbaric oxygen and topical oxygen. Presented at the 1999 UHMS Annual Scientific Meeting in Boston, MA.

12. Leslie CA, Sapico FL, Ginunas VJ, Adkins RH. Randomized controlled trial of topical hyperbaric oxygen for treatment of diabetic foot ulcers. *Diabetes Care.* 1998;11(2):111–115.

13. Feldmeier JJ, Hopf HW, Warriner RA 3rd, Fife CE, Gesell LB, Bennett M. UHMS position statement: topical oxygen for chronic wounds. *Undersea Hyperb Med.* 2005;32(3):157–168.

14. Warriner RA. Physiology of hyperbaric oxygen treatment. In: Larson-Lohr V, Josefsen L, Wilcox J, eds. *Hyperbaric Nursing.* 2nd ed. Palm Beach Gardens, FL: Best Publishing Company; 2011:13–31.

15. Thom SR. Hyperbaric oxygen: its mechanisms and efficacy. *Plast Reconstr Surg.* 2011;127(Suppl 1):131S–141S.

16. Thom SR. The impact of hyperbaric oxygen on cutaneous wound repair. In: Sen CK, ed. *Advances in Wound Care, Volume 1.* New Rochelle, NY: Mary Ann Liebert, Inc., Publishers; 2010:321.

17. Thom SR, Bhopale VM, Velazquez OC, Goldstein LJ, Thom LH, Buerk DG. Stem cell mobilization by hyperbaric oxygen. *Am J Physiol Heart Circ Physiol.* 2006;290(4):H1378–H1386.

18. Gallagher KA, Liu ZJ, Xiao M, et al. Diabetic impairments in NO-mediated endothelial progenitor cell mobilization and homing are reversed by hyperoxia and SDF-1 alpha. *J Clin Invest.* 2007;117(5):1249–1259.

19. Liu ZJ, Velazquez OC. Hyperoxia, endothelial progenitor cell mobilization, and diabetic wound healing. *Antioxid Redox Signal.* 2008;10(11):1869–1882.

20. Milovanova TN, Bhopale VM, Sorokina EM, et al. Hyperbaric oxygen stimulates vasculogenic stem cell growth and differentiation *in vivo. J Appl Physiol.* 2009;106(2):711–728.

21. Faglia E, Favales F, Aldeghi A, et al. Adjunctive systemic hyperbaric oxygen therapy in treatment of severe prevalently ischemic diabetic foot ulcer. A randomized study. *Diabetes Care.* 1996;19(12):1338–1343.

22. Kranke P, Bennett M, Roeckl-Wiedmann I, Debus S. Hyperbaric oxygen therapy for chronic wounds. *Cochrane Database Syst Rev.* 2004;(2):CD004123.

23. Guo S, Counte MA, Gillespie KN, Schmitz H. Cost-effectiveness of adjunctive hyperbaric oxygen in the treatment of diabetic ulcers. *Int J Technol Assess Health Care.* 2003;19(4):731–737.

24. Rakel A, Huot C, Ekoe JM. Canadian Diabetes Association Technical Review: the diabetic foot and hyperbaric oxygen therapy. *Canadian J Diabetes.* 2006;30(4):411–421.

25. Goldman RJ. Hyperbaric oxygen therapy for wound healing and limb salvage: a systematic review. *PM R.* 2009;1(5):471–489.

26. Löndahl M, Katzman P, Nilsson A, Hammarlund C. Hyperbaric oxygen therapy facilitates healing of chronic foot ulcers in patients with diabetes. *Diabetes Care.* 2010;33(5):998–1003.

27. Steed DL, Attinger C, Colaizzi T, et al. Guidelines for the treatment of diabetic ulcers. *Wound Repair Regen.* 2006;14(6):680–692.

28. Hopf HW, Ueno C, Aslam R, et al. Guidelines for the treatment of arterial insufficiency ulcers. *Wound Repair Regen.* 2008;14(6):693–710.

29. Fife CE, Buyukcakir C, Otto G, Sheffield P, Love T, Warriner R 3rd. Factors influencing the outcome of lower-extremity diabetic ulcers treated with hyperbaric oxygen therapy. *Wound Repair Regen.* 2007;15(3):322–331.

30. Apelqvist J, Elgzyri T, Larsson J, Londahl M, Nyberg P, Thorne J. Factors related to outcome of neuroischemic/ischemic foot ulcer in diabetic patients. *J Vasc Surg.* 2001;53(6):1582–1588.

31. Guo S, Counte MA, Gillespie KN, Schmitz H. Cost-

effectiveness of adjunctive hyperbaric oxygen in the treatment of diabetic ulcers. *Int J Health Technology Assess Health Care.* 2003;19(4):731–737.

32. Hailey D, Jacobs P, Perry DC, Chuck A, Morrison A, Boudreau R. *Adjunctive Hyperbaric Oxygen Therapy for Diabetic Foot Ulcer: An Economic Analysis* [Technology report no 75]. Ottawa: Canadian Agency for Drugs and Technologies in Health; 2007.

33. Löndahl M, Landin-Olsson M, Katzman P. Hyperbaric oxygen therapy improves health-related quality of life in patients with diabetes and chronic foot ulcer. *Diabet Med.* 2011;28(2):186–190.

34. Beard T, Watson B, Barry R, Stewart D, Warriner R. Analysis of adverse events occurring in patients undergoing adjunctive HBOT: 2009–2010. Presented at the 2011 UHMS Annual Scientific Meeting in Fort Worth, TX.

35. Larson-Lohr V, Norvell HC, eds. *Hyperbaric Nursing.* Flagstaff, AZ: Best Publishing Company; 2002.

36. Clarke D, ed. *Certified Hyperbaric Technologist Resource Manual.* Columbia, SC: National Board of Diving and Hyperbaric Medical Technology; 2011.

37. Workman WT, ed. *UHMS Guidelines for Hyperbaric Facility Operations.* Kensington, MD: UHMS; 2004.

38. Bielen R, ed. NFPA 99: Health Care Facilities Code. Quincy, MA: National Fire Protection Association; 2005.

Conclusion and Color Figures

Make a commitment to:

International

Interprofessional

Wound

Caring

Coming together is a beginning.
Keeping together is progress.
Working together is success.
— Henry Ford

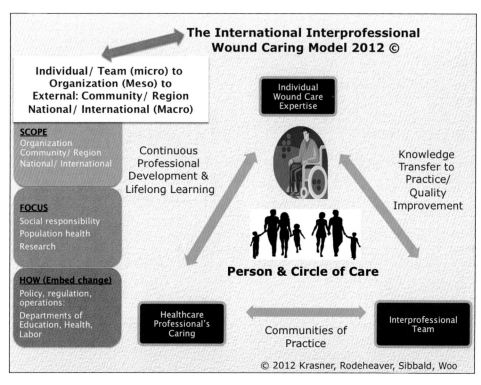

Plate 1. The International Interprofessional Wound Caring Model 2012. Chapter 1.1, p3.

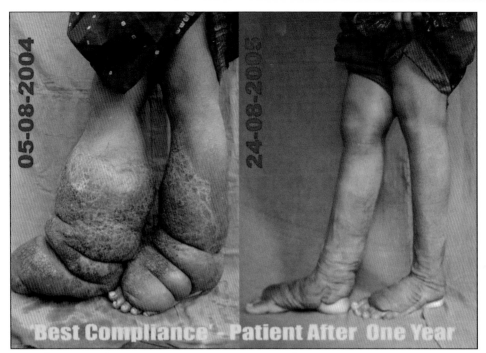

Plate 2. Integrated Dermatology treats lymphedema in Southern India: response to Ayurveda herbals, yoga breathing, movement, and massage. Chapter 1.2, p17.

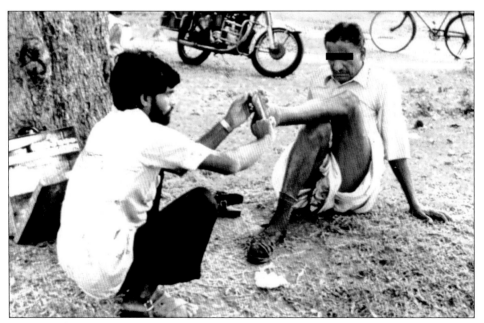

Plate 3. Effective management requires a carer with knowledge who carries appropriate therapies (essential drugs and devices) and has access to the patient. Chapter 1.2, p23.

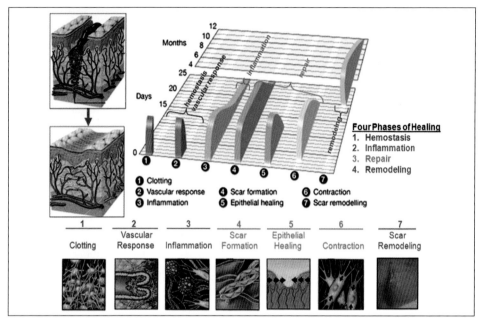

Plate 4. Sequence of wound healing. Normal skin wound healing proceeds through the 4 phases of hemostasis, inflammation, repair, and remodeling. Most chronic wounds get "stuck" in a prolonged inflammatory phase that prevents the wound from moving into an effective repair phase. Adapted from Schultz GS, Ladwig G, Wysocki A. Extracellular matrix: review of its roles in acute and chronic wounds. Available at: http://www.worldwidewounds.com/2005/august/Schultz/Extrace-Matric-Acute-Chronic-Wounds.html. Chapter 1.3, p25.

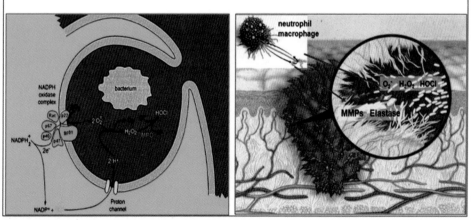

Plate 5. Neutrophils and macrophages perform critical functions in acute wounds by engulfing and killing bacteria and fungi by generation of ROS in endosomes and by releasing proteases that debride the acute wound bed. Chapter 1.3, p26.

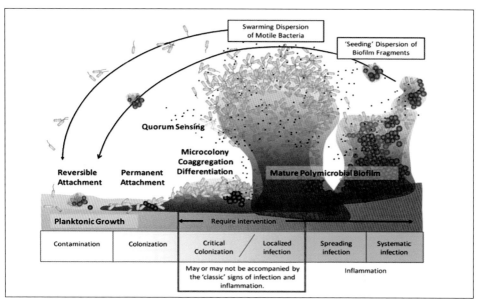

Plate 6. Biofilms in chronic wounds. Planktonic bacteria typically convert into biofilm communities when the levels of quorum molecules reach a threshold and change the pattern of bacterial gene expression. In the spectrum of bacterial bioburden, the concept of critical colonization probably reflects the presence of biofilms, which are not detected by standard clinical microbiology laboratory measurements. Reprinted from Phillips P, Sampson E, Yang Q, et al. Bacterial biofilms in wounds. *Wound Healing S Africa.* Available at: http://www.woundhealingsa.co.za/index.php/WHSA/article/view/17. Chapter 1.3, p28.

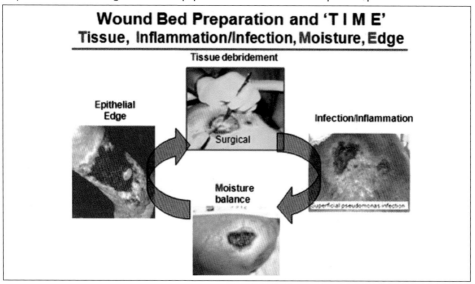

Plate 7. Imbalanced molecular and cellular environments of healing and chronic wounds. The molecular and cellular environment of acute healing wounds is dramatically different than that of chronic wounds and must be "rebalanced" to approximate the environment of healing wounds before healing can progress. Adapted with permission from Mast BA, Schultz GS. Interactions of cytokines, growth factors, and proteases in acute and chronic wounds. *Wound Repair Regen.* 1996;4(4):411. Chapter 1.3, p31.

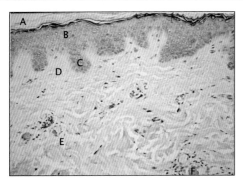

Plate 8. Normal skin: A) stratum corneum, B) epidermis, C) rete peg, D) papillary dermis, and E) reticular dermis. Chapter 4.17, p207.

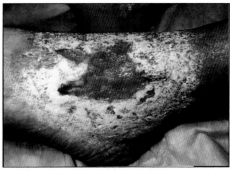

Plate 9. Zinc oxide ointment is placed around a venous ulcer to protect the ulcer margin. The residual material does not need to be removed but only the spaces require re-application. Chapter 4.17, p209.

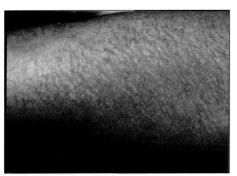

Plate 10. Contact irritant dermatitis. A cracked pavement appearance to the stratum corneum is seen over the underlying dermal erythema. Chapter 4.17, p210.

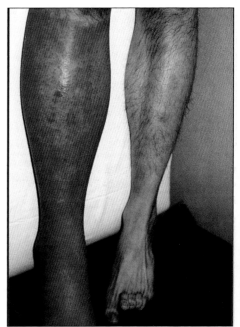

Plate 11. Contact allergic dermatitis. The right leg is swollen with bright red erythema mimicking cellulitis. The ointment applied under the compression bandage responsible for the reaction was lanolin. Chapter 4.17, p210.

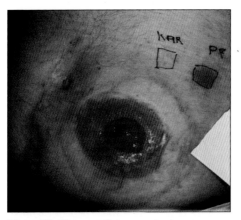

Plate 12. Contact allergy to ostomy paste was reproduced with a patch test applied on the abdomen above the appliance site. The patch test to karaya was negative. Chapter 4.17, p211.

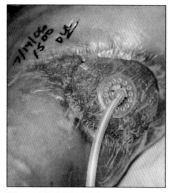
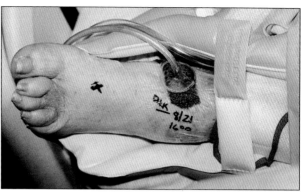

Plate 13. NPWT on thigh wound of IV drug abuser. Chapter 4.22, p276.

Plate 14. NPWT on debrided heel ulcer bridged to dorsum of foot. Chapter 4.22, p276.

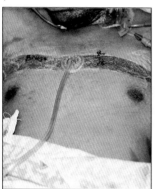
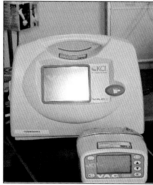
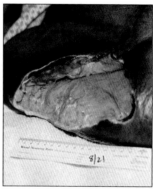

Plate 15. NPWT bridged axilla to axilla s/p excision for hidradenitis suppurativa. Chapter 4.22, p276.

Plate 16. VAC® ATS pump and VAC® Freedom pump (KCI®). Chapter 4.22, p276.

Plate 17. Infected dehisced surgical wound s/p bowel resection. Chapter 4.22, p276.

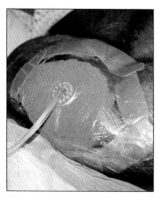
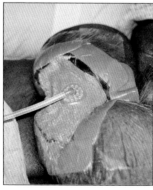
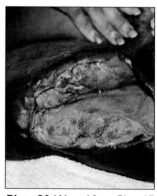

Plate 18. Granufoam Silver® (KCI®) dressing applied to wound from Plate 17. Chapter 4.22, p276.

Plate 19. Granufoam Silver® (KCI®) at 120 mmHg pressure. Chapter 4.22, p276.

Plate 20. Wound from Plate 17 with infection clear and wound granulating. Chapter 4.22, p276.

Your CHRONIC WOUND CARE 5
International Interprofessional Team of Editors

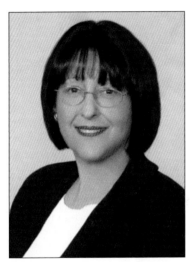

Dr. Diane L. Krasner, Nurse

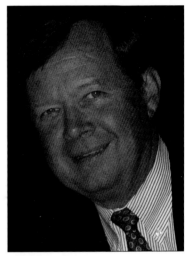

Dr. George T. Rodeheaver, Researcher

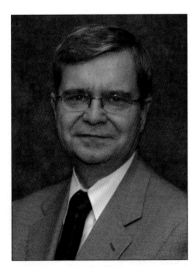

Dr. R. Gary Sibbald, Physician

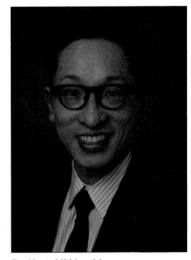

Dr. Kevin Y. Woo, Nurse

A

88, 103, 108, 144, 147, 173, 180, 183-4, 187, 193-4, 203, 206, 224, 241, 248, 250, 265-6, 287, 295

autolytic 187

enzymatic 33, 174, 187

mechanical 101, 187, 261-2

decubitus ulcer *see pressure ulcers*

dehisced wounds 272, 278, 281, 289, 295-6

dehydration 121, 124-5, 220, 254, 275, 292

depression 5, 53, 81-2, 84, 87, 92, 183-4, 236, 245-6

depth 37, 60, 101-5, 109, 147, 186, 226, 260, 281, 285, 295

dermatitis, contact allergic 210, 215, 318

dermatologists 14, 16, 21-2

dermatology 15, 17, 19, 21-4, 141, 219-20, 252

dermis 104-5, 189, 207-8

devices 14-15, 23, 32, 86, 105, 107, 114, 123, 133, 135, 152, 175, 188, 191, 217, 226, 231-3, 235-6, 239-40, 257-8, 262, 269, 272-7, 296, 298, 302, 315

DFUs *see diabetic foot ulcers*

diabetes 5, 14, 18, 48, 53, 57, 68, 80-1, 84, 88, 95, 119, 143, 161, 170, 178-9, 184, 187, 195-6, 200-1, 204-5, 217, 236, 245, 250, 253, 255, 267-9, 284, 286, 294, 304, 308-9

diabetic foot ulcers (DFUs) 13, 28, 32, 35, 44, 80-1, 84, 86, 103-5, 108, 110-11, 114-15, 140, 147, 155-6, 161, 163, 181, 184, 187, 192-4, 197, 229, 235-6, 241, 256, 262, 265, 267, 269, 277, 284, 298, 308

pain 84, 87, 183

diagnosis 3, 9, 14, 19, 22, 41, 45, 78, 102, 104, 114-15, 132, 148, 179, 182, 188, 193, 201-2, 217-20, 241, 244-5, 288

accurate wound 182, 193, 226

diet 120, 123, 126-30, 245

Dietary Reference Intake (DRI) 121, 129

dietitian 4, 122, 125, 145, 193, 254

registered 123-4, 182

disability 17, 51, 79

disfigurement 14, 19-21

documentation 60, 99, 101, 103, 105, 107-9, 111-13, 115, 146-7, 155, 162, 165, 169, 185, 203

donor sites 102, 104, 287, 299

skin graft 102

doxycycline 32, 35, 215

drainage 33, 190, 192, 202, 219, 226, 228, 238, 271, 295, 299

draining wounds 120, 125, 190-1

dressing adherence 228, 276

dressing change 79, 85, 90, 96, 101, 183-5, 190, 225, 229-30, 282

dressing formulary 229-30

dressing selection 62, 87, 94, 115, 179, 183, 190, 225, 229

dressings, occlusive 267

DRI (Dietary Reference Intake) 121, 129

drug holidays 72

E

ECM 26, 30, 235, 290, 292, 294-5

ECM proteins 26, 30, 33

economics 148, 150

eczema 96, 213-15

edema 34, 87-8, 109-11, 134, 147, 180, 183, 204, 226, 234-5, 237-8, 250, 262, 265, 288, 292, 295-6, 302

edge 26, 31, 65, 106, 186, 192-3, 203, 239, 255

education 16, 18, 21-2, 37-40, 43-5, 51-4, 56-61, 65, 68, 82, 86, 91, 94-5, 145, 155-6, 165, 168-9, 174, 185, 193, 240-1, 266

caregiver 55, 59-61, 142, 233, 240

family 58

healthcare 51

patient 42-3, 53, 62, 157, 184, 193, 219, 284

educational programs 45, 47, 53, 56, 59, 153, 155

effects

antimicrobial 188, 227, 249-50

bactericidal 259, 270

EGF (epidermal growth factor) 30

electrical stimulation (ES) 60, 136, 140, 197, 231, 255-7, 262, 265-9

electromagnetic fields 253, 257, 266-7

EMFs 257-8, 263, 265

emollient 20, 208, 212, 249

enablers 8, 41, 47-8, 161-2, 178

endpoints 14, 79, 131-2, 134-5, 286, 304

energy source 119-20

energy work 245-6, 248, 251

Enteral Nutrition 122, 124, 129